Skills for Practice in
Occupational Therapy

In memory of Chiara Lubich (1920-2008). An outstanding woman who taught so many people the most important skills for life.

For Elsevier:

Commissioning Editor: Rita Demetriou-Swanwick
Development Editor: Catherine Jackson
Project Manager: Kerrie-Anne Jarvis
Designer: Stewart Larking
Illustrations Manager: Kirsteen Wright
Illustrator: David Graham

Skills for Practice in Occupational Therapy

Edited by

Edward A.S. Duncan PhD BSc(Hons) DipCBT

Clinical Research Fellow, Nursing, Midwifery and
Allied Health Professions Research Unit,
The University of Stirling,
Stirling, Scotland, UK
and
Honorary Advanced Clinical Practitioner
NHS Forth Valley, Scotland, UK

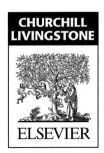

CHURCHILL LIVINGSTONE

ELSEVIER

EDINBURGH LONDON NEW YORK OXFORD PHILADELPHIA ST LOUIS SYDNEY TORONTO 2009

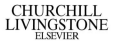

No part of this publication may be reproduced, stored in a retrieval system, or transmitted in any form or by any means, electronic, mechanical, photocopying, recording or otherwise, without the prior permission of the Publishers. Permissions may be sought directly from Elsevier's Health Sciences Rights Department, 1600 John F. Kennedy Boulevard, Suite 1800, Philadelphia, PA 19103–2899, USA: phone: (+1) 215 239 3804; fax: (+1) 215 239 3805; or, e-mail: healthpermissions@elsevier.com. You may also complete your request on-line via the Elsevier homepage (http://www.elsevier.com), by selecting 'Support and contact' and then 'Copyright and Permission'.

ISBN: 978 0 08 045042 1

British Library Cataloguing in Publication Data
A catalogue record for this book is available from the British Library.

Library of Congress Cataloging in Publication Data
A catalog record for this book is available from the Library of Congress.

Notice
Neither the Publisher nor the Editor assumes any responsibility for any loss or injury and/or damage to persons or property arising out of or related to any use of the material contained in this book. It is the responsibility of the treating practitioner, relying on independent expertise and knowledge of the patient, to determine the best treatment and method of application for the patient.

The Publisher

ELSEVIER your source for books, journals and multimedia in the health sciences
www.elsevierhealth.com

The publisher's policy is to use paper manufactured from sustainable forests

Working together to grow libraries in developing countries

www.elsevier.com | www.bookaid.org | www.sabre.org

ELSEVIER   BOOK AID International   Sabre Foundation

Printed in China

Contents

v

List of contributors

Katrina Bannigan
BSc BD PhD

Reader in Occupational Therapy,
Faculty of Health and Life Sciences,
York St John University College, York, UK

Charles H. Christiansen
EdD OTR OT(C) FAOTA

Executive Director, American
Occupational Therapy Foundation,
Maryland, USA

Christine Craik
MPhil DipCOT DMS MCMI FHEA

Director of Occupational Therapy,
Deputy Head (Learning and Teaching),
School of Health Sciences and Social Care,
Brunel University, London, UK

Edward A.S. Duncan
PhD BSc(Hons) DipCBT

Clinical Research Fellow,
Nursing, Midwifery and Allied
Health Professions Research Unit,
The University of Stirling,
Stirling, UK; Honorary Advanced Clinical
Practitioner, NHS Forth Valley

Kirsty Forsyth
PhD MSc OTR

Senior Lecturer,
Department of Occupational Therapy
and Art Therapy, Queen Margaret
University College,
Edinburgh, UK

Della Freeth
PhD BSc CertED FSS ILTM

Professor of Professional and
Interprofessional Education and
Head of Education Development Unit,
City University, London, UK

Priscilla Harries
PhD MSc DipCOT FHEA

Course Leader MSc Occupational
Therapy, Brunel University, London, UK

Tammy Hoffman

Lecturer in Occupational Therapy,
School of Health and Rehabilitation
Sciences, The University of Queensland,
Brisbane, Australia

Gary Kielhofner
DrPH OTR/L FAOTA

Professor and Wade-Meyer Chair,
Department of Occupational Therapy,
University of Illinois, Chicago,
Illinois, USA;
Adjunct Professor, London South Bank
University, London, UK

Alister C. Landrock
BDSDip BA PGDip

Lecturer, Department of Occupational
Therapy and Art Therapy, Queen Margaret
University College, Edinburgh, UK

Anne Landrock

Principal Teacher of Art and Design,
Glenwood High School, Fife, UK

Elizabeth Anne McKay
PhD

Head, Department of Occupational
Therapy, Faculty of Education and
Health Sciences, University of Limerick,
Limerick, Ireland

Jane Melton
MSc DipCOT

Consultant Occupational Therapist,
Gloucestershire Partnership NHS
Foundation Trust, UK

Steve Park
MS OTR/L

Postgraduate Fellow, Discipline of
Occupational Therapy,
Faculty of Health Professions,
University of Sydney, Sydney, Australia

Susan Prior

KTP Associate NHS Lothian Vocational
Rehabilitation KTP Project ADC
Basement, Royal Edinburgh Hospital,
Edinburgh, UK

Sharan R. Schwartzenberg
EdD OTR FAOTA

Tufts University, Professor,
Department of Occupational Therapy
(Boston School of Occupational Therapy),
Graduate School of Arts and Sciences
And Adjunct Professor, Department of
Psychiatry, School of Medicine,
Medford, Massachusetts, USA

Jenny Strong
PhD MOccThy BOccThy

Professor of Occupational Therapy,
School of Health and Rehabilitation
Sciences, The University of Queensland,
Brisbane, Australia

M. Clare Taylor
DipCOT BA(Hons) PGCert MA PhD

Principal Lecturer in Occupational
Therapy, Department of Occupational
Therapy, Coventry University, UK

Renee R. Taylor
PhD

Professor, Licenced Clinical Psychologist;
Department of Occupational Therapy,
University of Illinois, Chicago, USA

Foreword

As every occupational therapist appreciates, we are what we do. Our 'doing' defines us and reflects who we are, what we know and what we value. Within any practice context the skills brought to the interaction between the occupational therapist and those using the service are the visible interface of professional practice. In whatever way the occupational therapist views the profession, its philosophies and theories, is translated through the personal and professional skills that are the tools by which professional thinking is enacted. Clearly then to establish and develop the skills needed to execute occupational therapy practice is as important as developing the theoretical and professional reasoning that underpin our actions. This book explores and addresses the skills required by an occupational therapist working in today's diverse and demanding practice contexts.

In acknowledging that not all skills are visible the text begins by exploring the cognitive skills required to underpin practice. The skill of linking theory to practice, the perennial challenge of any developing practitioner who wishes to function as a professional, begins the process of exploring cognitive professional skills. These skills are explored alongside professional and leadership skills, a triad of 'doing' that any occupational therapist needs in order to practice effectively. Supported by a series of practical and realistic vignettes the text aims to help practitioners develop links between what they know and what they do. Writing a text about skills runs the risk of creating a workshop manual of instructions and guidelines, a trap this text avoids by reflecting the theoretical and evidence base of the skills' performance.

One of the strengths of any text that aims to portray a wide range of thinking and experience is the group of people who contribute to it. This text benefits from the experience of a range of occupational therapists, some of whom are tried and tested authors and others who are new to writing. Some contributors are based in academia, others in practice, some are UK based while others bring an international perspective. Such a breadth and depth of experience allows the reader to benefit from a huge range of thinking and experience.

This is truly a text for the 21st century, acknowledging as it does the international and inter-professional nature of occupational therapy practice. While many of the skills are universal for therapists and practitioners in a range of professions the strength of this text is its ability to deliver this knowledge directly to the practice context of occupational therapists.

Being seen as skilled is a tremendous accolade in any walk of life. Being skilled in professional practice is a status not achieved overnight or without considerable effort. I see that this text could act as a catalyst on the journey to skilled professional practice and hope very much that you draw from the experience of the contributors to help you along the way.

Annie Turner
Professor of Occupational Therapy
University of Northampton
May 2008

Preface

Skills for Practice in Occupational Therapy is all about what occupational therapists do and the skills they are required to have. Practice has changed considerably in recent years and is continually developing. Now, more than ever, practitioners are required to draw on a broad range of skills that involve different types of thinking, aspects of practice, research and evidence-based ways of working, as well as leadership and management expertise. Experience as a student, practitioner and clinical-academic has, over the last 18 years, reinforced in me the importance that practitioners are skilled for practice in each of these areas.

As I wrote in the Preface to *Foundations for Practice in Occupational Therapy*, I have always been struck by how poorly connected the theory and practice of occupational therapy actually are in the 'real world' of many practitioners' lives. To many the idea of truly connecting these two issues remains a utopian concept; one that is inculcated whilst students are at university, but never truly expected to be realized by many in practice. Yet this need not be the case. *Foundations* was designed to clarify at every opportunity the practical implications of the theory base being discussed, *Skills* strives to do the same in reverse: linking practice with theory and research wherever possible. Obviously this is achievable more in some chapters than others which are perhaps by their nature inherently pragmatic.

All texts such as this are influenced by the experiences and perspectives of the editor. Understanding these influences can help the reader to make sense of the structure and content of the book. I am very fortunate to have had a very rich undergraduate experience which had a defining impact on my development both as a clinician and academic. To date I have practised exclusively in a variety of mental health settings. My earliest clinical experiences after graduation were in community mental health teams in various areas of urban deprivation in Glasgow. After a few years I moved to help establish a new occupational therapy service in a high-security forensic psychiatric hospital. Both these settings provided excellent opportunities to develop and enhance a range of skills for practice. Along the way I have also been deeply (but not exclusively) influenced by two central theories for occupational therapy practice in mental health: the Model of Human Occupation and the Cognitive Behavioural Frame of Reference.

Research is central to effective and competent practice. In 2004 I was fortunate to gain a postdoctoral clinical-academic research fellowship in a leading national research unit for nursing midwifery and allied health professions in Scotland. I secured a permanent position in this unit as a clinical research fellow in 2006 and maintain my clinical role as an honorary advanced clinical practitioner in the occupational therapy services of NHS Forth Valley, Scotland. My current research includes both occupational-therapy-specific and multi-disciplinary-based projects. Ongoing studies include work in community and forensic mental health settings, community paediatrics, pre-hospital emergency care and palliative care.

Skills is the result of an international collaboration with eminent contributors from Australia, the USA and Ireland as well as the UK. As with all edited texts, the authorial voice and style of *Skills* changes from chapter to chapter. These differences in tone and depth have, by and large, been left unchanged in the editing process. *Skills* has brought together an expert group of academics and practitioners. To have muted their differences in style though authoritarian editing would have sterilized the text and left it a less interesting and varied contribution to the field.

Through the various chapters of this book I have aimed to provide an engaging, useful and practical introduction to the essential skills required by occupational therapists in contemporary practice. I hope it is found to be valuable by both students and practitioners alike and look forward to hearing some critical appraisal of this text and suggestions for ways in which it may be improved.

Edward A.S. Duncan
2008

Acknowledgements

Whilst the author (or editor) of a book has his name on the cover it is rarely, if ever, truly the work of one person alone, and even less so with an edited text. *Skills for Practice in Occupational Therapy* would not have been achievable without the significant contribution of many people, some of whom merit particular mention.

The contributors

This book has been contributed to by a range of exceptional therapists (both clinicians and academics) and colleagues each of who brought a wealth of personal and professional experience to their work. It has been extremely enjoyable to work with each of them and they each have my greatest respect and thanks for the contribution they have made.

The publishers

Elsevier, as always, have been extremely supportive in the book's development and production. In particular, thanks are due to Catherine Jackson who has patiently and wisely supported and guided me throughout the publication process.

Nursing Midwifery and Allied Health Professions Research Unit (NMAHP RU), The University of Stirling

I am fortunate to work in a multi-disciplinary environment where high-quality clinical-focused research is undertaken by a range of professionals. My thinking has been influenced by our collaborative research and energetic discussions about practice. This influence has undoubtedly impacted upon the structure and content of this book.

My family

There are not enough thanks sufficient for Anne, Catherine, Eleanor and Joseph. Without their love, understanding, support and patience this book would never have been realised.

Cover painting by Michel Pochet

The cover artwork for *Skills for Practice in Occupational Therapy* continues the theme that was first used in the 4th Edition of *Foundations for Practice in Occupational Therapy*. The picture is another image of the Forth Railway Bridge (Scotland), created during the same period and by the same artist as the image on the cover of *Foundations*. This remarkable cantilever bridge is a highly complex structure which spans the Forth Estuary, linking two sides of the same thing. It is, I feel, an effective representation of the vision I have of this book which highlights the multifaceted nature of the skills required in contemporary occupational therapy practice and endeavours to intricately link practice with its theoretical basis. Its Scottish significance is also close to my heart! The picture is the creation of Michel Pochet, a good friend, to whom I am very grateful that, once again, he has given permission for an image of his to be used in this way.

Michel Pochet, a Parisian born in Provence in 1940, spent his childhood under the hot sun and unique light of Corsica. At the age of 13 he wanted to become a painter, and to help nurture his talent, his mother returned to painting herself. She was a perceptive and unaffected watercolourist, and Pochet learnt his technique, which is still evident in his work, from her.

At 17, Pochet moved to Paris to study architecture at the School of Fine Arts, the best school of its kind in France. He continued to paint, sculpt, write poetry, novels and essays, his main subject being the relationship between God and beauty. Several of his books have been translated into Italian, Flemish, German, Portuguese, English and Spanish.

Michel Pochet lives and works in Rome, where he has founded an international artistic centre, the Centro Maria, to promote art 'in communion with God'. Details of the Centro Maria and Michel Pochet's work can be found at: http://flars.net/centomaria/.

Edward A.S. Duncan
2008

Introduction

Edward A.S. Duncan

The purpose and structure of this book

'Skills for Practice in Occupational Therapy' introduces the reader to the wide range of skills that occupational therapists require to have in order to practice effectively in contemporary health and social care environments. Each chapter is written with a practice skills focus in mind, but wherever possible this is directly linked to theory and existing evidence. The book is clearly targeted at and relevant for occupational therapy students who are developing these skills. But the direct practice relevance of the chapters also makes it a resource that should not be left on the student shelf, never to be opened after graduation, but become used as a resource for new and experienced practitioners alike.

Whilst this chapter provides a useful orientation to the book's purpose and contents as a whole, 'Skills for Practice in Occupational Therapy' is not intended to be read from cover to cover in chronological order. Readers will access different chapters at different stages depending on what they wish to know. However chapters have been extensively cross referenced, so the reader opening this book at one chapter may find themselves journeying through each section as they build up a bigger picture of what is required to deliver effective skills for practice.

The structure of each chapter, in the main sections of the book, is consistent. Chapters begin with a brief overview of the subject and chapter content, a highlight box is located at the front of each chapter to provide an even briefer and punchier synopsis. The body of the chapter then follows. Wherever possible, case vignettes are included to illuminate and illustrate the points being made. Each chapter concludes with a summary to bring together the key issues that have been presented and discussed.

What exactly do occupational therapists do?

The venue may differ (for example at a student house party; a family get-together, a meeting with a professional colleague, an interdisciplinary conference, or in a multidisciplinary team meeting...) but invariably the question is asked: 'What do you do?' or 'What is occupational therapy anyway?' One way of responding could be to recite a definition of the profession; telling the interested inquirer that occupational therapy,

- 'Is concerned with the key elements of occupational performance and identity: how a person identifies themselves and their future aspirations, their roles and relationships, together with their personal capacity for fulfilling these within their physical and social environment.
- Aims to enable and empower people to be competent and confident in their daily lives, and thereby to enhance well-being and minimize the effects of dysfunction or environmental barriers.'

And that occupational therapists:

- 'Use everyday occupations and tasks creatively and therapeutically to achieve goals that are meaningful to people and relevant to their daily life.
- Encourage people to collaborate in the therapeutic process in order to become partners with the therapist in the designing and directing of therapy' (Duncan 2006a: 6).

Such an approach, however, is not recommended: It would likely lead to bemused stares, a polite thanks, and a quick exit by the person concerned! So how can one appropriately respond to such questions? And why can such a straightforward question be so challenging to answer?

Often when asked, 'What do you do?', it is tempting to respond by saying what you are, rather than what you 'do'. And even when occupational therapists do respond by saying what they 'do', their description can belie the true depth and breadth of practice. Hagedorn (2000) discussed the challenges associated with being seen to do 'simple' things. Occupational therapy she stated is, by and large, a 'low tech' intervention in a 'high tech' modern healthcare environment. And when compared to 'high tech' interventions, such as three-dimensional imaging or steroid injections, may be viewed as merely 'common sense'. So, describing the depth and breadth of what occupational therapists 'do' is challenging. Part of the reason for this is that the 'visible' portion of practice is only a small percentage of what actually goes on. Hagedorn (2000) presented two differing images to illustrate this. First occupational therapy was compared to an iceberg, where only the tip of the vast mass is visible to the eye; but she felt this was an unattractive analogy as icebergs appear clumsy. Secondly, and more favourably, Hagedorn compared occupational therapy to a computer; each has an easy-to-use interface but is highly complex beneath the surface interface. However this image too could be criticized as being excessively mechanistic. Of course the appeals of imagistic analogies are subjective and different people will find them more or less helpful. But they can be useful strategies to convey that the message that the totality of what occupational therapists 'do' is not immediately apparent. (As an aside, I quite like the analogy of the common garden mint plant: highly useful and very adaptable, deeply rooted, fast spreading and very difficult to remove once embedded!)

Skills for practice

Vignette 1

A day in the life of an occupational therapist

Beth is an advanced clinical occupational therapist in an acute mental health inpatient service. She arrives at work at 8.30 am and is immediately greeted by a client who has been on the ward for a week. The client is worried about a visit that she will be receiving from her parents in the afternoon and wants to share her concerns with Beth, asking her what she should do: Beth spends some time listening to the client and arranges to see her later. Beth then attends the ward handover meeting with the nursing and psychiatric staff and discusses the relevance and urgency of several clients who the team have referred and wish to be assessed. The turnover on the ward is fast, so she may not have time to see them all and needs to judge which referrals are highest priority. Having completed the handover meeting, Beth then prepares and runs an open creative arts group for clients on the ward: this is always a challenging session as the needs of the group are varied, but the creative medium is popular throughout the ward and the group enables Beth to observe clients' range of functioning in a group setting. Once the group is completed and the notes are written up, Beth returns to the client she met first thing. The client shares some more details with Beth who decides to take a problem-solving approach to help the client generate her own solutions to the difficulties she foresees will arise when her parents visit.

Beth's next task is to carry out an initial assessment with a 26-year-old man (Chris), who was recently readmitted to the ward. Beth has heard that Chris is unhappy at being on the ward once again and is also aware that he is viewed by the nursing staff as being non-compliant with his medication and the ward routine. Beth's first aim is to engage with Chris and communicate with him that she wished to understand what he thought his difficulties were, and that she wanted to discover if there was anything he felt he wished to address. Her hope was that together they would be able to agree on what his functional problems were and develop an intervention plan they could both agree with and work towards.

Having spent longer than anticipated with Chris it was time to rush to her lunchtime journal club meeting. The journal club is a monthly interdisciplinary event that Beth had initially set up with a clinical psychologist. The club has now been attended by staff from various professional groups for over a year and some changes to practice have occurred due to discussions that have taken place. Beth had recently carried out an audit of the club and it was found to be well attended and highly valued. The findings of the audit had been submitted to a clinical effectiveness conference and her abstract was accepted for a poster presentation. Beth has now developed a draft poster and wants to show it to the journal club members to get some feedback before it is finalized.

Beth's afternoon begins with a clinical supervision session with her junior occupational therapist. This is quickly followed by a kitchen session with another client who is preparing to go home after an unusually lengthy admission (by this ward's standards). After this she attends the ward development meeting. This is a staff meeting for the senior staff members on the ward and plans new developments to its structure and routine. Beth is concerned about the level of therapeutic engagement as a whole and wants to encourage all staff to be more interactive with clients. However, she is very aware of ward politics and draws on all her leadership and personal management skills to be able to communicate these issues with the rest of the team. After the meeting, Beth returns to her ward office. This is the first chance she has had to read her emails. Amongst the usual stuff, two messages stick out: one of them is from the hospital's practice education facilitator to ask Beth if she would mind having an occupational therapy student, for 6 weeks, starting the following week? Another email is from a colleague in the local university with whom Beth is a co-grant applicant on a pilot research study application examining the effectiveness of an activity scheduling programme they have developed for clients with eating disorders: Beth needs to review the procedure that her colleague has suggested they use for recruiting participants. Half an hour before home time... Beth makes herself a well-deserved coffee and reaches for a copy of an article on using conceptual models in practice that she had recently seen in a journal...

3

This book is about what occupational therapists actually do: the skills they bring to practice. Skills are, 'the aptitudes and competencies appropriate for a particular job' (Chambers Dictionary 1994: 1617). Occupational therapists are now required to have and use a complex range of skills (see Vignette 1) to maintain their competence in a swiftly developing healthcare environment (Ryan et al 2003). It is for this reason that this book has been developed in four key sections that outline the broad range of skills required by practitioners to deliver best practice: Thinking, judgement and decision-making skills; Professional skills; Evidence-based and research skills; and Leadership, supervision and management skills.

'Skills for Practice in Occupational Therapy' addresses the aptitudes and competencies required by today's practitioners; and introduces these in a way that is accessible, relevant, closely linked to theory, and evidence based. If 'Foundations for Practice in Occupational Therapy' (Duncan 2006b) strove to link theory with practice, 'Skills for Practice in Occupational Therapy' endeavours to link practice with theory!

Whilst this book does contain practical advice and guidance on a range of issues, it is not designed to be a 'How to do' textbook that will take you step by step through an intervention or theoretical approach. Similarly, it does not purport to cover every necessary skill for practice. Instead the book covers a broad range of skills that are essential for today's practitioner. The chapters vary in theoretical and academic depth. Several of the chapters present complex areas of study that have been subject to research and theoretical development for many years: these chapters aim to introduce the topic to the reader, provide them with a foundation of knowledge in the area and signpost them to other resources to develop their knowledge further. Other chapters are inherently pragmatic. This diversity of depth and focus is appropriate as it reflects the differing types of skills that occupational therapists use in their everyday practice.

Thinking, judgement and decision-making skills for practice

Practitioners spend a lot of time thinking, judging/assessing, collaborating with clients, making decisions and reflecting on what they have done. Yet how often, and for how long, do people spend time to stop and consider why they made certain decisions, on what evidence they based their decisions, how successful their strategy of collaborating with clients is, and how evidence-based their judgements in practice are? These skills are central, yet largely invisible to competent and successful practice. Section 1 untangles the vast literature of this field and introduces the reader to a range of ideas, theories and evidence that highlight ways in which practitioners' thinking, judgements, decisions and reflections are influenced and can be enhanced.

Professional skills for practice

Section 2 focuses on the everyday skills practitioners use when intervening with clients. The chapters in this section focus on the core skills (Creek 2003) that occupational therapists use in practice:

- Assessment
- Use of activity/activity analysis (which includes environmental analysis)
- The therapeutic use of self
- Problem solving
- Group work.

Each of these skills assists practitioners to enable their clients to develop, maintain or explore their daily lives, enhance their well-being and minimize the effects of occupational dysfunction or environmental barriers. Additionally this section includes chapters on goal setting and report writing and record keeping; neglected but essential components of skilled practice. Each chapter, though practice focused, is closely linked to developments in evidence, theory and policy.

Evidence-based and research skills for practice

Section 3 addresses the importance of evidence-based and research skills in practice. Research is now the business of every practitioner (Bannigan et al 2007). In the UK, the College of Occupational Therapists has stated that, 'occupational therapists have a responsibility to contribute to the continuing development of the profession by utilizing critical evaluation, and participating in audit and research' (p. 17). A contemporary textbook on 'Skills for Practice in Occupational Therapy' cannot be without a section to guide practitioners in finding relevant research and appraising it for quality, examining how to implement the recommendations of research into practice, and evaluate how successful this has been. Further, occupational therapists now have to examine how they can undertake research in practice. Despite the very real challenges that face practitioners who wish to undertake research, it can be done. This section outlines various approaches that have been successful in undertaking clinically relevant research in practice and discusses the strengths and limitations of each. The section concludes with a chapter that contains important information on the skills that are required by practitioners in order to successfully present or publish their work.

Leadership, supervision and management skills for practice

Making good clinical judgements, having expert professional skills, finding and using the best evidence and engaging with research are all essential skills for practice. Yet, if a practitioner does not have high-quality personal and interpersonal skills their work will not reach its full potential. Section 4 addresses precisely these issues for practice. Every practitioner can be a leader; it is not an attribute that is solely attributed to people in authority, and being in authority does not mean that a person will be able to lead. First and foremost skilled leadership requires leadership of self. Amongst other attributes effective practitioners need to be authentic, have integrity and be trusted by others. But, even with these positive attributes (and others are necessary too) there is no escaping the demands of working in health and social care environments where practitioners frequently face challenging situations and people, and clients too! Therefore positive self management (looking after one's personal resources) is also vital for the individual who wishes to be an effective and skilled practitioner. When a practitioner can manage themselves, their influence on others will grow and so too will the range of issues that they have an impact on and influence in their work environment. Sometimes this will evidence itself through practitioners leading changes in a wider circle than their immediate professional discipline (as seen in Vignette 1). At other times it will be observable through the influence they have with their colleagues within their professional discipline; either informally or through formal structures such as student or clinical supervision.

Summary

So what do occupational therapists do? Perhaps this question cannot be truly answered through a catchy strap line. Competent occupational therapists are required to have a startling depth and breadth of knowledge, practical skills, and personal and professional attributes. 'Skills for Practice in Occupational Therapy' provides students and practitioners with an introduction and overview of the essential skills for practice. So, next time someone asks you what do you do....give them a copy of the book!

References

Bannigan K, Hughes S, Booth M 2007 Research is now every occupational therapists business. The British Journal of Occupational Therapy 70(3):95

Chambers 1994 The Chambers Dictionary. Chambers Harrap, Edinburgh

Creek J 2003 Occupational Therapy defined as a complex intervention. College of Occupational Therapists, London

Duncan EAS 2006a Introduction. In: EAS Duncan (ed) Foundations for Practice in Occupational Therapy, 4th edn., pp. 3–9. Elsevier/Churchill Livingstone, Edinburgh

Duncan EAS (ed) 2006b Foundations for Practice in Occupational Therapy, 4th edn. Elsevier/ Churchill Livingstone, Edinburgh

Hagedorn 2000 Tools for Practice in Occupational Therapy. Churchill Livingstone, Edinburgh

Ryan SE, Esdaile SA, Brown G 2003 Appreciating the big picture: You are part of it! The socio-political influences on health practice in the public and private sphere. In: G Brown, SE Esdaile, SE Ryan (eds) Becoming an Advanced Health Care Practitioner, pp. 1–29. Butterworth Heinemann, Edinburgh

Thinking, judgement and decision skills for practice

Using theory in practice

2

*Jane Melton,
Kirsty Forsyth and
Della Freeth*

★ Highlight box

- Making well-informed decisions and convincing others of their worth lies at the heart of professional practice.
- The use of conceptual models of practice is important in order to provide a practice framework for decision making, to make practice relevant for service users and for occupational therapists to develop expertise.
- The application of theory to practice is multidimensional and is influenced by the therapists' attributes, the support available within the environmental context plus the mechanisms that therapists have available and choose to engage in.
- Initial support to think clearly with the supportive framework of a well-grounded conceptual model or theory can help well-informed reflective practice to become a good habit and source of professional pride.
- Carefully considered practice development mechanisms and partnerships with academic colleagues can provide opportunities for therapists to better enable their service users to benefit from occupational therapy practice.

Overview

Occupational therapists react and respond in a variety of ways to the day-to-day occupation-focused decisions that need to be made in practice. The variety of responses are triggered and challenged by the environmental contexts, the conceptual thinking and technical ability of the practitioner, in addition to the presenting needs of the clients.

In this chapter we will illustrate the choices and issues that occupational therapists encounter when making decisions about the theories to support their occupation-focused, evidenced-based choices. To illustrate this we will provide a case overview of an organizational approach to practice scholarship. The voices of occupational therapists who are embracing the challenge and celebrating the benefit of using theory in their practice will be presented in the second part of the chapter together with a summary of measures to assist practitioners engage with theory in practice.

Historical context

Scholarly work to locate the theoretical concepts underpinning the practice of occupational therapy has gathered pace only in recent times (Duncan 2006). Despite these advances, there continues a debate in the profession about the perceived gap between theory and practice (Forsyth et al 2005a, Duncan 2006). Implied here is that practitioners have found it difficult to engage in or value theory (Mattingly and Fleming 1994) and that academics have detected that theory and research is not used routinely in practice (Fisher 1998, Wood 1998, Christiansen 1999). To support theoretically oriented occupational therapy practice, Kielhofner (2004) presented a contemporary, synthesized overview of the development, current position and future of knowledge available to support practice. In this valuable, in-depth précis Kielhofner describes the conceptual foundations of occupational therapy, outlines the historic difficulty that the field has experienced in infusing theory into practice and makes suggestions for further development. Despite this contribution calls continue for the profession to embrace the use of theory in practice in order to raise standards and to meet the growing opportunities presented to empower those who require occupational therapy intervention (Forsyth et al 2005a). We aim to support this position through the presentation of this chapter.

Introduction

First we examine the nature and importance of putting theory into practice. We acknowledge that therapists find this challenging. We argue that using a scholarship of practice philosophy which supports conceptual models of practice, supports effective occupational therapy by shaping theory-driven actions and drawing from the available evidence base. We suggest that the use of conceptual models of practice is important in order to provide a practice framework for decision making, to make practice relevant for service users and for occupational therapists to develop expertise.

We then turn to a case study of applying the scholarship of practice approach to encourage the use and development of theory in daily practice. Through the explanation of practitioner quotes we will argue that the application of theory to practice is multidimensional and is influenced by the therapists' attributes, the support available within the environmental context and the mechanisms that therapists have available and choose to engage in. We conclude with suggestions of practical ideas that therapists can consider when seeking to develop their practice through the understanding and application of occupational therapy conceptual theory.

What are theories and why do they matter?

Theories are connected sets of ideas that form the basis for action. Theories explain the way things are and predict what will happen if we make changes. Because they provide explanation and prediction theories can be scrutinized, debated and tested. This is important because it is the way in which knowledge and understanding move forward, guiding actions by making them better-informed.

Let us stray outside occupational therapy for a short while to look at a vivid example without being weighed down by professional knowledge or 'baggage'. Worries about climate change are spawning many competing and complementary theories. These theories are not irrelevant intellectual exercises. Mankind is genuinely concerned about the possible existence and consequences of global warming. The explanations and predictions provided by these climate-related theories are highlighting the importance of changing behaviour and attitudes; and further, suggesting the nature of the required changes. This generates (heated!) debate which challenges and refines the theories: their explanations and predictions. We begin to think about things differently and do things differently: these changes affect the course of the future.

The alternative is not thinking very much about things that appear to be OK for the moment, or that feel too big or too difficult to change. This often entails doing more or less the same as in the past and achieving similar results to the past. This becomes a problem when it is combined with changing circumstances. In our example of climate change the central problem is an acceleration effect: the rapid growth of damaging behaviours caused by rapid 'development'. In health and social care the changing circumstances are linked to relatively rapid changes in the age profile and family structures of the population; healthcare developments that enable more people to live for much longer with significant impairments; changed social expectations about the delivery of care and so on. We need to scrutinize what we do now to discover our implicit explanations of how things work and fit together, unearthing our views about what is really important. This enables predictions and informed choices to be made.

To complete our use of the climate change example; there is a theory which might be summarized as follows: *There is a role for 'green' taxation of air travel in efforts to combat global warming.* Broadly, the elements of explanation in this theory are twofold:

- Travel is price-sensitive
- Air travel makes a significant contribution to global warming by depositing carbon emissions and other pollutants high in the atmosphere.

Many testable predictions can be made about the effects of increasing taxation of air travel, for example:

- The volume of air travel will fall
- The rate of increase in damage to the atmosphere (and consequently climate) will slow
- Jobs will be lost in airlines
- Local tourism and the use of other forms of transport will increase
- Reduced business travel will change the ways in which business is transacted.

We are not expecting anyone to be convinced by this scant account of green taxation: far greater scientific and economic rigour would be required. The point is simply that the theory provides testable explanations and predictions that can be debated and can guide actions.

Debate about really big questions should be communal so that many perspectives are brought into the process of refining ideas and actions. Debate in day-to-day occupational therapy practice will sometimes be social (e.g. within multidisciplinary team meetings, during clinical supervision or as part of continuing professional development (CPD) or when reconfiguring services) but often the debate will be inside the head of the therapist during 'reflection' or 'critical thinking' (see Chapter 5).

Good therapists never stop debating with themselves and others about how things fit together, what should be regarded as important, what interventions are predicted to be most effective, how their earlier interventions worked out and so on. If we stop thinking about explanations, predictions and the consequences of actions, the development of our professional practice ceases and it gradually becomes outdated, out of touch with changed circumstances and less effective for clients. Without thinking with underpinning theory professional practice is guesswork (Higgs et al 2001). Thus it is no surprise that the Health Professions Council (2003) has identified that registrant occupational therapists must be able to use 'the established theories, models, frameworks and concepts

11

of occupational therapy' in order to demonstrate their clinical proficiency at formulating and delivering plans to meet service user need. These theories and models provide a rigorously built framework to help us to choose what we should do and explain these choices to others. Making well-informed decisions and convincing others of their worth lies at the heart of professional practice. In most cases your therapeutic interventions will be thwarted if your client cannot see their worth. In addition you will not be able to provide the service that you would wish to provide for clients if you cannot convince colleagues and other stakeholders that your actions and plans are well informed.

Every discipline develops a specialized knowledge base, important concepts, models and theories to help busy practitioners make rapid but well-informed decisions about their practice. Examples of specialized knowledge in occupational therapy include the relationship between a person's belief in their ability to undertake a task on their performance ability or how a person with motor limitations can be augmented to maximize their function by adapting their environment (Kielhofner 2004). Particular perspectives on key concepts in occupational therapy might embrace occupational performance and volition. Finally, some examples of models or theories that synthesise the knowledge and concepts in occupational therapy are the Model of Human Occupation (MoHO) (Kielhofner 2008) and the Canadian Model of Occupational Performance (Townsend and Polatajko 2007). We argue that the ability to think within a defined framework of conceptual ideas assists the therapist in a number of ways. These include:

- having a structure upon which to locate thinking, reasoning and the construction of practice based decisions
- guidance in selecting research evidence, assessments and interventions that most appropriately link with the essence of occupation therapy practice
- having a language with which to articulate the occupational needs of the client
- having resources with which to build professional know-how into expertise and
- better matching of service user needs and aspirations with the provision of therapy.

So are there problems with integrating theory into occupational therapy practice?

In short, yes – at least for the present. Despite the acknowledged importance of infusing practice with insights derived from research evidence, conceptual models and pertinent theories (Cusick 2001, Duncan 2006), practitioners have expressed disillusionment with the relevance of theory to their practice (Closs and Cheater 1999, Kielhofner 2005) while academics observe that existing knowledge in the field is not being systemically applied in practice (Fisher 1998, Wood 1998, Christiansen 1999). Therapists might, therefore, be viewing theory as more 'ornamental' than 'instrumental' to their practice. Why might practitioners not find theory relevant to their everyday work?

There is little doubt that the definition of 'theory' poses challenges in many disciplines (Nixon and Creek 2006). Other issues include the demands and constraints of practice settings that leave limited time for reflection and innovation (Oxman et al 1995, McCluskey and Cusick 2002). Moreover, traditional models of theory building are based on 'technical rationality', the idea that practical action flows naturally from basic knowledge (Schön 1991). In fact intermediate work is required to reformulate basic knowledge in ways that make its relevance and application to practice more certain and obvious (see Chapter 15).

We too have heard therapists proclaim that they are uncomfortable with theory. The reasons for this are expressed in different ways. Some therapists suggest that:

- The language appears 'lofty' or detached from their clients' world
- They find it difficult to 'fit' theory to their practice

- The theory is not culturally sensitive
- They feel pressured to understand a multitude of theory bases and apply them in practice leading to confusion or apprehension
- Understanding or using theory routinely is too difficult or time consuming in their practice context
- It is unnecessary to consider theory, particularly in a busy clinicians schedule
- The whole notion of putting theory to clinical work is too 'scary'
- Theory limits their creativity as therapists
- They don't want their practice to be like everyone else's or to be prescriptive.

In addition, the need to learn, appraise, synthesize and use the various theory bases which apply to occupational therapy practice can be overwhelming. For instance, the differences in some of the conceptual definitions can be minimal and might challenge the reader to wonder why separate frameworks were established. Equally, the differences can be huge and challenge the reader to wonder whether they relate to the same therapeutic intervention at all.

So what do all these concerns about applying theory to occupational therapy practice indicate? Almost certainly, we should view the knowledge, conceptual and theoretical bases of occupational therapy as not yet as fully developed as practitioners need. Work needs to be done to better articulate key conceptual models and theories. Accessible presentation will encourage use and scrutiny, in turn encouraging development of both theory and practice. Secondly, habits and confidence are important. Initial support to think clearly with the supportive framework of a well-grounded conceptual model or theory can help well-informed reflective practice to become a good habit and source of professional pride.

A potential way forward: Scholarship of Practice

There is growing recognition that the kind of knowledge required for decision-making in practice is different from the kind of knowledge that is generated to explain phenomena; that is, knowing about something is not the same as knowing how to do something (Schön 1991, Higgs et al 2001). In response to this, the 'Scholarship of Practice' has been used recently in some occupational therapy services in the UK and is defined as delivering and generating evidence for practice through a partnership between academia and practice (Forsyth et al 2005a) (see Figure 2.1). In this way theory is built in practice and considerations include *both* the generation of theory and the use of theory in practice. In addition the Scholarship of Practice pays attention to building tools for practice such as standardized assessments or visual representations that synthesize ideas and act as reminders. Scholarship of Practice gradually builds conceptual models of practice that are informed by challenges from practice, reflective wisdom, evidence from research and the abstract thinking of theory building.

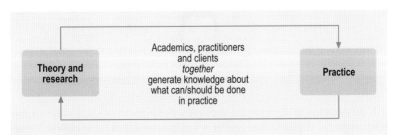

Figure 2.1 A scholarship of practice.

13

Focusing on conceptual models

It has been argued that conceptual models of practice link theory to practice within a scholarship of practice philosophy (Kielhofner 2004, Duncan 2006). Relatively abstract and general theories are formulated into concepts and propositions which support practice-based action and skills, providing guidance as to how to use theory in practice. Thus a conceptual model of practice includes both theory in addition to practice-based tools for application of theory. Most disciplines will have more than one conceptual model and these will function to help professionals understand complex practice-based challenges and how to formulate decisions about bespoke intervention packages for individuals. The aim here is to ensure skilled practice action (Figure 2.2). One example of a conceptual model which describes occupational therapy concepts is the Model of Human Occupation (MoHO) (Kielhofner 2008). The MoHO seeks to explain how human occupation is motivated, patterned and performed. It assists occupational therapists to understand their client's ability to perform their occupations with their own temporal, physical and socio-cultural environment. Within the framework conceptualized in the MoHO, 20 assessment tools have been developed, to date, for clinical practice application. The literature about these concepts has over 25 years of history which adds weight to the claim that the model provides professional knowledge that is a comprehensive and evidence-based framework for occupational therapy practice.

Conceptual models are useful as tools for thinking and become a key element for problem setting and problem solving (Parham 1987, Munoz et al 1993). Where a clinician is challenged to make sense of an uncertain situation that initially makes no sense (Schön 1991) a robust, relevant and well-understood model of practice can assist. It offers a means of identifying and rationalizing what is being observed and a set of ideas within which to frame practice decision-making. Thus the articulation of specific professional knowledge and service user outcomes can be made with greater clarity.

Maximizing a person's opportunity to gain benefit from intervention is generally and rightly the purpose of a clinician's decision making in practice (Lloyd Smith 1997, Tickle-Degnen 1998). Included here is the goal to make interventions cost effective and based on the best available evidence (Law et al 2001). If therapists are able to use models of practice judiciously and reflectively it follows that they will be better positioned to understand and use the associated practice skills of assessment and intervention. A robust conceptual model of practice facilitates constructive critique of 'custom and practice' and the integration of research evidence. This can result in occupationally conceptualized, theoretically based, evidence-informed thinking.

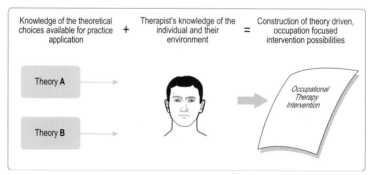

Figure 2.2 An equation to illustrate the importance of theoretical knowledge synthesised with understanding of the individual and their environment in order to deliver the best practice solutions for and with each service user.

Models of practice can bring a fresh perspective, stimulating a practitioner's understanding of a person's occupational need at a higher level of sophistication and creativity. It seems logical then for occupational therapists, who are working with people who have challenges with their occupational participation through illness or disability, to use a set of conceptual ideas to help them to understand and formulate the information that they are gathering about a client's needs. No therapy would however be complete without the therapist being able to communicate the purpose, process and outcomes of intervention to service users and colleagues. A conceptual practice model, used thoughtfully, will help this communication to be clearly articulated thus raising the profile of the clients' requirements and the best practice solutions available via occupational therapy intervention.

So how can this be achieved?

Conceptual models of practice have a structure that is supportive of reflective and theoretically formulated practice. What can facilitate and support therapists' use of conceptual models within everyday clinical work? We now turn to a case study of applying the scholarship of practice model. The main points that will be drawn out through the case study will be that therapists can consider their own attributes and attitudes towards the use of theory in their practice; that leaders within an organisational context can support the use of theory to enhance practice standards and that therapists can expect, develop and use various mechanisms to extend their understanding and practical application of theory for practice.

Lessons from a case study In this case study we use quotations from practitioners to illustrate the supports that can assist therapists to develop skills in the use of conceptual models of practice. The practice setting illustrated is Gloucestershire Partnership NHS Foundation Trust (GPT). Occupational therapists who work in this service have been collaborating with the UK Centre for Outcomes Research and Education (UK CORE). This collaboration provides support in the use of a particular conceptual model of practice as the main informing body of knowledge. After appraising the available theoretical perspectives, occupational therapists in GPT selected the Model of Human Occupation (Kielhofner 2008) to underpin their practice.

Whilst we use illustrations from this practice area, we hope that the supporting mechanisms illustrated will be relevant for the majority of therapists in most settings. We want to emphasise that therapists can still be successful in developing skills to use theory in practice even if some elements of the case study are not present within their context. Our illustrations here are about:

i. The attributes that therapists can strive to develop in order to be successful at using theory in practice
ii. Helpful elements of the environmental context
iii. Specific mechanisms which support therapists use of theory in practice

(i) The attributes that therapists can develop to be successful at using new or developing theories in practice Little research has been undertaken to examine the attributes of occupational therapists who are successful in implementing new ideas. Chard (2006) touches on the matter in her research by suggesting that the attitudes of single-mindedness, tenacity and the ability to re-conceptualise new ways of working seem to be the most important characteristics for applying innovation. Arguably, therapists who have the ability to be clear about their role can more easily adapt to change as they will have confidence in the boundaries of their knowledge and expertise. Perhaps the first feature of the therapist who can drive forward the development of their practice is ability and desire to be proactive, taking personal responsibility for the learning and

development required for theoretically oriented practice. Without this intrinsic motivation to adapt and advance their practice therapists might be perceived as disinterested or resistant (Rogers 2003) (see Vignette 2.1).

Vignette 2.1

Example of an occupational therapist who is able to articulate her position about the use of theory in practice thus illustrating her single-mindedness, tenacity and clarity about her way of working

'I mean its about knowing what you can do as an occupational therapist, who you are as an occupational therapist, what your place is in the world of [field of work], and what you can offer people really, your role in the team. But then also what resources you have and to be able to use those effectively, in terms of both who you see and then what the next steps are with them... I am able to talk about what I do and why and to be a very strong advocate for what I do and if someone says well "why are you doing that?" I can now say "and here's the evidence for it and this is what we're doing and why".'

(ii) Helpful elements of the environmental context It appears to be the social environment in particular that might act as a support to therapists' development of theoretically orientated practice. Where there is management support for investment in updating practice a multitude of learning opportunities can be created by knowledgeable professional leaders. Having confidence in occupational therapy leaders to support theoretical developments over time is pivotal to foster a facilitative environment (Chard 2000) (see Vignette 2.2).

Vignette 2.2

Example of an occupational therapist articulating her observation of the work context, particularly the occupational therapy leadership support for her use of theory in practice

'I'd say it [the organisation] definitely does support it [practice development]. Obviously the professional side of occupational therapy very much supports it and that's very, very strong. And that's not just on MoHO but it could be Sensory Integration or whatever.'

(iii) The specific mechanisms which support therapists' use of theory in practice We will offer comment upon five mechanisms which some therapists have used successfully to bring theory into their practice. They include:

1. Obtaining the available theory to support practice
2. Accessing appropriate continuing education
3. Using professional supervision
4. Practising in practice
5. Setting practice standards.

1. Obtaining the available theory to support practice

Having the knowledge about what contemporary theories are available to support practice action is fundamental to theoretically oriented practice. Therapists have a responsibility to keep up to date with practice developments (College of Occupational Therapists 2005) and therefore have a responsibility to seek out innovation. It appears though that not all occupational therapists are independently investing time to find out about the theoretical or evidence-based developments that will support their own advancement in practice despite the fact that they are conscientious about their responsibilities (Metcalf et al 2001, Taylor 2007). This suggests that occupational therapists might find emerging knowledge more accessible if it is repackaged in a variety of ways. For example, 80% of the sample of occupational therapists surveyed in one study appealed for brief summaries of relevant practice information to be provided for them rather than them having to search the literature themselves (Bennett et al 2003).

Accessing theoretical concepts is also facilitated by clinicians having contemporary tools available in the workplace. These include acquiring theoretically based, practice-oriented textbooks; web-based information; and assessment manuals that summarize theoretical underpinnings. In addition clinical forums or special interest groups for discussion of relevant theories and their application with knowledgeable practice and academic leaders serve to underpin knowledge within practice.

We have observed that practitioners working collaboratively with academics have prompted the creation of resources which help to collectively explain the theory that the service is adopting. For example in GPT, an animated, power point picture was developed, locally known as 'the pin-man' which has been consistently used to illustrate case study material allowing therapists to engage with 'thinking with theory' in a practical way (Figure 2.3) (see Vignette 2.3).

Vignette 2.3

Example of an occupational therapist articulating the way in which she has been obtaining the available theory to support her practice

'It [theory] makes it a lot clearer and when I feel a bit confused or a bit too laid back and not as organised as I would like to be, I can just take a step back and look at the case and what I am doing with people and try to put it into the context of the Model of Human Occupation or I use the little 'pin-man' to see how that applies to somebody.'

2. Accessing appropriate continuing education

Occupational therapists commonly discuss the benefits of attending training courses for specific new techniques (Curtin and Jaramazovic 2001). Attending external training courses can be a costly process and it is clear that not all knowledge gained in attending courses is used in the practice setting (Chard 2004). A question can be posed about the prudence of investing service resources in education delivered this way if some therapists are not subsequently able to integrate knowledge into practice. It could be argued that learning as a local group is more effective in transferring new knowledge into practice. Common action points can be negotiated amongst participants and subsequent change managed in practice. Therapists can not only develop knowledge about the new practice development but can also develop skills by becoming competent in sharing that knowledge locally with their colleagues. Building and sharing practice-based knowledge within the practice area assists the organisation to have a community of practice scholars.

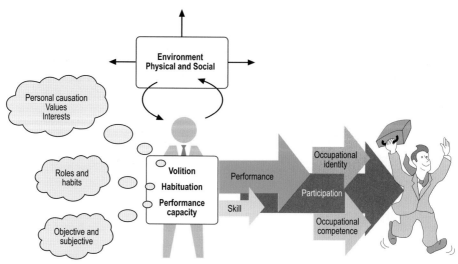

Figure 2.3 An example of a locally produced powerpoint tool used in practice to explain theoretical concepts. *'The MOHO Pin-man' Adapted from: The Model of Human Occupation (MOHO) Kielhofner (2002).*

By adopting a strategic approach to the continuing education opportunities for occupational therapists, working in partnership with academic colleagues who are schooled in understanding the theory of occupational therapy, GPT have been able to offer locally delivered, problem-based learning courses (Forsyth et al 2005b). The skills of practitioners within the Trust have been drawn upon to provide a variety of workshops, didactic and experiential teaching. This has enabled therapists to engage with theory and its associated assessments. Specifically, the mechanism where therapists have a short time out of clinical work to concentrate on learning in a small group and then have a set time to implement before reporting back upon their new practice learning has been a successful system (see Vignette 2.4).

Vignette 2.4

Example of an occupational therapist articulating the way in which she has benefited from locally constructed and delivered continuing education

'I've recently attended another session which was the Volitional Questionnaire training and I've also attended the follow up session in January. This morning I've also had a meeting with someone else about doing the "train the trainers" for the Model of Human Occupation Screening Tool. So I'd say that's been quite a dramatic development actually for learning. As I say, I've always used the Model of Human Occupation right from being a student but since the Scholarship of Practice [practice development initiative] has been in place I've certainly developed an awful lot more skills and competency in using the assessments and I'm now feeling confident enough to train other people to do that too. It is quite a big change.'

3. Using professional supervision

Clinical supervision practised well can be helpful in enhancing occupational therapy practice (Sweeney et al 2001) (see Chapter 22). Indeed, practice based on the idea of 'reflection in action' or reflective practice has been argued to be an underpinning mechanism of professional problem solving (Schön 1991, Roberts 2002) (see Chapter 10) and developing professional craft knowledge (Smith 2001). It is perhaps no surprise then that occupational therapists are expected to participate in professional supervision in order to ensure the quality of practice (Department of Health 1998, College of Occupational Therapists 2005). The mechanism that we propose here is a particular, structured technique of reflecting on clinical scenarios using occupational therapy theory as part of a discussion with colleagues who have experience at using theory in practice. Examples from the literature (Wimpenny et al 2006) support the message from our case illustration which shows that the routine of thinking within a particular theoretical framework can be strengthened if therapists have the opportunity to reflect on their practice in this way (see Vignette 2.5).

Vignette 2.5

Example of an occupational therapist articulating the benefits with her understanding of occupational therapy theory that she has felt from engaging in professional supervision

'you can only do so much yourself, you can sort of "download your head" but then it's only your view on things and then I think it's important to have the opportunity to talk through things. It often clarifies things a lot more than just thinking it through by yourself.'

4. Practise in practice

Occupational therapists and other healthcare practitioners with clinical responsibilities locate their priorities within direct client care (LeMay et al 1998, Metcalf et al 2001). Undertaking theoretically orientated initiatives can be perceived as an 'added extra' to core practice rather than as an essential component to best practice (Melton et al 2003). Research has demonstrated that some services enable therapists to access new therapeutic initiatives but that those services do not necessarily have any overt governance or support for the new learning to be followed through in practice (Chard 2004). By changing the culture to expect therapists to put new knowledge appropriately into action, services can demonstrate the use of theory and evidence to practice, enhance the practice skills of staff and use resources to best effect. Thus, this position supports therapists to use their time in 'hands on' practice as a priority whilst also expecting that the practice is developed (see Vignette 2.6).

Vignette 2.6

Example of an occupational therapist articulating her perception of the value and use of 'practise in practice' to support her learning

'Mmmm, the thing that immediately comes to mind is how important it is to actually put it [new knowledge of theory and assessments for practice] into practice ... I think that whilst you can go a long way in isolation in taking on broad theory, when you get to the tools and when you get to the application you really need to be in regular contact with clients with whom you're applying that.'

5. Setting practice standards

The development and use of practice guidelines has been heralded as a strategy to improve standards of practice and enhance professional development (Cusick and McCluskey 2000). In order for this to be undertaken successfully practitioners ideally need to agree to the standards and form their practice actions accordingly. Time has been invested in GPT to document both pictorial and narrative care pathway standards that occupational therapists are expected to follow, where appropriate, in their practice. Taking a corporate approach to practice development, occupational therapists and support staff in GPT have been assisted to develop theoretically based assessment and intervention pathways to guide their practice. These practice standards do not in any way remove the therapist's responsibility for clinical reasoning with the information that they generate through assessment procedures. Rather the information that they gather and have available acts as a supporting mechanism to generate intervention goals with service users. In addition the care pathways form a structure to facilitate the appropriate use of the assessment tools developed within a theoretical framework and foster the interpretation of assessment results to be articulated within the associated theoretical base (see Vignette 2.7).

Vignette 2.7

Example of an occupational therapist articulating her use of practise standards to support her practice and development

'The care pathway has just become part of supervision and it's really worked. We've sat down and especially when we've done caseload management and we say, "well what are we doing with people" in terms of articulating what you're doing and why you are doing it. I know I'm doing it for the right reasons.'

Summary of measures to assist practitioners engage with theory in practice

- Be proactive and take responsibility for learning and developing your practice.
- Take responsibility for finding out what the practice-based theories are and how they might connect with your practice.
- Acquire the most contemporary version of the literature explaining the theory; use the internet to seek out current innovation in theory development.
- Contribute to web-based discussion forums with questions and comments.
- Seek out other therapists as part of local CPD who can debate the application of the theory within practice, forming groups of special interest to debate and discuss the application of theory to practice.
- Practise formulating the strengths, needs, aspirations and occupational goals of your service users using the theory base.
- Network with academics who are schooled in understanding the theory of occupational therapy.
- Interpret and articulate the results of the standardized assessment tools that you use in practice in association with the appropriate occupational therapy theoretical base.
- Build and share practice-based knowledge within your practice area.

We conclude with a final remark from an occupational therapist from GPT who has successfully engaged in the mechanisms for client-centred, theory-driven, occupational therapy practice development (see Vignette 2.8).

Vignette 2.8

'I have to say that my clinical reasoning is probably very much informed by the Model of Human Occupation at the moment and if I think about before that it was probably not underpinned by anything terribly much if I'm honest. I think that I was one of those people who didn't really think too much about it. I'd see the person, I'd ask about how they were going in terms of their occupational function like their Activities of Daily Living and their interests and their worth and stuff and how their going with that and I might have looked at things that were issues for them that they want to work on. I don't know that I was as client focused as I am now in terms of trying to draw out what is really meaningful for them and where their motivation and their personal causation particularly lie. I think it was more that I might have just made more assumptions than I do now. I wouldn't necessarily have looked at the depth that I do now.'

Summary

Throughout this chapter we have argued that there is the potential for positive outcomes and benefits for service users, therapists and services as occupational therapists grasp the challenge of integrating theory into their practice. The extent of this challenge is not underestimated in the busy schedule of occupational therapists in practice. We have illustrated though that with carefully considered practice development mechanisms and partnerships with academic colleagues, therapists can seek opportunities which enable their service users to benefit from occupational therapy practice which is underpinned by appropriate, occupation-focused theory.

References

Bennett S, Tooth L, McKenna K, et al 2003 Perceptions of evidence-based practice: A survey of Australian occupational therapists. Australian Journal of Occupational Therapy 50:13–22

Canadian Association of Occupational Therapists 1997 Enabling Occupation: an Occupational Therapy Perspective. CAOT Publications ACE, Ottawa

Chard G 2000 An investigation into the use of the Assessment of Motor and Process Skills (AMPS) in clinical practice. British Journal of Occupational Therapy 63(10): 481–488

Chard G 2004 Implementing the Assessment of Motor and Process Skills (AMPS) in the workplace: a comparison of the experiences of occupational therapists and new graduates. British Journal of Occupational Therapy 67(2):54–64

Chard G 2006 Adopting the Assessment of Motor and Process Skills into practice: therapists' voices. British Journal of Occupational Therapy 69(2):50–57

Christiansen C 1999 Defining lives: Occupation as identity: An essay on competence, coherence and the creation of meaning. American Journal of Occupational Therapy 53(6): 547–558

College of Occupational Therapists 2005 Code of Ethics and Professional Conduct. College of Occupational Therapists, London

Closs SJ, Cheater FM 1999 Evidence based nursing practice: a clarification of issues. Journal of Advanced Nursing 30:10–17

Curtin M, Jaramazovic E 2001 Occupational therapists' view and perceptions of evidence-based practice. The British Journal of Occupational Therapy 64(5):214–222

Cusick A 2001 The research sensitive practitioner. In Higgs J, Titchen A (eds) Professional Practice in Health, Education and the Creative Arts, pp. 125–135. Blackwell Science, Cornwall, UK

Cusick A, McCluskey A 2000 Becoming an evidence-based practitioner through professional development. Australian Occupational Therapy Journal 47:159–170

Department of Health 1998 A First Class Service. Quality in the NHS. HMSO, London

Duncan EAS (ed) 2006 Foundations for Practice in Occupational Therapy 4th edn. Elsevier, London

Fisher AG 1998 Uniting practice and theory in an occupational framework. American Journal of Occupational Therapy 52(7):509–521

Forsyth K, Summerfield Mann L, Kielhofner G 2005a Scholarship of practice: making occupation-focused, theory driven and evidenced-based practice a reality. British Journal of Occupational Therapy 68(6):1–9

Forsyth K, Melton J, Summerfield Mann L 2005b Achieving evidence based practice; An innovative process of continuing education through practitioner-academic partnership. Occupational Therapy in Health Care 19(1–2):211–227

Forsyth K, Duncan EAS, Summerfield Mann L 2005c Scholarship of Practice in the United Kingdom: an occupational therapy service case study. Occupational Therapy in Health Care 19(1–2):17–29

Health Professions Council 2003 Standards of Proficiency, Occupational Therapists, p. 11. HPC, London

Higgs J, Titchen A, Neville V 2001 Professional practice and knowledge. In Higgs J, Titchen A (eds) Practice Knowledge and Expertise in the Health Professions, pp. 3–9. Butterworth Heinemann, Oxford, UK

Kielhofner G 2002 The Model of Human Occupation, Theory and Application, 3rd edn. Lippincott, Williams and Wilkins, Maryland

Kielhofner G 2004 Conceptual Foundations of Occupational Therapy, 3rd edn. FA Davis Company, Philadelphia

Kielhofner G 2005 Scholarship of Practice: creating discourse between theory, research and practice. Occupational Therapy in Health Care 19(1–2):7–16

Kielhofner G 2008 The Model of Human Occupation, Theory and Application, 4th edn. Lippincott, Williams and Wilkins, Maryland

Law M, Baum C, Dunn W 2001 Measuring Occupational Performance, Supporting Best Practice in Occupational Therapy. Slack, NJ

Le May A, Mulhall A, Alexander C 1998 Bridging the research–practice gap: exploring the research cultures of practitioners and managers. Journal of Advanced Nursing 28(2):428–437

Lloyd-Smith W 1997 Evidence-based practice and occupational therapy. British Journal of Occupational Therapy 60(11):474–478

Mattingly C, Fleming M 1994 Clinical reasoning: Forms of inquiry in a therapeutic practice. F A Davis Press, Philadelphia

McCluskey A, Cusick A 2002 Strategies for introducing evidence-based practice and changing clinician behaviours: a manager's toolbox. Australian Journal of Occupational Therapy 49(2):63–70

Melton J, Forsyth K, Summerfield Mann L 2003 Delivering evidence-based practice: no money, no time, no skill? [editorial]. The British Journal of Occupational Therapy 66(10):439

Metcalf C, Lewin RJP, Wisher S et al 2001 Barriers to implementing the evidence base in four NHS therapies. Physiotherapy 87(8):433–441

Munoz JP, Lawlor M, Kielhofner G 1993 Use of the MoHO: a survey of therapists in psychiatric practice. Occupational Therapy Journal of Research 13(2):117–139

Nixon J, Creek J 2006 Towards a theory of practice. British Journal of Occupational Therapy 69(2):77–80

Oxman A, Davis D, Hayes R et al 1995 No magic bullets: a systematic review of 102 trials of intervention to help health professions deliver services more effectively or efficiently. Canadian Medical Association Journal 153:1423–1443

Parham D 1987 Toward professionalism: the reflective therapist. American Journal of Occupational Therapy 41(9):555–561

Parham LD 1986 Applying theory to practice. In: American Occupational Therapy Association Occupational Therapy Education: Target 2000. AOTA, Rockville, MD

Roberts AE 2002 Advancing practice through continuing education: the case for reflection. British Journal of Occupational Therapy 65(5):237–241

Rogers EM 2003 Diffusion of Innovation, 5th edn. The Free Press New York,

Schön DA 1991 The Reflective Practitioner: How Professionals Think in Action. Ashgate Publishing, England

Smith DL 2001 Facilitating the development of professional craft knowledge. In: Higgs J, Titchen A (eds) Practice Knowledge and Expertise in the Health Professions, p. 172–177. Butterworth Heinemann, Oxford, UK

Sweeney G, Webley P, Treacher A 2001 Supervision in occupational therapy, Part 3: accommodating the supervisor and the supervisee. The British Journal of Occupational Therapy 64(9):426–431

Taylor MC 2007 Evidence-Based Practice for Occupational Therapists, 2nd edn. Blackwell Publishing, Oxford, UK

Tickle-Degnen L 1998 Using research evidence in planning treatment for the individual client. Canadian Journal of Occupational Therapy 65(3):152–159

Townsend E A, Polatajko J H 2007 Enabling Occupation II. Advancing an Occupational Therapy Vision for Health, Wellbeing and Justice through Occupation. Canadian Association of Occupational Therapists, Ottawa, Canada

Wimpenny K, Forsyth K, Jones C et al 2006 Group reflective supervision: thinking with theory to develop practice. British Journal of Occupational Therapy 69(9):1–6

Wood W 1998 It is jump time for occupational therapy. American Journal of Occupational Therapy 52:403–411.

Judgement and decision-making skills for practice

3

Priscilla Harries and
Edward A.S. Duncan

 Highlight box

- Practitioners form judgements and make decisions in everyday practice.
- Making judgements and decisions are two of the key cognitive tasks used in professional thinking.
- These judgements and decisions can have a considerable impact on the quality of client care.
- It is important that students and practitioners understand the different manners in which judgements and decisions can be understood in practice.
- Practical examples are included to help the reader consider the different factors involved in judgement and decision making.

Overview

Why is judgement and decision making important and worthy of inclusion in a book that focuses on Skills for Practice? Few practitioners would contest the notion that they possess knowledge upon which they base their decisions in practice. What the basis of this knowledge is and how they use it in practice is, however, much less clear. Making judgements and decisions are two of the key cognitive tasks used in professional thinking. This chapter teases out how practitioners think in practice, form judgements and make decisions; each of which when made well enables people to take wise action and ultimately enhance the effectiveness of a service's provision.

The chapter begins by looking at definitions for key terms in the area. It then continues by presenting some of the early occupational therapy studies of clinical reasoning; discussing what this research has told us about the way occupational therapists think, as well as the limitations of the research methods they used. Two related but differing theories of judgement and decision making, that have developed from cognitive psychology, are then presented: cognitive continuum theory and dual process theory. The contribution of each of these theories to practice is examined.

The chapter then considers how practitioners can apply judgement and decision-making skills in practice and exercises are provided to illustrate the challenges and processes of judgement and decision-making tasks. To conclude, the chapter discusses the impact of practitioners' personal and professional values on judgement and decision making in practice.

Definitions

Researchers studying different cognitive tasks have used a wide variety of terms to describe different types of thinking such as reasoning, judgement, problem solving and decision making (Gale and Marsden 1985). Reasoning implies the drawing of conclusions. Reasoning may be deductive, when the conclusion is logically drawn based on factual information, or inductive, when the conclusion drawn is only possible and needs to be tested in light of further information (Eysenck 1993). A judgement requires a person to consider an item of information or an option and to assign a weight, based on the perceived level of importance. Problem solving involves generating alternatives to select from (see Chapter 10). Decision making occurs when a person makes a selection from possible alternatives that have been considered. In occupational therapy the term 'clinical reasoning' tends to be used to cover all these thinking processes but each term can be defined independently and can be used with a distinct meaning.

What tends to clarify the meaning of the terms is understanding the theoretical and methodological orientation of the researcher. Those most interested in the outcome of thinking tend to compare how information has been used with the decision that has been taken. They are most interested in judgement and decision making. Such researchers tend to use quantitative methodologies characteristic of the schools of judgement analysis and decision analysis. They are interested in identification of statistical weightings of judgements or the calculation of the probability that a particular decision has been, or will be, made. Research using judgement analysis has been conducted in occupational therapy by Unsworth (1995, 1996, 1997, 2001), Harries and Harries (2001a, 2001b) and Harries and Gilhooly (2003a, 2003b). To date decision analysis research has not been published in occupational therapy literature.

Researchers more interested in describing the actual processes of thinking, as opposed to the decision outcome, tend to focus their attention on reasoning and problem solving. These latter researchers tend to use qualitative methods such as those informed by phenomenological and ethnographic theories. To date these have accounted for the majority of occupational therapy clinical reasoning research studies.

The early studies[*]

Joan Rogers used her Eleanor Clark Slagle lecture of 1983 to talk about the ethics, science and art of clinical reasoning. Rogers (1983) defined clinical reasoning as, '...the scientific, ethical and artistic dimensions' of practice (p. 616). Emphasizing that these are inextricably linked.

Later, Mattingly and Fleming (1994) conducted an influential research project of American occupational therapists' clinical reasoning. It was the first major study to explore the reasoning strategies used by occupational therapists and used an ethnographic and action research approach: interviewing, observing and videoing 17 occupational therapists over a 2-year period (Mattingley and Fleming 1994). The researchers identified reasoning 'tracks' or styles and linked these to reasoning strategies. Their findings

---

[*] From Harries and Harries 2001a, with permission of the College of Occupational Therapists.

emphasized that occupational therapists' reasoning was, 'largely tacit, highly imagistic and deeply phenomenological' (Mattingly 1991, p. 797).

Since the work of Mattingly and Fleming (1994), there has been a burgeoning of research in occupational therapy examining the clinical reasoning of occupational therapists (see Fondler et al 1990, Fleming 1991a, Creighton et al 1995, Alvernick and Sviden 1996, Fortune and Ryan 1996, Fossey 1996, Hagedorn 1996, Munroe 1996, Crabtree and Lyons 1997, Hooper 1997, Chapparo 1999, McKay 1999, Paterson et al 2002, Paterson 2003). This literature has been presented and discussed in greater depth by Patterson and Summerfield-Mann (2006). Whilst there are a few exceptions, the defining characteristics of this body of research are that the methods are qualitative, the sample sizes are generally small, and the participant populations are predominantly north American.

A few key points can be generalized from these and other studies of a similar format in nursing and other professions (Fawcett et al 2001, Sefton 2001, Upshur et al 2001, Rycroft-Malone et al 2004). Generally, these studies view clinical reasoning (or decision making) as being formed of several components including the use of knowledge, self reflection by the clinician (a component of meta cognition), clients' needs, expectations or desires, and shared decision making. Crucially, the vast majority of these studies view the components of clinical reasoning as being of equal value – like pieces of a jigsaw that are each as important as the other.

Although qualitative approaches were chosen to try to give a holistic understanding of thinking in terms of context, they appear to be limited in terms of their ability to represent the holism of actual thinking. Their lack of validity relates specifically to the difficulty the approaches have in reliably accessing experts' well-practised intuitive thinking.

Analytical versus intuitive thinking

The first major study of thinking processes in clinical situations was the study of medical problem solving by Arthur Elstein and his colleagues (Elstein et al 1978). Their study used three methods of data collection: direct observation of problem solving using simulated clinical problems, concurrent think aloud and retrospection (whilst viewing video footage). Elstein et al (1978) identified hypothetico-deductive reasoning as the strategy for diagnosis formation in medicine. Occupational therapists also identified hypothetico-deductive reasoning through the 'occupational dysfunction' diagnosis (Fleming 1991b). However, when comparing differences between novices and experienced practitioners' diagnosis formation strategies, Elstein found that there were other forms of thinking (Elstein et al 1990). As experts had the advantage of previous experience they had developed a store of 'scripts' (Abernathy and Hamm, 1994). If a client had a familiar problem practitioners used pattern matching to trigger the direct automatic retrieval of an appropriate script. Therefore experts confronted with a familiar problem used a rapid and automatic form of processing that was acknowledged as intuitive reasoning (Abernathy and Hamm 1994).

The more practised in a thinking process a practitioner is, the more intuitive it may become. People are aware of how a motor task such as driving can become partially subconscious; in the same way cognitive tasks can become partially automatic when they have been well practised. It is therefore difficult to verbalize thinking pertaining to a high level of expertise; and post hoc rationalization can reduce the verbalization to a report of a lower-quality thinking process.

Ethnographic and information-processing methods

Ethnographic and information-processing methods appear to have had difficulty in establishing thoughts used in clinicians' intuitive thinking. These methods have to rely heavily on the reasoner's awareness of how information has been used to make judgements; they have been limited in their ability to access the more unconscious, rapid and unrecoverable reasoning at the intuitive end of the continuum (Ericsson and Simon 1980). In the early studies intuitive reasoning was not given much attention, for example in the occupational therapists' study, intuitive reasoning was only nominally identified and described as 'difficult to map' (Fleming 1991a).

Whilst these studies were being conducted, other theorists were concurrently drawing into question the efficacy of using verbal reports to access thinking. If intuitive thought was 'non-recoverable' the issue of whether decision-makers would have any access into their thinking became apparent (Nisbett and Wilson 1977). With regard to accessing the thinking of experts in particular, verbal reports were recognized by some as inefficient and misrepresentative (Hoffman 1987). Concurrent verbalisations, at best, only got to the content of working memory, or the information attended to (but not necessarily how it is used) and retrospective verbalisations were prone to forgetting and post-hoc rationalisation (Ericsson and Simon 1980). However it is not clear cut. Some recall can be valuable and measures are being taken to maximise the accuracy of recall methods. Unsworth (2004) has begun to use head-mounted video cameras to record occupational therapists' interventions. This approach has been shown to enhance the accuracy of memory during retrospective recall.

Roberts (1996) and Robertson (1996) recognised the influence of expertise on occupational therapists' reasoning. The AOFT/AOTA study had focused on hypothetico-deductive strategies in problem identification tasks. These can be verbalised more easily and hence are reported more effectively. Roberts, however, demonstrated that reasoning varied according to the level of expertise and the nature of the task. In her research, 38 practitioners wrote down their thoughts immediately after reading three referral letters. Although some of the reasoning may have been lost before the participant began to write down their thoughts, interesting findings were made. Some practitioners initially used rapid formulations of the issues involved (pattern matchers/heuristic reasoners). They mentioned their recognition of the scenario and recalled previous cases. Others searched for cues and reasoned using various hypotheses, sometimes not reaching any specific formulation. They appeared to have less experience to draw on. The rapid formulators did not show intuitive reasoning exclusively. Evidence of hypothetico-deductive reasoning was also seen when considering some aspects of the case. In these instances participants were thought to have been less familiar with the information. This would concur with the view that reasoning strategies result from interaction between both the experience of the practitioner and the nature of the task.

The value of experience

In Elstein's 1978 study, differences between novice and expert thinking were explored. They identified that it was the extent of clinical experience in a particular domain that was key to expert thinking. Experts were able to interpret data more accurately when testing hypotheses than novices. This finding had implications for medical education, as contrary to what had been thought, it was not the reasoning strategies themselves that can improve clinicians' problem solving but the domain-specific knowledge that is important. Pre-registration problem-solving training would, therefore, not create experts: lifelong learning would be necessary to achieve mastery of knowledge domains. Education subsequently made a move away from problem-solving training and toward problem-based learning (Norman and Schmidt 1992). This new method of education increased clinical knowledge through facilitating exposure to clinical case scenarios.

Cognitive continuum theory

In order to better understand why certain thoughts are difficult to access, it is necessary to gain a deeper understanding of how and why differing modes of thought occur. Hammond's Cognitive Continuum Theory (CCT) can be valuable in understanding these issues (Hammond and Brehmer 1973).

Hammond's CCT described a range of cognitive modes from intuitive to analytic with quasi-experimental processing as a mid-point. Hammond felt that in more intuitive reasoning, strategies such as pattern recognition and heuristics (rules of thumb) were used: information available (cues) is immediately linked to known patterns (Larkin 1979). This is therefore a largely subconscious, rapid, automated process and is essentially 'non-recoverable' (Hammond and Brehmer 1973). At the other end of the continuum, analytical thought occurs. In this mode of thought, hypothetico-deductive reasoning is used: a slower, step-by-step method of thinking that is highly conscious. In hypothetico-deductive thinking, cues are used to generate possible hypotheses and further cues used to test these hypotheses.

Many theorists have agreed that when less practised in a cognitive task, analytical processing is more likely to be used but when more practised in a task, and the information is familiar, intuitive strategies are more likely (Benner 1984, Elstein et al 1990, Norman et al 1994). In addition to the role of expertise, the Cognitive Continuum identified the influence of task characteristics on reasoning strategy. Task characteristics, such as stability and availability of task information are thought to have a strong influence on the possible types of cognitive processing (Shanteau 1992). Therefore the mode of cognitive processing (i.e. thinking) used tends to be a result of the combined effect of level of experience of the practitioner and the characteristics of the task.

Dual-process theories of thinking

Dual-processing theory (Stanovich and West 2003) is a more recent decision-making theory that has developed from cognitive psychology. Whilst bearing similarities to CCT (as both differentiate between intuitive and analytical thinking), there is an important difference in approach. Dual-processing theory posits that the two cognitive systems (the intuitive, which is automatic, holistic and fast; and the analytical, which is deliberate, rational, explicit and slow) are in fact two different systems; not a single continuum as proposed in Hammond's CCT. Functional magnetic resonance imaging has indicated that these systems are in fact neurologically different (Goel et al 2000). In dual-processing theory, the fast, automatic form of processing is referred to as System 1 (S1) and the slow, deliberate form as System 2 (S2) (Stanovich and West 2000).

Dual-processing theory can be understood in the following way. S1 delivers judgements through largely subconscious reasoning (tacit knowledge) and only the outcome is conscious; whilst, S2 is a highly conscious and logical reasoning process. S2 type reasoning enables practitioners to think about hypothetical situations, analyse potential future possibilities and other features of a situation that are not immediately apparent. S2 type thinking uses central working memory (Gathercole 2003), focuses on one task at a time, and is correlated with general intelligence (Stanovich and West 2000). S2 type reasoning is viewed as having evolved more recently than S1 and, interestingly, is a faculty that only humans have (Evans 2003).

Parallels between the components of clinical reasoning, for instance the work of Mattingly and Fleming (1994), and dual-process theory are easy to make. Concepts such as tacit knowledge and intuitive reasoning appear closely linked to the holistic nature of S1, whilst knowledge and research drawn from an objective basis are more closely associated with the objective reasoning of S2.

Paley et al (2007) drew comparisons between clinical reasoning and empirical knowledge using dual-process theory. Whilst their paper focused on nursing research, the arguments are valid for other areas of health-care research, including occupational therapy. In order to draw comparisons with dual-processing theory they referred to the type of reasoning associated with intuitive reasoning and 'artful practice' as N1 and objective knowledge drawn from quantitative research as N2.

Paley et al (2007) however highlight that there is one major difference between the N1/N2 distinction and the S1/S2 distinction; whilst the majority of occupational therapy clinical reasoning literature regards N1 and N2 as equal partners. Cognitive dual-processing theory, on the other hand, emphasises that the principal function of S2 is to override, monitor, suppress the invalid inferences of S1 (Kahneman and Frederick 2002, Evans 2003, Evans and Over 2004). Therefore, while occupational therapy literature, to date, generally views N1 and N2 as equally valid ways of thinking, it is clear that S2 ways of thinking are epistemologically superior.

Heuristics and biases

The heuristics and biases research literature explains why there is a disparity between S1 and S2 ways of thinking (Kahneman et al 1982, Gilovich et al 2002). This research shows that people often make mistakes when the clinical experience (S1) is not controlled by measurable objective evidence (S2). The reasons behind this are outlined in greater detail by Paley et al (2007).

Interestingly S1 type thinking is not only responsible for clinical errors in thinking, but can also explain some academic errors as well. For example how people view and understand scientific research can be compromised by their prior beliefs about its findings (Koehler 1993). Resch et al (2000) and Kaptchuk (2003) have both established that well-designed studies can be dismissed because they either indicate an unconventional intervention is effective, or that a well-respected intervention is ineffective. Conversely poorly designed studies can sometimes be accepted as they appear to support widely held beliefs. This principle is not only restricted to experimental research. Generally any method will be regarded as valid if its conclusions are believed, and as invalid if its conclusions are disagreed with (Fugelsang and Thompson 2000, Roberts and Sykes 2003, Fugelsang et al 2004).

So what does knowledge of S1 and S2 tell us about N1 and N2 types of thinking in occupational therapy? It means that intuitive clinical reasoning is likely to make mistakes (due to S1 type weaknesses in thinking) when it is not corrected by the more structured and objective approach of S2 thinking processes. The impact of thinking errors associated to S1 type thinking are not limited to occupational therapy or nursing, etc. Stanovich (2003) has stated that through such errors, 'physicians choose less effective medical treatments; people fail to accurately assess risks in their environment; information is misused in legal proceedings; millions of dollars are spent on unneeded projects by government and private industry; parents fail to vaccinate their children; unnecessary surgery is performed; animals are hunted to extinction; billions of dollars are wasted on quack medical remedies; and costly financial misjudgements are made' (p. 292). Dual-processing theory demonstrates that tacit knowledge and experience (S1/N1) cannot be viewed equally to knowledge that is rigorously researched and empirically based (S2/N2). To continue to view N1 and N2 forms of knowledge as equal, Paley at al (2007) state, is to celebrate the possibility of error in practice.

It could be said that the notion that we should, 'base our practice on "generalisable evidence" demolishes our traditional practice. Such worldviews urge us to swap our ideas of crafting care around the unique complexity of the individual, for a generalisation about what worked for most people in a study' (Barker 2000: 332). This is an argument that has proven popular in health-care literature in general and occupational therapy is no exception. The structure of this argument is as follows: 'Quantitative studies refer to populations; practitioners care for individuals; therefore, quantitative studies are irrelevant to clinical practice. This is similar in form to: epidemiological studies of cancer refer to populations; individuals make decisions; therefore, epidemiological studies are irrelevant to my decision to smoke. Both of these arguments dismiss the concepts of probability and risk, and would make a nonsense of actuarial procedures and insurance. In any case, the experience on which the nurse, [or occupational therapist] draws when working with an individual is also population-based: the population of clients she or her colleagues have previously seen. If the population defined by a research study is irrelevant to the unique individual, so is the population defined by clinical experience' (Paley et al 2007: 697).

So, how can we use our knowledge of dual-processing theory in practice? S1 is how most practitioners reason, most of the time. But if practitioners use S2 type thinking it will monitor and improve this intuitive form of reasoning (Degani et al 2006). It is this rationale that supports evidence-based practice, helps practitioners to question their judgements about practice and encourages the search for more evidence-based ways of thinking and working.

Three factors, however, inhibit the use of S2 thinking in clinical practice. First, there appears to be a natural resistance to the use of S2 type thinking and there is a general reluctance to accept the idea that practitioners make S1 type errors in reasoning. Secondly, evidence-based decision making and S2 type thinking do not come naturally. And thirdly, S2 type thinking requires time and space – something that challenges everyone (Paley et al 2007).

The idea that intuitive reasoning and holistic practice (S1/N1), is equal in weight and status to scientific evidence (S2/N2), is persuasive. But this should not get in the way of delivering the highest quality services to clients. And to achieve this practitioners need to employ S2 type strategies. There is, of course, no single answer to this issue, but there is one possibility that may offer a solution: the use of conceptual models of practice.

Conceptual models of practice

Within occupational therapy, structured use of conceptual models of practice such as the Canadian Model of Occupational Performance and Engagement (Townsend and Polatjko 2007) or the Model of Human Occupation (Kielhofner 2007) could be viewed as approaches that adopt S2 supervisory functions in practice. Their conscious use ensures that all necessary factors have been considered and given due priority when working with a client. When viewed in the light of the evidence that supports the supervisory nature of S2 over S1, conceptual models such as MOHO and CMOP-E which have evolved through rigorous research, do not provide an illusion of safety as Smith (2006) suggested. They are not a panacea for perfect practice. But they do ensure that the inherent biases and mental shortcuts of practitioners, masquerading under the guise of 'artful practice' or clinical reasoning (and which typify S1 type thinking), cannot be carried away unabated, drawing clients into decisions that are ill-considered and lacking in reliable evidence to support their validity.

Conceptual models of practice, as an answer to the dual-processing dilemma, are only one option and their endorsement here should not be taken to suggest that these models are viewed as perfect or infallible. But some do provide an evidence-based structure to follow which limits the possibilities for personal S1 type biases, and conceptual models continue to be researched and refined.

Applying judgement and decision-making skills in practice

Judgement and decisions skills have to be learnt for every stage of the occupational therapy process from referral through to evaluation. Through the use of scenarios as well as real life experience, reasoning skills can be exercised in relation to specific domains. The following examples are designed to improve your reasoning in practice.

Imagine you are an occupational therapist in an adult community mental health team. You may consider taking some general referrals which have been sent to your team and some which have been sent directly to you. These referrals fall into the second category: they have been sent directly to you. Look at the referral in Figure 3.1 and indicate the degree of priority you feel the referral warrants. In practice you would also be likely to see the client before making a fully informed judgement. However, for this task just use your initial impressions of whether you would work with the client. So how much priority would you give it? Put a cross on the line at the bottom of the referral to give your decision.

In doing this task you will have decided how much attention to give to the differing types of information. You will have judged how important those types of information are to the decision of prioritisation. You will have used your skills of judgement and decision making. If you have experience of this field the referral may have reminded you of someone similar whom you, or a colleague, have worked with. In that case you may have been influenced by your previous experience. Has any knowledge of current government policy influenced your thinking? For example some governments require services to focus on clients with severe enduring mental health needs. If you do this task with colleagues or fellow students discuss:

- Did you know what to look for?
- What types of referral information were most important and why?
- Was any type of information irrelevant and why?
- How well did you agree in relation to your judgements?
- Were any types of information used in relation to each other (non-linear cue use)?
- How closely did you agree in relation to your final prioritisation rating (decision making)?
- Have you drawn on any prior experience of a client who was similar (use of scripts)?

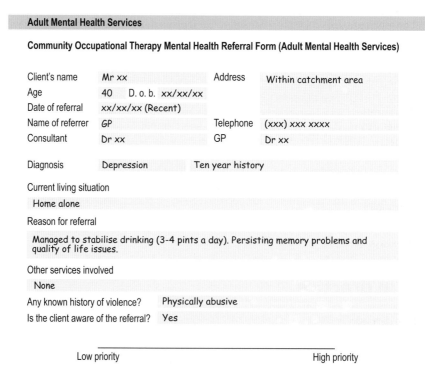

Figure 3.1 An example of a community occupational therapy mental health referral.

A common comment is that it is difficult to make a decision without knowing what other referrals might look like. This is linked to the phenomenon of calibration. Experience is needed to know how to appropriately calibrate judgements and decisions. So look at this second referral (see Figure 3.2). Go through the same process. Which referral is given higher priority?

In order to learn from those who have experience in the judgements and decisions of their domains we need to study experts in their specific specialities. How would occupational therapists with many years of experience in the field of community mental health make these types of judgements and decisions? Research was conducted in the UK with 40 experienced occupational therapists on 120 referrals of this type. It was found that four different judgement policies were being used. Policies differed according to whether the practitioner aimed to work in a generic or occupationally orientated way (Harries and Gilhooly 2003a). A website has been developed to train novices to follow the occupationally orientated expert judgement policies. The website allows the novice to practise on a set of referrals in order to know how to calibrate their decisions. Training information is then provided about the expert policies and then a second set of referrals is given for prioritisation. Feedback on how the decision maker has done in relation to the expert group is then provided. The training package has been shown to be effective in developing novices' referral prioritisation skills (Weiss et al 2006) and is a now a freely available evidence-based educational tool to be found at www.priscillaharries.com (Harries 2006). (Email priscilla.harries@brunel.ac.uk for the passwords.)

It is well documented that when experienced, people are better at judging what is important and what is not (Shanteau et al 1991), they are better at balancing the client's perspective with the realities of the environment and they have a vision of people's capacity for change. When a practitioner is new to a clinical or social domain it is difficult to make wise judgements or decisions; it is easy to feel overwhelmed as all new information can seem important. Experience is the only way to move forward; each time

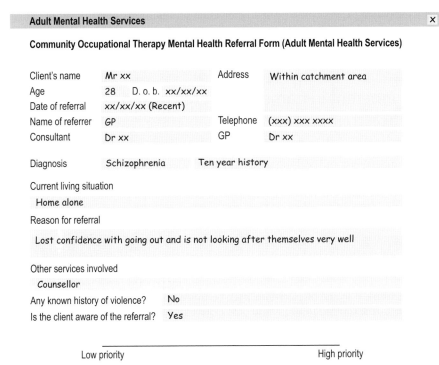

Figure 3.2 Another referral example.

one moves to a new domain one has to start from the beginning and learn what is important in the new field. This new knowledge facilitates the store of 'scripts' in memory (Abernathy and Hamm 1994); these scripts are based on knowledge of similar clients and the narratives that have been heard. Recognition can then be used to pattern match between what has been experienced and any familiar situation which later arises.

Memory and recognition

Research on memory has been conducted to identify how experienced clinicians organise memory 'chunks' and how recall mechanisms facilitate recognition of previously encountered scenarios (Norman and Schmidt 1992). Groen and Patel (1985), identified that novice problem solvers reasoned backwards from hypotheses generation to data, whereas experts reason forward using 'if .... then' rules (propositional reasoning). It is apparent that to use these propositional rules experts have to draw on their well-structured knowledge bases (Johnson-Laird and Shafir 1993). However when an expert is confronted with an unfamiliar problem they will revert back to methods of hypothesis testing (Elstein et al 1990). The use of scripts should not limit how a practitioner works with people but be used to develop an awareness of what is important to pay attention to and what change is possible.

Values

How someone decides what is important when assigning weights or selecting an option is linked to ones' personal and professional values and the values of the setting in which the judgements and decisions must be made. In discussing how judgements have been made, values individuals hold can be brought to light. Some of these are from personal experience, some from professional experience. Where practitioners vary in their values, judgements will be made differently. In a health system that promotes parity and adherence to protocol, it is important to get to the core of an individual's thinking in order to identify thinking methods that result in best practice. Is it more important to help someone with managing self care needs or to gain a work role? Do clients need to socialise? These issues are not black and white and the client themselves or carers are often able to help to focus priorities.

Values inherent in frames of reference and theoretical frameworks

The differing theoretical frameworks that occupational therapists draw on are key to the process of judgement and decision making. These influence how phenomena are viewed and therefore where importance is placed both in terms of what is viewed as an issue that needs addressing and how best that issue might be addressed. They view people from different perspectives and require attention to be given to different aspects of that person. Each frame of reference or theoretical framework has a different value system.

Psychoanalytic, client-centred, cognitive behavioural, biomechanical, developmental, social and occupational frames of reference (see Duncan 2006a) each hold links to what is viewed as important. The client-centred frame of reference for example requires the client to be heavily involved in the decision-making process (see Chapter 4) whereas the biomechanical frame of reference may be more practitioner-led. Psychoanalytical theories require attention to be paid to past experiences whereas cognitive-behavioural theories focus on the here and now. The value systems also vary between the conceptual models of occupational therapy practice. Research from the major conceptual models support their use as being relevant to a multiplicity of needs whether it be a person's social withdrawal or muscle weakness. And the use of conceptual models of practice does

Vignette 3.1

Jean

Jean was seen at home by the occupational therapist from the community mental health team. The GP had referred the client due to her high anxiety levels, limited IQ and a recent bereavement. Due to her anxiety Jean had also lost her job. During the interview the practitioner noticed how anxious and underweight Jean is. She also observed that there was a lack of food in the house. One aspect that the occupational therapist now wants to assess, through observation and interview, is why Jean is not eating enough to sustain her weight. Depending on the issues that present, the practitioner will choose interventions that are informed by differing theoretical frameworks. Each theory holds differing values which alter the focus of the intervention.

not restrict practitioners from also using a variety of frames of reference (such as the bio-mechanical, or client-centred frame of reference) depending on the presenting problem. However, not all occupational therapists practice in this way and many select their theoretical basis of practice from a range of frames of reference without necessarily using a conceptual model of practice as an occupational filter (Mallinson and Forsyth 2000). In these cases practitioners aim to select a frame of reference that best fits the client's need and the context for the intervention; taking into account the strength of the theory's evidence base and of the cost effectiveness of its use.

In the above example, Jean is not eating because she may have anorexia nervosa, an occupational therapist may view her needs from a psychoanalytical perspective. Her unresolved emotional conflict could be thought to be the result of prior life experiences. Her withdrawn childlike state could be seen as a sign of emotional underdevelopment. A practitioner could involve the client in projective art, drama therapy and creative group work to facilitate the psychosocial development of her emotional maturity. The ability to express oneself, to develop a sense of self-efficacy and self-esteem would be necessary before Jean will develop the wish to eat. Once partial psychosocial capacity is achieved, the practitioner would add an educational perspective, for example teaching skills in cooking, budgeting, and giving advice as Jean resumes social and work activities.

If however, Jean was not eating because she had severe rheumatoid arthritis, her needs would be viewed from a very different perspective. Her difficulties may be due to the physical weakness, pain and limited range of movement that can cause problems with cutting up food, opening cans and turning on taps. In this case a biomechanical and compensatory perspective may be taken (McMillan 2006). Joint protection advice would be provided to try to reduce the risks of further hand function deterioration. Altering kitchen work surfaces may be suggested, to allow heavy pans to be slid rather than lifted, so that ulna deviation is not exacerbated. Splints may be made by the practitioner to stabilise the radiocarpal and metacarpal phalangeal joints in a functional position. Fatigue management advice may be given to ensure periods of rest are balanced with periods of activity. Equipment such as tap turners, stair rails and elastic shoelaces may be provided to maximise independence and thereby provide some privacy for dressing and bathing occupations. Advice and support to engage in valued leisure or work occupations would also be essential to ensure that Jean has a good quality of life.

If however a client with a physical disability has developed depression as a result of their capacity to cope with their disability, psychological theories may also be needed. Cognitive-behaviour theories would be used to promote positive thinking and to change/challenge cognitive distortions. However, an occupational therapist would not conduct cognitive-behaviour therapy in isolation but would use it alongside occupational engagement (Duncan 2006b). The benefits of engaging in a valued occupation that assists the client to recognise their own skills and potential can help to reinforce positive thinking. The key is to find occupations that are matched to the individual's capacity and value system, thereby ensuring a sense of self-efficacy and achievement.

Some practitioners and theorists advocate selecting an occupational therapy conceptual model of practice before seeing a client to ensure the occupation focus of the intervention (Forsyth and Kielhofner 2006; see Chapter 7); others do not. Regardless, the reasons for clients' needs have to be determined before it is known which specific frame of reference will be most valuable in guiding interventions. Some initial assessment is therefore needed before a theoretical frame of reference (such as the biomechanical or cognitive behavioural) is chosen. This will then influence the method of the full assessment and inform which issues need to be explored further. For example if Jean has not been eating through a:

- Lack of strength to open packets, turn on taps, hold cutlery (for example due to pain from rheumatoid arthritis) the practitioner may use a biomechanical frame of reference and compensatory approach – instructing in joint protection techniques and providing aids and adaptations.
- Lack of motivation (for example due to low mood due to recent loss of her partner and work role) the practitioner may use a cognitive-behavioural frame of reference – advising on positive-thinking strategies and planning graded, achievable goals.
- Lack of knowledge (for example budgeting difficulties, anxiety about abilities due to being recently bereaved) the practitioner may take an educational approach – practising using transport, road safety, menu planning, shopping, cooking.
- Low IQ and limited skills (for example due to mild learning disability and recent loss of a parent/carer) the practitioner may take a developmental approach – educating Jean from her current level of ability up to her maximum level of capacity.
- Poor insight, denial and bizarre eating behaviour for example due to anorexia nervosa, the practitioner may take a psychodynamic approach examining reasons for low self-esteem through therapeutic art sessions.

Therefore the way in which practitioners reason using conceptual models of practice and frames of reference can have a significant impact on the judgements and decisions in practice.

Summary

This chapter has highlighted the importance of judgement and decision-making skills in practice. Occupational therapy clinical reasoning literature has been presented and discussed. Two judgement and decision-making models (the CCT and dual-process theory), drawn from cognitive psychology were described and discussed. These models highlight the difference between intuitive reasoning which characterises what is known as 'artful practice' and rational reasoning which is a more logical, deliberate and conscious form of reasoning and characterises evidence-based ways of working. Historically the types of knowledge generated through 'artful practice' and more evidence-based methods have been looked upon with equal worth within occupational therapy. However both the CCT and dual-process theory highlight the superiority of the judgement and decision making that come from the logical, deliberate method (S2/N2); whilst recognising that most people tend to be naturally intuitive decisions makers in practice (S1/N1). The chapter presented conceptual models of practice as one possibility that could increase the amount of S2 type judgement and decision making in practice. Practical examples were also given to illustrate the complexity of judgement and decision making in practice.

References

Abernathy CM, Hamm RM 1994 Surgical scripts: master surgeons think aloud about 43 common surgical problems. Hanley & Belfus, Philadelphia, PA

Alvervik A, Sviden, G 1996 On clinical reasoning: patterns of reflection on practice The Occupational Therapy Journal of Research 16(2): 98–110

Barker P 2000 Reflections on caring as a virtue ethic within an evidence-based culture. International Journal of Nursing Studies. 37: 329–336

Benner P 1984 From novice to expert: excellence and power in clinical nursing practice. Addison-Wesley, Menlo Park, CA

Chapparo C 1999 Working out: working with Angelica-interpreting practice. In: SE Ryan, EA McKay (eds) Thinking and reasoning in therapy: Narratives from practice. Stanley Thornes. Cheltenham, UK

Crabtree M, Lyons M 1997 Focal points and relationships: A study of clinical reasoning. British Journal of Occupational Therapy 60(2): 57–64

Creighton C, Dijkers M, Bennett N et al 1995 Reasoning and the art of therapy for spinal cord injury. American Journal of Occupational Therapy 49: 311–317

Degani JAS, Shafto M, Kirlik A 2006 What makes vicarious functioning work? Exploring the geometry of human-technology interaction. In: A Kirlik (ed) Adaptive Perspectives on Human–Technology Interaction, pp. 179–196. Oxford University Press, New York

Duncan EAS 2006a (ed) Foundations for Practice in Occupational Therapy, 4th edn. Elsevier/ Churchill Livingstone, Edinburgh, UK

Duncan EAS 2006b The cognitive behavioural frame of reference. In: EAS Duncan (ed) Foundations for Practice in Occupational Therapy, 4th edn, pp. 217–232. Elsevier/ Churchill Livingstone, Edinburgh, UK

Elstein AS, Shulman LS, Sprafka SA 1978 Medical problem solving: an analysis of clinical reasoning. Harvard University Press, Cambridge, MA

Elstein AS, Shulman LS, Sprafka SA 1990 Medical problem solving: a ten year retrospective. Evaluation and the Health Professions 13(1): 5–36

Ericsson KA, Simon HA 1980 Verbal reports as data. Psychological Review 87(3): 215–251

Evans J 2003 In two minds: dual-process accounts of reasoning. Trends in Cognitive Science 7(10): 454–459.

Evans J, Over D 2004 If. Oxford University Press, Oxford, UK

Eysenck M 1993 Principles of Cognitive Psychology. Lawrence, Hove, UK

Fawcett J, Watson J, Neuman B et al 2001 On nursing theories and evidence. Journal of Nursing Scholarship 33(2): 115–119

Fleming MH 1991a The therapist with the three-track mind. American Journal of Occupational Therapy 45(11): 1007–1014

Fleming M H 1991b Clinical reasoning in medicine compared with clinical reasoning in occupational therapy. American Journal of Occupational Therapy 45(11): 988–996

Fondiller ED, Rosage LJ, Neuhaus BE 1990 Values influencing clinical reasoning in occupational therapy: An exploratory study. Occupational Therapy Journal of Research 10: 41–55

Forsyth K, Kielhofner 2006 The Model of Human Occupation: Integrating Theory into Practice and Practice into Theory In: EAS Duncan 2006 (ed) Foundations for Practice in Occupational Therapy, 4th edn., pp. 69–108. Elsevier/ Churchill Livingstone, Edinburgh, UK

Fortune T, Ryan S 1996 Applying Clinical Reasoning: A caseload management system for community occupational therapists. British Journal of Occupational Therapy 59: 207–211

Fossey E 1996 Using the Occupational Performance History Interview: Therapist reflections. British Journal of Occupational Therapy 59: 223–228

Fugelsang JA, Thompson VA 2000 Strategy selection in causal reasoning: when beliefs and covariation collide. Canadian Journal of Experimental Psychology 54: 13–32

Fugelsang JA, Stein C, Green A et al 2004 Theory and data interactions of the scientific mind: evidence from the molecular and the cognitive laboratory. Canadian Journal of Experimental Psychology 58: 86–95

Gale J, Marsden P 1985 Diagnosis: process not product. In: M Sheldon, J Brooke, A Recotr (eds) Decision-Making in General Practice. Macmillans, Basingstoke, UK

Gathercole S 2003 (ed) Short-Term and Working Memory. Taylor and Francis, Hove, UK

Gilovich T, Griffin D, Kahneman D 2002 (eds) Heuristics and Biases: The Psychology of Intuitive Judgement. Cambridge University Press, Cambridge, UK

Goel V, Buchel C Frith C et al 2000 Dissociation of mechanisms underlying syllogistic reasoning. Neuroimage 12(5): 504–514

Groen G J, Patel VL 1985 Medical problem-solving: some questionable assumptions. Medical Education 19: 95–100

Hagedorn R 1996 Clinical decision making in familiar cases: A model of the process and implications of practice. The British Journal of Occupational Therapy 59: 217–222

Hammond KR, Brehmer B (eds) 1973 Quasi-rational and distrust: implications for international conflict. Human Judgement and Social Interactions. Rineholt & Winston, New York

Harries P 2006 Editorial: The development of a web-based tool for training referral prioritization skills. International Journal of Therapy and Rehabilitation 13(6): 777

Harries PA, Harries C 2001a Studying clinical reasoning, part 1: have we been taking the wrong 'track'? British Journal of Occupational Therapy 64(4): 164–168

Harries PA, Harries C 2001b Studying clinical reasoning, Part 2: applying social judgement theory. British Journal of Occupational Therapy 64(6): 285–292

Harries P, Gilhooly K 2003a Identifying occupational therapists referral priorities in community health. Occupational Therapy International 10(2): 150–164

Harries P, Gilhooly K 2003b Generic and specialist occupational therapy casework in community mental health. British Journal of Occupational Therapy 66(3): 101–109

Hoffman RR 1987 The problem of extracting the knowledge of experts from the perspective of experimental psychology. AI Magazine: 53–67

Hooper B 1997 The relationship between pre-theoretical assumptions and clinical reasoning. American Journal of Occupational Therapy 51: 328–338

Johnson-Laird PN, Shafir E 1993 The Interaction between reasoning and decision-making: an introduction. Cognition 49: 1–9

Kahneman D, Frederick S 2002 Representativeness revisited: attribute substitution in intuitive judgment. In: T Gilovich, D Griffin, D Kahneman (eds) Heuristics and Biases: The Psychology of Intuitive Judgment, pp. 46–71. Cambridge University Press, Cambridge, UK

Kahneman D, Slovic P, Tversky A (eds) 1982 Judgment under Uncertainty: Heuristics and Biases. Cambridge University Press, Cambridge, UK

Kaptchuk TJ 2003 Effect of interpretive bias on research evidence. British Medical Journal 326: 1453–1455

Kielhofner G 2007 Model of Human Occupation, 4th edn. Theory and Practice. Lippincott Williams & Wilkins, Baltimore, MD

Koehler JJ 1993 The influence of prior belief on scientific judgments of evidence quality. Organizational Behavior and Human Decision Processes 56: 25–28

Larkin J H (ed) 1979 Information processing and science instruction. Cognitive Process Instruction. Franklin Institute, Philadelphia, PA

Mallinson T, Forsyth K 2000 Components of the Occupation Filter. In: EAS Duncan 2006 (ed) Foundations for Practice in Occupational Therapy, 4th edn., p. 86. Elsevier/Churchill Livingstone, Edinburgh, UK

Mattingly C 1991 What is clinical reasoning? American Journal of Occupational Therapy, 45(11): 979–986

Mattingley C, Fleming MH 1994 Clinical reasoning: forms of inquiry in a therapeutic practice. Davis, Philadelphia, PA

McKay EA 1999 Lilian and Paula: a treatment narrative in acute mental health. In: SE Ryan & EA McKay (eds) Thinking and reasoning in therapy: Narratives from practice, pp. 53–64. Stanley Thornes, Cheltenham, UK

McMillan I 2006 Assumptions underpinning a biomechanical frame of reference in occupational therapy In: EAS Duncan 2006 (ed) Foundations for Practice in Occupational Therapy, 4th edn., pp. 255–276. Elsevier/Churchill Livingstone, Edinburgh, UK

Munroe H 1996 Clinical reasoning in community occupational therapy. British Journal of Occupational Therapy 59(5): 196–202

Nisbett R, Wilson T 1977 Telling more than we can know: verbal reports on mental processes. Psychological Review 84: 231–259

Norman GR, Schmidt HG 1992 The psychological basis of problem-based learning: a review of the evidence. Academic Medicine 67(9): 557–565

Norman GR, Trott AL, Brooks LR et al 1994 Cognitive differences in clinical reasoning related to postgraduate training. Teaching and Learning in Medicine 6: 114–120

Paley J, Cheyne H, Dalgleish L et al 2007 Nursing's ways of knowing and dual process theories of cognition. Journal of Advanced Nursing 60(6): 692–701

Paterson ML 2003 Professional Practice Judgement Artistry in Occupational Therapy Practice. Unpublished PhD thesis. The University of Sydney, Australia

Paterson M, Summerfield-Mann L 2006 Clinical Reasoning. In: Duncan EAS (ed) Foundations for Practice in Occupational Therapy 4th Edn. Elsevier/Churchill Livingstone, Oxford, UK 315–335

Paterson M, Higgs J, Wilcox S et al 2002 Clinical reasoning and self-directed learning: Key dimensions in professional education and professional socialisation. Focus on Health Professional Education: A Multi-Disciplinary Journal 4(2): 5–21

Resch KI, Ernst E, Garrow J 2000 A randomized controlled study of reviewer bias against an unconventional therapy. Journal of the Royal Society of Medicine 93: 164–167

Roberts AE 1996 Approaches to reasoning in occupational therapy: a critical exploration. British Journal of Occupational Therapy 59(5): 233–236

Roberts MJ, Sykes EDA 2003 Belief bias and relational reasoning. The Quarterly Journal of Experimental Psychology 56A(1): 131–154

Robertson L 1996 Clinical reasoning, Part 2: novice/expert differences. British Journal of Occupational Therapy 59(5): 212–216

Rogers J 1983 Clinical reasoning: The ethics, science, and art. American Journal of Occupational Therapy, 37: 601–616

Rycroft-Malone J, Seers K, Titchen A et al 2004 What counts as evidence in evidence-based practice? Journal of Advanced Nursing 47(1): 81–90

Sefton AJ 2001 Integrating knowledge and practice in medicine. In: J Higgs, A Titchen (eds) Practice Knowledge and Expertise, pp. 29–34. Butterworth Heinemann, Oxford, UK

Shanteau J 1992 Competence in experts: the role of task characteristics. Organizational Behavior and Human Decision Processes 53: 252–266

Shanteau J, Grier M, Berner E 1991 Teaching decision making skills to student nurses. In: J Baron, RV Brown (eds) Teaching decision making to adolescents, pp. 185–206. Lawrence Erlbaum, Hillsdale, UK

Smith G 2006 Telling tales – How stories and narratives co-create change. The British Journal of Occupational Therapy 69(7): 304–311

Stanovich K 2003 The fundamental computational biases of human cognition: heuristics that (sometimes) impair decision making and problem solving. In: JE Davidson, RJ Sternberg (eds) The Psychology of Problem Solving, pp. 291–342. Cambridge University Press, New York

Stanovich K, West RF 2003 Evolutionary versus instrumental goals: how evolutionary psychology misconceives human rationality. In: Over D (ed) Evolution and the Psychology of Thinking: The Debate, pp. 171–230. Psychology Press, Hove, UK

Townsend E, Polatajko HJ 2007 Enabling Occupation II: Advancing an Occupational Therapy Vision for Health, Well-being, & Justice through Occupation. Canadian Association of Occupational Therapists, Ottawa, Canada

Unsworth CA 1996 Team decision making in rehabilitation. American Journal of Physical Medicine and Rehabilitation 75: 483–484

Unsworth CA 2001 Studying clinical reasoning. British Journal of Occupational Therapists. 64(6): 316–317

Unsworth CA 2004 Clinical reasoning: How do pragmatic reasoning, worldview and client-centredness Fit? The British Journal of Occupational Therapy 67(1): 10–19

Unsworth CA, Thomas SA, Greenwood KM 1995 Rehabilitation team decisions on discharge housing for stroke patients. Archives of Physical Medicine and Rehabilitation 76: 331–340

Unsworth CA, Thomas S A, Greenwood KM 1997 Decision polarization among rehabilitation team recommendations concerning discharge housing for stroke patients. International Journal of Rehabilitation Research 20: 51–69

Upshur REG, VanDenKerkhof E, Goel V 2001 Meaning and measurement: an inclusive model of evidence in health care. Journal of Evaluation in Clinical Practice 7(2): 91–96

Weiss D, Shanteau J, Harries P 2006 People who judge people. Journal of Behavioral Decision Making 19: 441–454

Shared decision-making skills in practice

4

Edward A.S. Duncan

 Highlight box

- Client-centred practice is easy to discuss but challenging to deliver.
- Practitioners, consciously or unconsciously use a variety of decision-making models in practice.
- Shared decision making is a valuable decision-making model for occupational therapists.
- Shared decision making requires at least two participants, the sharing of information and the making of a decision that is agreed by all parties.
- There are a variety of strategies that can be used to increase the likelihood of shared decision making taking place.
- It is important to measure your decision-making skills in practice, as many think they deliver shared decision making, but few actually do.

Background

Whilst client-centred therapy was first developed by Carl Rogers (Rogers 1939), it was not perhaps until the development of health promotion in the 1980s when the role of people in controlling and developing their own care became more prominent in international health care (WHO 1984). Within occupational therapy, client-centred practice was initially driven by Canadian Occupational Therapists (Canadian Association of Occupational Therapists/Department of National Health 1983), but has since become internationally recognized and embedded in ethical codes of conduct (COT 2005, COTEC 1996). Parker (2006) described practitioners views of client-centred practice as ranging from 'quite simple' to 'daunting'. But what is client-centred occupational therapy?

The relationship between client-centred occupational therapy and the shared decision-making model

Various definitions of client-centred occupational therapy exist. Law et al (1995) provided the first definition describing it as, 'an approach to providing occupational therapy which embraces a philosophy of respect for and partnership with people receiving services. It recognises the autonomy of individuals, the need for client choice in making decisions about occupational needs, the strengths clients bring to an occupational encounter and the benefits of client therapist partnership and the need to ensure that services are accessible and fit the context in which a client lives' (p. 250). Key features of client-centred occupational therapy that emerged from the work of Law et al (1995) included:

- Autonomy and choice
- *Partnership* (author's emphasis)/responsibility
- Enablement
- Contextual congruence
- Accessibility
- Respect for diversity.

Later, Sumsion (2000) conducted research with British occupational therapists and developed the following definition of client-centred occupational therapy,

> 'Client-centred occupational therapy is a partnership [author's emphasis] between the client and the therapist that empowers the client to engage in functional performance and fulfils his/her roles in a variety of environments. The client participates actively in negotiating goals which are given priority and are at the centre of assessment, intervention, and evaluation. Throughout the process, the therapist listens to and respects the clients' values, adapts the interventions to meet the clients' needs and enables the client to make informed decisions' [author's emphasis] (p. 308).

Building on this definition, Parker (2006) drew out the following key features of client-centred occupational therapy:

- The individual
- *Partnership* (author's emphasis)
- Respect and listening
- Empowerment
- Goal negotiation
- Language
- *Informed decision making* (author's emphasis).

Clear similarities can be seen between the key features highlighted by Law et al (1995) and Parker (2006). Of particular relevance to the subject of this chapter, however, is the concept of 'Partnership', which is clearly highlighted in both definitions and summary features, and 'informed decision making' which appears in Sumsion's (2000) definition and in Parker's (2006) summary.

Delivering client-centred practice is easier said than done. Maitra and Erway (2006) conducted a study of client and occupational therapist perceptions of client-centred practice. They aimed to, 'conduct a comparative study of the perceptual involvement of clients and occupational therapists in the *shared decision* making [author's emphasis] process in health care facilities in the United States' and secondly, 'to investigate whether there is a difference in the *shared decision making* [author's emphasis]' (p. 300). Whilst a relatively small study (11 occupational therapists and 30 clients were interviewed) interesting findings arose. The study indicated that whilst practitioners did involve clients in the process of goal setting and treatment planning, a perceptual gap existed between the samples in relation to practitioners' use of client-centred practice and shared decision making: Clients did not always feel as if they participated in shared decision making, whilst practitioners believed they delivered it. Maitra and Erway's (2006) work is of interest as it nicely highlights the daily challenges of undertaking client-centred practice and clearly links the concept of client-centred practice to the centrality of partnership working and shared decision making by practitioners and their clients.

Decision-making models

Whilst occupational therapy literature is now replete with literature about client-centred practice, very little has been written about shared decision making. Yet a great deal has been written about shared decision making in the broader health-care literature (see for example Bekker et al 1999, Charles et al 1997, Bugge et al 2006), and is of relevance to occupational therapy practice today.

Shared decision making is one of many decision-making models in the health-care literature. Before describing shared decision making in more detail, it is worth considering some of the other major models of decision making in practice. Principle amongst these are the paternalistic model, the physician (or in this context practitioner) as agent model, and the informed decision-making model (Charles et al 1997).

Paternalistic model

The paternalistic model of decision making assumes that patients (as the word itself suggests) are passive recipients of care. This model is clearly outlined in the work of Talcott Parsons (1902–1979), an American sociologist, who conceptualized the sick role (Parsons 1952); which clearly positions professionals as experts and patients (as the word itself suggests) as passive receivers of care. However, this definition is, as the vast literature of informed and shared decision-making literature within medicine illustrates, no longer an accurate blanket description of medical decision making in practice. Occupational therapists too followed this model for some time (Wilcock 2002) until professional philosophical tensions moved the profession largely away from this model of decision making. However, whilst the profession's overarching philosophy of care has changed, paternalistic practice can still be found – even in practitioners who express the desire to be client-centred (Daniëls et al 2002).

The following models of decision making have emerged, to a certain extent, as a reaction to the paternalistic model (Levine et al 1992, Deber 1994).

Practitioner as agent model

In the practitioner as agent model (a phrase adapted from the more commonly referred to physician as agent model (Charles et al 1997)) the professional retains overall control of the decisions that are made. However, in this model there is a clear expectation that the practitioner will work to gain a comprehensive understanding of their clients' preferences, desires and values and form their action plan on the basis of what they consider the client would desire. Despite the good intentions of a practitioner to deliver the care that a client desires, this model of decision making remains incongruous with the philosophy of current occupational therapy practice. However there may be times when this model is the closest one is able to get towards partnership working (see Vignette 4.1).

The informed decision-making model

'An informed decision is one where a reasoned choice is made by a reasonable individual using relevant information about the advantages and disadvantages of all possible course of action and in accord with the individual's beliefs' (Bekker et al 1999: 1). Within an informed decision-making model, a practitioner's role is primarily about information sharing from the practitioner to the client, but it is argued that whilst clients wish to gain as much information about their condition or interventions as possible (Bekker et al 1999), they do not consistently wish to be solely responsible about the decisions they make (Charles et al 1997). Informed decision making has potential, and has been provided, in occupational therapy practice (see Vignette 4.2), but it is not ideal for everyone: some clients will lack capacity to make informed decisions (Sumsion 2000), whilst others lack the desire and will not wish to take on such responsibility.

Vignette 4.1

Mark is a 9-year-old boy with severe learning difficulties. He lives at home with his parents, his 13-year-old sister and 11-year-old brother. Mark attends his local special needs school and his teacher has reported that he wanders around, has difficulty concentrating and frequently interrupts other children from their tasks. In the playground he often appears isolated from others. The school has requested an occupational therapy assessment to see how best to help Mark.

The occupational therapist visited Mark at school. As Mark has significant communication difficulties it was not possible to meaningfully interview him to understand his perspective and views. Instead the occupational therapist observed him in the classroom and playground over several sessions and interviewed his teacher. The occupational therapist also visited Mark at home, observed his behaviour over two sessions and interviewed his family. Mark's family reported that he is able to participate in a range of activities at home and when the occupational therapist watches Mark at home being given support by his siblings he is observed to be able to maintain his concentration for longer periods in play-type activities. The occupational therapist discusses options with Mark's family and teacher and with their agreement develops an intervention plan that engages Mark in small-group work within the classroom and supported play with peers in the playground. After 2 weeks of implementation of this plan, Mark is observed by the occupational therapist to be concentrating for longer periods in the classroom and socializing more in the playground. Mark's teacher reports that he appears more settled and disturbs the other children less.

Vignette 4.2

Barry is an 86-year-old gentleman. He has lived alone since the death of his wife 6 years ago. His main interests are his garden, his cat and meeting his friends once a week for a pub lunch. Barry was admitted to his local hospital after falling at home. He fell in the kitchen after tidying up his dinner and had lain all night on the floor until being discovered by his daughter when she arrived the following morning to take him shopping. On arrival at hospital it was noted that Barry's blood sugar levels were poor (he has diabetes), he had fractured his left hip, and was badly shaken by the experience.

Barry has made a better physical recovery than expected and both he and the physiotherapists are happy with the progress he is making. His daughter and some of the clinical team, however, remain concerned that he will not be able to cope with living at home independently and fear he will fall again.

The occupational therapist carries out an assessment with Barry using the Canadian Occupational Performance Measure (Law et al 1994). This assessment highlights that getting out of bed, walking distances, and bending down are some of the main occupational performance difficulties he is currently experiencing. Barry rates these activities highly (8–9) as they are necessary for him to continue to carry out the activities he is used to. Barry rates his current performance of these activities as 3, 2, 2, respectively and his satisfaction as a consistent 2. The occupational therapist also presents Barry with some key figures and facts about the known dangers of returning home, for a gentleman of his age, after having a fractured hip. Barry considers all this information, but decides that despite his occupational performance difficulties and the potential dangers of returning home alone, that he will in fact return to his house. For Barry the risk of future falls does not outweigh the risk of loss of identity, role and routine that he feels giving up his home would entail. The occupational therapist designs an intervention plan to assist Barry to improve his areas of occupational performance difficulties and visit his house to carry out an environmental assessment.

45

The shared decision-making model

The shared decision-making model is increasingly put forward as the ideal decision-making process (Charles et al 1997). It is the middle ground between paternalism and practitioner as agent, which both take control away from the client, and informed decision making; which, while empowering the client through the provision of information also transfers the responsibility of interventions decisions: a responsibility many prefer not to have (Charles et al 1997).

It is important that practitioners ask clients what sort of involvement they wish to have in their care and intervention (that is whether they wish practitioners to make (and communicate) decisions for them), whether they as clients wish to make informed decisions based on information from practitioners, or whether to participate in a shared decision-making model of care.

Certain features of a decision-making process are required for it to be classified as a 'shared' decision. A shared decision must:

* Involve at least two participants
* The sharing of information, and the making of a decision (which should include an option to do nothing) must be made and agreed upon by everyone (Charles et al 1997).

Shared decision-making interventions

But how do you practise shared decision making? There are a wide variety of interventions that, when used appropriately, assist in making shared decisions. Three key interventions that are typically considered to support shared decision making are described in depth elsewhere in this book: goal setting (Chapter 8), the therapeutic use of self (Chapter 9) and educational skills (Chapter 11). However there are various features of all therapeutic relationships that can either build or diminish the potential for shared decision making in practice. (Braddock et al 1997, Edwards and Elwyn 1999, Elwyn et al 2000, 2005a).

Establishing a partnership and decision-making preference

The first stage in developing shared decision making is to establish a therapeutic partnership with the client (see Chapter 9 for further information). This is particularly important when working with people who have long-term conditions. As Montori et al (2006) highlighted, a key characteristic of shared decision making in practice with people who have long-term conditions is 'ongoing partnership between the clinical team (not just the clinician) and the patient' (p. 25). Once the relationship has been established, then practitioners should work to understand what type of role the client wishes to have within the relationship: Do they wish to see the professional as agent? Do they wish to be informed decision makers? Do they wish to partake in shared decision making? These issues have to be communicated and understood very carefully: Clients are unlikely to immediately understand what you mean if you were to ask them a question such as 'What type of decision-making capacity do you wish to have in this relationship?'! This information needs to be gained through careful discussion with the client. It can often be more helpful to understand clients' preferred format by presenting a series of options (see Vignette 4.3). However it should also be remembered that clients may prefer different types of decision-making models depending on the nature of the decision being made, their current health status, and the consequences of the decision in question. Clients decision-making preference is a dynamic concept that has to be continually understood and responded to by practitioners.

Defining the problem

Problem definition is, in effect, a process of assessment (see Chapter 6 for further information). It is through the assessment process that practitioners and clients exchange information about a particular situation or problem. Assessment, and therefore problem definition, requires a two-way exchange of information. The practitioner must provide all the information about relevant intervention options, and clients should share all their relevant history and their values relating to the potential intervention options presented by the practitioner. However, despite the relatively straight forward nature of the information exchange described above, research highlights that both practitioners and clients do not always share all the relevant knowledge with each other (Bugge et al 2006). Whilst a study of the non-exchange of information has not been conducted within the context of occupational therapy, its occurrence across a broad range of clinical environments (Bugge et al 2006) suggests that it will be no different in an occupational therapy context either (see Vignette 4.4).

In Bugge et al's (2006) study the following reasons were given by clients and practitioners for not exchanging relevant information during clinical encounters.

Vignette 4.3

Bethany is a 20-year-old woman. She is currently taking a year out of her psychology degree at University. She was diagnosed with chronic fatigue syndrome 8 months ago. Her symptoms commenced following a glandular-fever-type illness and her recovery has been hampered since by severe and disabling fatigue, lack of concentration, low mood and poor concentration.

The occupational therapist visited Beth at home to carry out an assessment of her needs. Due to Bethany's condition it was necessary to carry out the assessment over several sessions, as Bethany was only able to concentrate for short periods of time and tired quickly. Initially Bethany was very hesitant of becoming involved with the occupational therapist as she was concerned that she would be 'made' to do things she didn't want to, or didn't have the energy to complete. The occupational therapist spent her initial meetings with Bethany listening to her talk about her life, condition, the difficulties she currently faced and her hopes and desires for the future. As well as information gathering, a central task of these sessions was to build up Bethany's trust in the occupational therapist. Towards the end of the fourth session Bethany told the occupational therapist that whilst she did want to get better, she remained hesitant to engage in any active intervention as she feared she would lose control and become more sick. The occupational therapist reassured Bethany that her approach, and the approach of her team, was very much one of working together with clients. Bethany was told that she had control of how she wished to involve her clinical team; if she wished them to tell her what to do, to give her advice, or to collaborate in making decisions together, as a core part of the whole team. Bethany appeared keen to work together with the team: she found the idea of them telling her what to do scary, but also did not want the responsibility of making all the choices herself. Bethany was reassured that she could be actively involved in all the decisions about her care and she would not be made to do anything she didn't want to.

Hesitantly at first, Bethany agreed to commence goal setting with her occupational therapist. Goals were set weekly and agreed upon together by both Bethany and her occupational therapist. It took several weeks of trial and error to set achievable goals that were in Bethany's words 'challenging enough, but not too much'. This was achieved through Bethany giving good feedback to the occupational therapist, in whom she had built increasing trust, and deciding together what the next appropriate goal should be.

Clients' rationale for not exchanging information:

- The environment was unconducive to sharing information: for example there were other people present during the meeting.
- The practitioner's behaviour put clients off: for example practitioners appeared hurried, uninterested or not listening to the client.
- Clients wanted to present a particular self-image.
- Clients did not believe that certain pieces of information were important.

Practitioners' rationale for not exchanging information:

- The environment was unconducive to sharing information: like clients, practitioners were also put off by the presence of others in the room: for instance they would not ask clients potentially embarrassing questions if others were present.
- Practitioners lacked knowledge about certain interventions.
- Practitioners decided not to share information about other interventions because they believed, without checking, that such interventions were not desired by the client.

None of these reasons seem outwith the realm of possibility within an occupational therapy encounter. It is therefore essential that all possible steps are taken to ensure that all the necessary information is exchanged between a client and their practitioner. A key step to ensure accurate problem definition is the active employment of the therapeutic use of self (see Chapter 9) as well as techniques such as active questioning of the client to see if they wish to ask anything that you have not already discussed.

Vignette 4.4

Tim is a 54-year-old married businessman with two grown-up children. Two months ago he had a stroke that left him with muscle weakness (especially in his left arm), slightly slurred speech and some loss of sight. Tim received stroke rehabilitation as an inpatient and was discharged 2 weeks ago. He has now been referred for continued community stroke rehabilitation at home. The occupational therapist visits Tim at home to see how he is doing. Tim's wife Sheena is present throughout the visit. During the interview they all discuss Tim's activities of daily living, leisure activities and return to work.

What neither Tim nor his occupational therapist mention is Tim's sexual relationship with his wife.

The occupational therapist knows, from the discharge notes that she received, that Tim did mention worries about this at an early stage, to an occupational therapist during a kitchen session, but that this had not been taken forward by her or any member of the clinical team. The visiting occupational therapist does not mention it as she is uncertain of how to raise the subject (or indeed if she should raise the subject) in the presence of his wife, furthermore she is not sure what she could recommend, or even if Tim still has concerns in this area of life.

Tim is indeed still concerned about his sexual relationship with his wife. In fact it is his main concern; he has been able to discuss or began to address all the other issues. Tim does not mention it because he is unsure what his wife would think of him for discussing these issues with a younger lady (the occupational therapist), was unsure of how to raise the subject and maintain his composure and was not even certain if the occupational therapist was the right person to talk to as the one in the hospital had not appeared that interested when he mentioned it during a kitchen session one day! The occupational therapy interview ends and a continuing rehab package is agreed by both the practitioner and Tim. His sexual dysfunction issues were not discussed and remain Tim's biggest source of anxiety and concern.

Including the client in the decision-making process

At first glance, including clients in a shared decision-making process seems like an obvious statement to make; it wouldn't be shared if you didn't! Indeed occupational therapy ethical guidelines state that (except in exceptional circumstances, such as mental health legislation), 'Clients have a right to make choices and decisions about their own health care' (p. 6). Yet how easy is it to truly achieve this in practice? Several studies illustrate the negative perceptions of clients' involvement and participation in their own rehabilitation and illustrate the challenges of achieving true participation in practice (Doolittle 1992, Becker and Kaufman 1995, Daniëls et al 2002). Such is the discrepancy of philosophy and practice, that achieving true client participation in the decision-making processes of their care has been claimed to be more 'rhetoric than reality' (Lewis 2003: 4). However the challenges of involving clients in meaningful participation must remain the goal of every practitioner. True participation and shared decision making are more likely to occur when practitioners ensure clients understand their problems, explore their worries, fears or expectations, discuss options and make collaborative decisions.

Ensuring clients understand their problems and the decisions required

It is vital that clients, as well as practitioners, understand their problems and what, if any, decisions are required. In order to achieve this, practitioners must ensure that they communicate with all clients in a manner that builds confidence and rapport (see Chapter 9) and in language that is easy to follow and in the preferred media of the client (see Chapter 11). Building positive therapeutic engagement and educating clients are both essential skills that are required if a client is to understand their problems and the decisions that are required. However the routine nature of building therapeutic relationships and educating clients' results in the complexity of truly achieving this is in practice being often overlooked (see Vignette 4.5).

Exploring clients' worries, fears and expectations

Engaging in therapeutic assessment and interventions can be anxiety provoking for clients. Anxiety negatively affects a client's ability to concentrate. This in turn can reduce clients' abilities to exercise choice and engage in partnership working. Practitioners can help to reduce clients' level of anxiety by explicitly eliciting and discussing with clients their worries, fears and expectations, about their health and care generally, and of occupational therapy in particular. Time and space should be given throughout sessions to allow clients to ask questions. It can also be useful to explicitly ask clients if they have any concerns (see Vignette 4.6).

Vignette 4.5

Carlo is a 10-month-old boy. He was born 4 weeks early and was noted to have low birth weight with asymmetric growth retardation on delivery. A diagnosis of mild cerebral palsy was made at a later date following an MRI scan.

Carlo's development is being closely monitored by a paediatric community physiotherapist, paediatric community occupational therapist and consultant paediatrician. Carlo had been seen by his physiotherapist for several weeks before the occupational therapy service receives a referral and arranges to visit him. The occupational therapist visits Carlo's home at the same time as the physiotherapist, in order to carry out some joint working and to lessen the burden of health-care professionals visiting the house each week. However, whilst Carlo's parents were informed why the physiotherapist was visiting, they never received an explanation as to why the occupational therapy referral had been made and this was not clearly explained by the occupational therapist when she visited.

During a series of joint visits the occupational therapist assesses Carlo's motor, process and communication skills and observes his response to a variety of stimuli. However, because of the nature of these visits, the occupational therapist never explained to Carlo's parents exactly why she was there, what she was looking for, and what she had to offer that was different to the physiotherapist. Because of this, Carlo's parents were puzzled about her role and what she was doing when she visited. To them, despite the complexity of analysis that the occupational therapist was undertaking, it just appeared as if she was there to hold toys for the physio!

Vignette 4.6

Teresa is a 44-year-old woman who has suffered from depression for the last 12 years. She has been 'signed off' sick from her work for the last 3 months and has been referred to a return-to-work project by her job centre. Her initial appointment at the project is with an occupational therapist. When the occupational therapist commences his initial interview (a standard format of questions the project asks all new referrals) Teresa appears very anxious and responds to the practitioner's questions with the minimal of information. At a certain point the occupational therapist stops what he is doing and puts down his forms. He suggests to Teresa that it may be most helpful if she could start first of all by telling him all she thought he should know about her life and illness and how she felt about being referred to the project. Teresa responded well to this strategy and spoke openly about her life before she was diagnosed with depression as well as the impact the illness had had on her life and the life of her family. Teresa discussed how work had previously been a very important part of her life: not only financially, but also socially. Teresa had worked as a seamstress in several clothing factories and had enjoyed the 'buzz' and collegiality of working in these settings. Since being 'signed off' work, Teresa has missed these aspects and would love to regain these aspects of her life. Having engaged Teresa more fully within the interview, and having seen her relax as she spoke, the occupational therapist then asked Teresa if she had any particular views or concerns about attending the project. Teresa reported that she had lost a great deal of confidence since being 'signed off' and feared that if she returned to work (and in the process lost her government benefits) she may not manage to maintain her productivity at levels she used to, which could result in her dismissal and significant loss of income upon which she and her family depended. The occupational therapist was then able to discuss the work of the project in further detail and how they had managed similar situations in the past.

Discussing different intervention options

Practitioners should discuss with their clients the differing therapeutic options that are available. Interventions have at least two options, as the option to do nothing is always available and ethically should be supported if that is the desire of the client (COT 2005). Discussing options enables clients to fully participate in the decision-making process and can also reduce the fear of the unknown, as clients who discuss available options will have a greater knowledge of what each intervention entails. A useful method of discussing potential interventions with clients is to discuss the 'pros and cons' (or advantages and disadvantages) of each option (See Chapter 10 for further information) (see Vignette 4.7).

Making decisions

Having worked your way through each of the stages above, it is necessary to make choices and decisions about the direction of intervention. Fortunately few of the decisions made by occupational therapists and their clients in practice have irreversible consequences; though some decisions (for example major environmental alterations to a client's house or the decision to enter a nursing home) will be less easily reversed than others (for instance developing an activity schedule with a client who is depressed). Nevertheless making decisions for and with clients is a significant event. Clients should be asked if they wish further time to consider intervention options and (wherever possible) it should be made clear that such decisions are open to review and can be altered if the client wishes to at a later date.

Vignette 4.7

Lucy was referred to occupational therapy by her consultant psychiatrist following discussion at the weekly community mental health team meeting. She is 27 years old and lives with her parents and two younger brothers. She was recently discharged home after being admitted to an acute psychiatric ward for 2 months after being diagnosed with bipolar disorder and concern from her consultant psychiatrist and family that she may self harm.

During the occupational therapy initial interview it became clear that Lucy was upset by her medical diagnosis and her recent experience of admission. Following her discharge Lucy felt that it was difficult to get back into her old routine and she had lost confidence in doing things she previously found simple. Until 6 months ago Lucy had attended college, where she had been studying business management. Lucy reported that she had previously been enjoying the course. When asked about her other interests she replied that she enjoys watching television, swimming and using the internet. Lucy stated that in the future she hoped to run her own business.

The occupational therapist discussed the idea of Lucy returning to study as a goal they could work towards. Lucy was initially hesitant about working towards this as she was unsure if she would be able to manage – though at the same time she was unable to say what she did want to do. Lucy agreed with the occupational therapist that it would be a good idea to look at the pros and cons of working towards returning to college. Together Lucy and her occupational therapists sat down and drew up a list of the pros and cons of working towards returning to college. Having done this, Lucy felt that doing nothing would only lead her to increase her isolation, whilst she said she could see from the pros and cons sheet that working towards returning to college would not bind her to that choice, but would help her to take her first steps towards recovery and regaining the life she once had. She was still uncertain that she would make it back to college, but agreed that it was worth working towards just now.

51

Measuring shared decision making in practice

Given the centrality of the client in occupational therapy, and the policy imperatives to increasingly involve clients in their care, shared decision making has now become increasingly relevant in health care and occupational therapy is no exception.

Occupational therapy is internationally recognized as having a client-centred philosophy, yet research into the practitioner–client partnership has shown that delivering client-centred practice is challenging and there is a dissonance between the theory of client-centred practice and partnership working in practice (Daniëls et al 2002, Maitra and Erway's 2006).

The previous section described shared decision making, as a method of ensuring client-centred practice, and outlined ways in which practitioners can work to ensure that clients are involved in their care to the level they wish to be and are facilitated to participate in shared decision making with practitioners when so desired. As shared decision making is both a recognized 'good' of practice and a challenging concept to deliver, practitioners should measure the degree of participation and shared decision making they deliver in practice as a routine core process measure. In this way they will truly be able to state whether or not they are being client-centred.

Client feedback

Client's satisfaction with their involvement, participation and shared decision making should be routinely included as part of practitioners' process evaluations. Ideally this should occur whilst the practitioner and client are still working together, so that changes can be made if the client does not feel that there is an adequate partnership. It can feel awkward asking clients for feedback on one's clinical performance. But questions such as, 'Is there anything I am not doing that you would like me to do?' can provide opportunities for clients to raise concerns about your style of partnership working. This can be achieved through interview, though clients may not feel free to be honest in their evaluation, or by questionnaire which provides some distance between the practitioner and client and may enable some clients to be more honest. Client's evaluations of practitioners are, however, fraught with difficulty as they may feel pressured to be overly positive or not report concerns they have for fear it would further affect their relationship. More objective measures of shared decision making are therefore highly desirable.

The OPTION scale

The OPTION scale is an objective observational measure of shared decision making in practice (Elwyn et al 2005b). It has been developed to evaluate the extent to which shared decision making occurs within a therapeutic encounter. Whilst originally developed in primary care, the tool has been developed as a measure of any health-care consultation (Elwyn et al 2005b) and would be suitable to measure an occupational therapy contact when options are being considered and/or decisions made: for example during an intervention planning session.

In order to score the OPTION scale practitioners are required to record a session, with the clients permission, which is then listened to and rated using the OPTION scale.

Rating the OPTION scale

The OPTION scale measures the extent to which a client is involved in the decision-making process within a session (Elwyn et al 2005b). The scale itself consists of 12 items which are each rated over a five-point scale ranging from 'The behaviour is not observed' to the 'behaviour being exhibited to a very high standard' (Elwyn et al 2005b: 93). The psychometric properties of the measure have been researched and it has been shown to be a reliable and valid method of measuring the degree of shared decision making that occurs in a clinical encounter (Elwyn et al 2005b). Further, research into the OPTION scale has highlighted that, '...practitioners with no previous training in shared decision making achieve very low levels of patient involvement in decision making' (Elwyn et al 2005b: 58).

Summary

Client-centredness has been the clarion call of occupational therapists since the early 1980s. Occupational therapy has built itself up to be focused on individual client autonomy, based on client choice, and centred on partnership working (Law et al 1995, Sumsion 2000, Parker 2006, Sumsion 2006). However delivering client-centred occupational therapy has been acknowledged as daunting (Parker 2006) and the perceptual gap that exists between the rhetoric and the reality of practice has been researched and reported (Daniëls et al 2002, Maitra and Erway 2006).

Different models of decision making, and their contribution to client-centred practice, have been described within this chapter. Whilst some models of decision making (such as the informed decision-making model) should rightly be recognized as being client-centred, shared decision making (Charles et al 1997) was presented as a model which is gaining wide endorsement and popularity as a useable method of working in partnership with clients in a wide range of settings. A range of shared decision-making interventions, with practice scenarios to illuminate the concepts being discussed were then presented.

Shared decision making, though increasingly researched within health care in general, has been surprisingly under researched within the context of occupational therapy. As an approach to decision making it has a great deal to offer clinicians who wish to narrow the gap between the rhetoric and reality of client-centred occupational therapy practice.

References

Becker G, Kaufman SR 1995 Managing an uncertain illness trajectory in old age: patients' and physicians' views of stroke. Medical Anthropology Quarterly 9: 165–187

Bekker H, Thornton JG, Airey CM et al 1999 Informed decision making: an annotated bibliography and systematic review. Health Technology Assessment 3(1)

Braddock CH, Edward KA, Hasenberg MH et al 1997 Informed decision making in outpatient setting: time to get back to basics. The Journal of the American Medical Association 282: 2313–2320

Bugge C, Entwhistle V, Watt IS 2006 The significance for decision making of information that is not exchanged by patients and health professionals during consultations. Social Science and Medicine 63: 2065–2078

Canadian Association of Occupational Therapy/Department of National Health and Welfare 1983 Occupational therapy guidelines for client centred practice. Canadian Association of Occupational Therapists, Toronto, Canada

Charles C, Gafni A, Whelan T 1997 Shared decision-making in the medical encounter: what does it mean? (or it takes at least two to tango). Social Science and Medicine 44(5): 681–692

College of Occupational Therapists 2005 The Code of Ethics and Professional Conduct for Occupational Therapy. College of Occupational Therapists. London

Council of Occupational Therapists in the European Countries 1996 Code of Ethics and Standard of Practice. Available at: http://cotec-europe.org/organisation/ethics.htm Accessed on 21 November 2007

Danëls R, Winding K, Borell L 2002 Experiences of occupational therapists in stroke rehabilitation: Dilemmas of some occupational therapists in inpatient stroke rehabilitation.

Scandinavian Journal of Occupational Therapy 9: 167–175

Deber R 1994 Physicians in health care management: 7. The patient–physician partnership: Changing roles and the desire for information. Canadian Medical Association 151: 171

Doolittle ND 1992 The experience of recovery following lacunar stroke. Rehabilitation Nursing 17: 122–125

Elwyn G, Edwards A, Kinnersley P et al 2000 Shared decision making and the concept of equipoise: the competence of involving patients in health care choices. British Journal of General Practice 50: 892–897

Elwyn G, Hutchings H, Edwards A et al 2005a The OPTION scale: measuring the extent that clinicians involve patients in decision making tasks. Health Expectations 8: 34–42

Elwyn G, Edwards A, Wensing M et al 2005b Shared Decision Making. Measurement using the OPTION instrument Cardiff University, Cardiff, UK

Law M, Baptiste S, Carswell A et al 1994 Canadian Occupational Performance Measure. Canadian Association of Occupational Therapists, Toronto, UK

Law M, Baptiste S, Mills J 1995 Client-centred practice: what does it mean and does it make a difference? Canadian Journal of Occupational Therapy 62(5): 250–257

Levine MN, Gafni A, Markham B et al 1992 A bedside decision instrument to elicit a patient's preference concerning adjuvant chemotherapy for breast cancer. Annals of Internal Medicine 117(1): 53–58

Lewis L 2003 Is 'participation' all just rhetoric? Mental health nursing. Available at: http://findarticles.com/p/articles/mi_qa3949/is_200311/ai_n9322083 Accessed on 21 November 2007

Maitra KK, Erway F 2006 Perception of client-centred practice in occupational therapists and their clients. The American Journal of Occupational Therapy 60(3): 298–310

Montori VM, Gafni A, Charles C 2006 A shared treatment decision making approach between patients with chronic conditions and their clinicians: the case of diabetes. Health Expectations 9(1): 25–36

Parker 2006 The client-centred frame of reference. In: EAS Duncan (ed.) Foundations for Practice in Occupational Therapy, pp. 193–216. Elsevier/Churchill Livingstone, Edinburgh, UK

Parsons T 1952 The Social System. Free Press, Glencoe, UK

Rogers CR 1939 The clinical treatment of the problem child. Houghton Mifflin, Boston, UK

Sumsion T 2000 A revised definition of client-centred practice. British Journal of Occupational Therapy 63(7): 15–21

Sumsion T 2006 Client-Centred Practice in Occupational Therapy. Churchill Livingstone, Edinburgh

Wilcock A 2002 Occupational for Health. Volume 2. A journey from prescription to self health. College of Occupational Therapists, London

World Health Organisation 1984 Discussion document on the concept and principles of health promotion. Canadian Public Health Association Health Digest 8L: 101–102

Reflective practice: doing, being and becoming a reflective practitioner

5

Elizabeth Anne McKay

Highlight box

- Engaging in thinking about your thinking is key to being a reflective practitioner.
- Participating with others in reflective processes can bring about changes in practice and service delivery.
- Reflective models/methods can facilitate your reflective ability – try them out to discover which you prefer.
- Sharing practice stories with peers and MDT members enables understanding of each others' perspectives and offers new opportunities for working together.
- Reflection can occur before action, in the midst of action, or following action – it is important that action follows reflection.

Overview

Reflection and reflective practice are terms that we all hear in our daily practice; we could assume that we all consider that they mean the same thing to all – this may not be the case. This chapter returns to the basics regarding reflection and reflective practice, its historical development and its importance and relevance to professional practice today are explored. The concept of doing reflection, being reflective and becoming a reflective practitioner are integrated throughout the chapter. The terms will be defined and the key theorists discussed. The significance of reflection to individual and importantly, teams of practitioners will be highlighted as a method for bringing about change in service delivery. Types of reflection, models and methods to facilitate reflection are explored. Throughout the chapter 'promoting reflection' activities are introduced; these can be done individually or with peers and offer strategies for enhancing doing reflection. The chapter concludes with highlighting signs and outcomes of reflection practice.

Introduction

I am delighted that this chapter is near the start of this text: why you ask? The answer is that often reflection is seen as only a retrospective activity (something to do after the event) but that is only part of the story. Reflection is much more than just looking back; that is to say having reflected on an experience or an event what does it mean for you now: in what ways will your thinking or behaviours be different? Reflection importantly, is about shaping your future thinking and actions.

By being near the beginning of this text it sets in place the notion that reflection is something that can be used prior to events as well as post experiences. So as you read, whether you are a reader of books from beginning to end, or a dipper into selected chapters – reflection should be part of the process so that you can make meaning of the chapter material in relation to your knowledge and experiences. As you read consider: What does this mean for me? Could this be useful to my practice now or in the future? What could I bring into my practice or my team's practice now?

We are all familiar with the concept of the reflective practitioner; the reflection process is something built throughout your professional career. Therefore, it is good to establish this habit early on whether you are a student, a novice therapist or an expert practitioner. Throughout this chapter there are *Promoting Reflection* exercises for you to work on individually or with others. By completing these you will be developing or enhancing your reflective abilities. By the end of this chapter you will be able to:

- Define reflection
- Discuss why it is imperative to professional practice
- Be aware of a range of models of reflection
- Be familiar with a range of strategies to promote your reflection including story telling and critical incidents.

This chapter will consider the theoretical basis of reflection and why it is important to individual occupational therapists and teams. The chapter will present various models to facilitate reflection and discuss activities for 'doing' reflecting in and on practice to assist the development of becoming and being a reflective practitioner. Try the exercise in Box 5.1 below.

To assist you to become a reflective practitioner two therapists will be presented throughout the chapter at different stages in their career: David and Caroline.

David is 25. He is 6 months from qualifying from his pre-registration Masters in Occupational Therapy. David worked previously as a residential care worker with teenagers and he has a degree in Sociology. He is currently finishing his research thesis and he has one more placement to complete to qualification. David is single.

Michelle is an expert practitioner having worked for 15 years with children. She is recognized by the profession as a specialist in autism. She has worked in Australia and the USA. She has decided that she would like to take her professional development further and is considering returning to education. She is 36 years old, married with two boys aged 7 and 10 years old.

So why is reflection important?

Reflection is an essential component for the competent and capable therapist practising in the 21st century. Developing reflective practitioners is now a requirement for pre-registration health programmes in the UK (Quality Assurance Agency for Higher Education 2001). Furthermore the Health Professions Council (HPC) (2004) incorporates reflection into the Standards of Proficiency for Occupational Therapists specifically Section 2.2 states that the registrant must 'be able to audit, reflect on and review

Box 5.1

Before we begin I would like you to think back on some personal experience from the past 3 months. Take a few minutes to remember it, what happened, who was involved, when and where did it take place, why? Now take some time to recall what you felt and thought about that at the time: concentrate on the thoughts and the feelings.

Now

How do you think and feel about that event. What has changed, what did you learn from that event – how does it impact on your life today?

practice' (p. 5); furthermore, this is expanded in section 2c2 to 'understand the value of reflection on clinical practice and the need to record the outcome of such reflection' (p. 13). Reflective practice is identified as a key component of work-based learning to maintain a registrant's continuing professional development as part of their lifelong learning (HPC 2006). Practitioners are expected to self-reflect critically on personal performance and adopt a reflexive approach to problem solving. Reflecting on performance and acting on reflection is a professional imperative. Eraut (1994) highlights that the failure not to engage in regular reflection is professionally irresponsible.

Today, it is important that professionals are not only competent to practise but also that they are educated for capability (Fraser and Greenhaugh 2001). By that, I mean that given ever-changing practice contexts; against a backdrop of health and social care systems and processes that are constantly scrutinised for cost effectiveness: practitioners have to think and operate at the higher cognitive level, that is they have to engage in self-evaluation and critical analysis of self. Practitioners require to compare their practice against their own experience and knowledge of theory in their specialist area; thus reflection is about the process of therapy not just about evaluating an intervention with a client (Kuit et al 2001). Reflection is a bridge to linking the theory–practice gap; reflection on your own practice is an essential skill for lifelong learning.

Developing the capability and capacity to adapt to meet changing needs is key to educating practitioners, therefore most professional educational programmes incorporate the factors Cowan (2006) identifies below as essential for developing capability into their curricula. Curricula will include opportunities for learners to:

- Demonstrate competence through active learning methods.
- Develop capacity to cope through solving problems they have identified.
- Create their abilities through doing, making and organising.
- Initiate and engage with others.
- Negotiate their learning needs with educators.
- Be assessed appropriately for the activity undertaken.

Through engagement in such activities throughout their pre-registration education both in university and also importantly, in practice settings, entry-level practitioners are enabled to begin their professional careers more ready to negotiate the reality of the practice world.

Individual reflection on 'doing' practice

Whilst the factors above are embedded in pre-registration education, at an individual level therapists, whether novices or experts, still require to develop their critical thinking abilities through purposefully engaging in thinking about why and what it is they do in practice? What were they trying to achieve? How well it was done? And how can their practice be different or improved in the future? Critical thinking is achieved through active learning methods including the development of reflective processes; it is through reflection we integrate our thoughts and actions. The reflective process involves us in thinking about and critically analysing our actions with the goal of improving our professional performance and therefore our practice. Engaging in reflective practice requires individuals to assume the stance of observer of their own practice. This allows them to be able to identify the assumptions and feelings underlying their practice, to speculate about how these assumptions and feelings affect practice and how these can be modified for future practice (Osterman 1990). Practitioners are the experts in what they learned from their varied professional experiences; whether these are through practice, reading, course attendance or research. Being reflective involves you as an active participant not a passive recipient (Kinsella 2000).

Multiple voices reflecting on 'doing' practice

The reflective process is often regarded as an individual activity; for example we often hear of being a reflective practitioner, but rarely about a reflective team. However, there are compelling reasons for reflection to be done in collaboration with others: it is through working together as a team, or as a community of practitioners, that we can work to transform practice (Freire 1972). As all our continued professional development occurs in cultural, social and political contexts, the health and social care teams in which occupational therapists work are rich grounds for learning. Teams can share and discuss practice, to make change to improve services for clients through collective reflection and subsequent collaborative action. Through working with others we are open to the possibility of change: our ways of understanding can be explored, challenged and alternatives created. Winpenny et al (2006) offer an illuminating account of group reflection. Through sharing our practice stories with others we become participants in our joint practice: gaining additional perspectives of a situation or an event and discovering new meanings or insights. This is necessary, if we only reflect individually we run the risk of navel gazing. Bolton (2001) stresses this 'reflective practice work can ... become politically, socially as well as psychologically useful, rather than a mere quietest navel-gazing exercise' (p. 3). Boud (2006) too, highlights that there is a need for new methods of reflection that move the focus from the individual learner in the workplace to systems that support team and organisational reflection and action in the workplace: namely, productive reflection. Productive reflection should lead to action with and for others for the advantage of all involved including the service users, the organisation and wider society (Cressey and Boud 2006).

In summary, active reflection can enable individual practitioners and teams to monitor, evaluate and adapt their performance: as a result their professional practice can be enhanced and the quality of service delivery to clients improved.

What is reflection?

Reflection is one of those words that is often used indiscriminately and that has many different meanings according to the user's perspective. In a recent exercise, practitioners were asked for their personal definitions of reflection: a sample is included below (see Box 5.2).

The practitioners above identified key aspects of reflection: reviewing their performance, examining it in detail, relating to their past knowledge and experiences and future actions. Their definitions concentrate on retrospective reflection or 'reflection on action'. Similarly, when students completed this exercise the majority of their views of reflection were also retrospective (see Box 5.3).

Box 5.2

Therapists' definitions of reflection

- Looking back on 'thinking' about something that has happened or something you have done, thinking how would I have done it differently or how would I deal with the same situation again?

- A systematic process to look at a situation in detail, to explore ideas for why the outcome occurred to learn new ways of dealing with this.

- To give thought to your actions/behaviour in order to improve/acknowledge what is going well.

- Reviewing your actions, appraising the efficacy of it, the theory behind it. Your decision to do it.

- Looking back on a past experience to see what you learned or didn't learn from it.

- Looking at an event/issue and considering all aspects of it in terms of your past experience, knowledge base and evidence.

Box 5.3

Students' definitions of reflection

- Reflection is important to look back…what have you done right and what treatment you could improve in the future

- Reflection enables the person to return to the experience and analyse those experiences both good and bad.

- To look back on your treatment and change it to adapt to different individuals – if it worked.

Defining reflection

For clarity, it is useful to go back to dictionary definitions. Kirkpatrick (1988) defines 'Reflect' as '…to give an image of as in a mirror' (p. 1087). The idea of holding a mirror up to gain a picture of practice is useful but limited as it only focuses on a specific frame in time. 'Reflect' is also defined as 'to consider meditatively' (p.1087), this develops the process from looking at – to thinking about in a more in-depth and in an intentional manner. Kirkpatrick (1988) goes on to describe 'Reflection' as '…the action of the mind by which it's conscious of its own operations' (p. 1087). Here an individual is actively thinking about or examining their thinking: this process is meta-cognition (Eraut 1994).

In relation to learning from experience, Boud et al (1993) defined reflection as a term that describes the processes used in exploring experience as a method of enhancing understanding. Osterman (1990) considered reflection as the essential part of the learning process as it results in making sense of or extracting meaning from the experience. More recently reflection is defined as the consideration of an experience or of learning to enhance understanding or to inform action (Fry et al 2006). All incorporate essential elements such as enhanced understanding, or a means of making meaning, however, Fry et al (2006) make explicit the informing action component that is vital to take practice forward.

An overview of reflective practice

The notion of reflective practice is now embedded in educators' and practitioners' thinking. It is found frequently in occupational therapy literature and elsewhere in nursing (Somerville and Keeling 2004), medicine (Fraser and Greenhaugh 2001) and education (Cowan 2006). It is however not strongly supported by empirical evidence. Nonetheless it maintains a strong component of education and practice. Dewey (1910) initially discussed reflection. Others have developed this concept over time, most notably, Schön (1983, 1987), Kolb (1984), Boud and Walker (1991), Fish et al (1989, 1991) and, Johns (1998). Several models of reflection will be highlighted; these have been selected as occupational therapists and other health practitioners most often use them. The work of Brookfield will be presented and the importance of story telling as a reflective method will be examined (Mattingly 1991). In relation to occupational therapy specifically the work of Alsop and Ryan (1996), Kinsella (2000) and most recently Brown and Ryan (2003) are all worthy of further investigation by the reader.

Kolb's (1984) work on the learning cycle will be considered first, as it is a useful starting point to examine experiential learning and how to develop understanding further. It provides a foundation from which reflective practice can be promoted (see Figure 5.1).

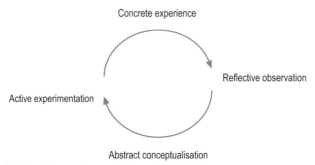

Figure 5.1 Kolb's learning cycle

To illustrate the essentials of Kolb's work complete the task in Box 5.4.

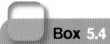

Box 5.4

In pairs, think about a recent clinical event that occurred in your practice, or whilst on placement. Take turns and tell your story of that event.

Note at all stages partners may ask for clarification or ask questions. With stages three and four partners may offer alternative courses of actions for consideration.

1. Tell your story – describe your **experience.**
2. Share your **reflections** on that experience.
3. What **ideas/practical actions did you do/or consider** to advance from that experience?
4. How did you/will you **experiment** with your ideas/or practical actions?

Through completion of this task you have completed one full turn of Kolb's cycle. Stages three and four provide further input into concrete experience and the learning cycle begins again. New understanding or learning is dependent upon the integration of such experiences in relation to practice theory through reflection.

The influence of Schön

It is impossible to examine reflective practice without recognising the work of Donald Schön who brought reflective practice, the reflective practitioner to the fore; as well as the concepts of 'reflection in action' and 'reflection on action' (Schön 1983, 1987).

Schön examined the relationship between professional knowledge and professional competence; he proposed that practitioners should examine artistry in their own profession through observing and learning through reflection. Such 'reflection on action' or practice is core to professional development as recognised experts in a profession demonstrate artistry that cannot be taught through traditional methods (Fry et al 2006). Furthermore, when working with non-complex cases or situations Schön proposed that experts demonstrate near automatic performance or 'knowing in action'. As experts in their specialist area, they know more than they can say or make verbally explicit, they are skilled and spontaneous in their performance but are often unable to articulate the dynamics of their practice fully. When questioned about their practice: they often describe the rules and procedures that underpin their practice – not what they did or what guided their thinking, such rules and procedures remain static and unchanged and do not reveal how or why they performed in that manner.

This process of rethinking some part of our 'knowing in action' leads to on the spot experimentation when the practitioner acts and thinks simultaneously or 'reflection in action'. This process involves the practitioner in reshaping their actions in the midst of the action. Schön considered that 'reflection in action' was often a consequence of surprise when engaged in an experience that challenged our usual assumptions or knowledge. This process may also be recognized as 'thinking on your feet' (Fish et al 1991) (Box 5.5).

Box 5.5

Can you recall the last time you were aware of 'thinking on your feet' in your practice? Revisit that event, what prompted you to 'think on your feet' and why? What was the outcome?

Schön proposed a 'reflection in action' coaching method for practitioners to use with learners, whether students or new staff, in their workplace to acquire new skills and insights. It involves three stages:

1. Follow Me – The coach explains and demonstrates a task breaking it down at various points and then giving time for questions/clarifications. This facilitates the learner to see the whole task completed and to understand the process and their relationship to it.
2. Joint experimentation – This stage helps the learner formulate what they want to achieve and by working together through demonstration/questioning the coach/learner explore different ways of producing and completing the task.
3. Hall of mirrors – Here the learner and coach continually shift their perspectives with a task, taking turns to move the task to completion; with each giving their input/view of the task, this gives a two-tier view of their interaction which encompasses acting/questioning/reflecting/acting through this process the learner completes the task.

Some aspects described above may be familiar strategies to you, you probably do not use the language described above. Nonetheless, using this method allows the learner and the coach to work collaboratively in developing 'reflection in action'.

Types of reflection

In discussing reflection it becomes clear that there are some debates in the literature. These often centre on reflection and its relationship to meta cognition (Eraut 1995). Kember (2000) proposes that meta-cognition involves some self-reflection to monitor one's own thinking. What is important is that reflection needs time, space, structure and support to be developed. Three distinct types of reflection in relation to continuing professional development can be identified in the literature namely (Kinsella 2000, Cowan 2006, Fade 2007):

1. Looking forward (prospective or anticipatory reflection or '*reflection for action*')
2. Looking at present (spective or '*reflection in action*')
3. Looking back (retrospective or '*reflection on action*')

To illustrate the above consider the following. You are contemplating a change of job, you browse the professional journals and websites: this gives you an idea about what is out there, the jobs available, the location and type of clients and the range of staff you might be working with (Anticipatory). You go on a visit to a particular job location: while there, you stop to think about how you would complement or fit into this team. What could you offer here and in what ways would this post help your career? What would it be like to work here? (Reflection in action). Once the visit is completed you review the experience: Who did you meet? What might you contribute? What was it like? (Reflection on action). Now you have to decide to apply or not to apply.

Let's return now to David and Michelle:

David has just been informed that his final placement will be in a forensic mental health setting in a specialist hospital. What are his anticipatory reflections? These may include thoughts regarding: anxiety about the setting or client group, what are the clients like? What have they done? What will the environment be like? What can I bring from my past experiences to this placement? What others can you think of?

Michelle has decided to explore further study options. She has a BSc (Hons) and has completed practice-related courses throughout her career. Now she is interested in Master level study. She is unaware of what the possible routes may be to a Master level qualification. In anticipation of returning to study she is examining her work and life balance. What would be feasible for her? What skills or knowledge does she already have? How can she structure her family life to ensure she can cope with returning to study? Is funding available? Will she be able to have study leave? And will her manager support her decision? What others can you think of?

Often we engage in anticipatory reflection without being aware of doing it; however conscious forward thinking can help you prepare for a particular event or help you to decide on possible courses of action. As Cowan (2006) states this type of reflection can 'establish goals for subsequent learning or development by identifying needs, aspirations and objectives which will subsequently be prominent in the mind' (p. 51) (Box 5.6).

Box 5.6

I know that I often use anticipatory reflection prior to going to meetings, especially if I know that the meetings may be difficult or contentious. How do you use or how can you use anticipatory reflection in your practice?

Models of reflection

This next section explores a number of models that can aid your ability to reflect on your own or with peers or team members. They offer you strategies and structures to guide and develop your skill as a reflective practitioner. These models offer a logical framework to make sense of complex information. Alternatively, there are other methods that are also useful to explore to enhance your reflective abilities such as the use of metaphors, literature (medical humanities), drawing and photography (Mattingly 1998, Murray et al 2000, Denshire 2005, McIntosh and Webb 2006).

The model developed by Boud and colleagues (Boud et al 1985, Boud 1991) states that reflection is grounded in the *personal foundation of experience* of the learner (Boud and Knights 1996) that is, the belief that all experiences to date have contributed to shaping who that person is now. Furthermore, it also includes the notion of *intent*, what is the learner's intent in relation to the learning experience as this gives a particular focus for that learning context (Fig. 5.2).

Preparation	Experience	Reflective process
Focus on		
Learner	Milieu	Return to experience
Milieu	Noticing and intervening	Attend to feelings
Skills/strategies	*Reflection in action*	Re-evaluation of the experience
The experience you bring to the event	Personal foundation of experience	
	Intent	

Figure 5.2 Boud et al (1985) Model for promoting learning from experience

Preparation

Boud's model places emphasis on preparation prior to a learning event, and this mirrors anticipatory reflection, as discussed previously. However, here there is a more in-depth approach to consideration of the learner, the milieu or the environment that the event will take place, and importantly the learner's skills set and strategies. Giving time to consider strategies, which one may use in that event can help preparation and flexibility when in the situation. David's experience illuminates this aspect (see Box 5.7).

Experience

The middle section of the model deals with the learning experience. Learning occurs in context, which encompasses both the human and physical environment, we learn through our interactions within the environment. When in a specific context it is important to notice what is happening to ourselves in relation to the external factors, learners can be assisted to do this by others highlighting aspects that may be important. For example, a practitioner may draw the learner's attention to how a client is positioned in a group task, or to how they are sitting in their chair. You may intervene in an *external* way (do something) for example: you talk with someone; or it may be that you assist someone to complete a task as you become aware that they are having difficulties. Alternatively you may intervene *internally* (think something) for example noting some follow-up activity, such as reading more about a condition or a treatment. Self-vigilance for the person

Box 5.7

David's preparation

In David's final placement his intent to learning may differ if he feels this is his last hurdle to professional practice or alternatively this is an area in which he feels he would like to specialize, in the future.

David as learner

Thought has to be given to the skills and strategies that David has and the experiences he can draw on from his past (both personal and professional), as well as his knowledge in relation to the setting, e.g. forensic psychiatry. David recognizes that he has had some experience working with clients in a mental health community team, but this was in a very different setting. Similarly, he has worked with teenagers who were challenging so he may be able to utilize some of those experiences. He has to consider what other skills and strategies he can take into this learning experience?

The milieu

This involves thinking about the placement setting thoroughly the types of clients, the scope of occupational therapy, environment, staff and security.

For example, if David considers what it is like to work in a secure environment this will heighten his awareness of possible risks and safety. He may discuss this issue with his fellow students who have been to that, or similar placements previously and who may offer useful practical advice. Alternatively he may ask his educator for advice when he starts the placement.

involved is key, being aware of how they are acting and modifying their actions in the midst of experience is 'Reflection in action'. Here too David's experience helps us understand this aspect further (see Box 5.8).

The final aspect of the model is the reflective processes; this is 'reflection on action'. Following the event the learner returns to the experience reviewing and describing what happened in as much detail as possible. The learner needs to attend to their feelings – how it felt for them. They must re-evaluate the experience – What it means now? What may it mean for their future actions or behaviour.

The strands of reflection

Another model commonly used by practitioners that was developed by Fish et al (1991) is entitled 'strands of reflection'. This model differs from Boud et al (1985) in that it concentrates on providing a structured and systematic method to review an event or experience: there is no implicit anticipatory reflection component. From my experience of working with practitioners this model is often regarded positively and seems to offer a useful method to assist them in detailed and contextualised 'reflection on action'.

To aid the use of the model it is useful to think of your experiences, like a rope that is made up of several strings or strands; these strands are woven together and build a stronger or richer perspective to the reflective process. Within the model, four key strands come together to help reflection in an organised manner: factual strand, retrospective strand, sub-stratum strand and the connective strand. Together they provide a means of reflecting upon your practice. They are not intended to be used independently; they seek to facilitate practitioners to interpret their practice experiences. By separating the four strands, each can be looked at closely and then all four can be reformed as a whole from which the practitioner can move forward.

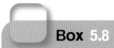

Box 5.8

David's reflecting on 'reflection in action'

At a supervision session in week 6 of an 8-week placement, David's supervisor asks him to discuss why he changed the format of a group session he had conducted the previous day. David explained that he had planned to do a group collage with a number of the men on the ward. He had decided to hold the session in the ward treatment area, as he was aware that some people could not be engaged in treatment sessions off the ward. He had chosen to do a group collage about football, as it was a constant subject on the ward, with most men contributing on their team and its progress through the season.

The group collage was an activity that had many levels of engagement and would also allow for those who had difficulty attending and concentrating for long periods, an opportunity to dip in and out of the session as they needed to.

He explained that his original plan for the session was that each would work for 10 minutes on their own football themes and that this would then progress to each member contributing their individual work to the group collage; followed by a discussion of everyone's work. However, David observed that at 10 minutes into the task the four men were really engaged with creating their own collage, he felt that if he had stopped them to move to the group task this would disrupt their engagement with the task. He decided to go with the flow of the activity and take his lead from them. Approximately 20 minutes into the task most seemed to have completed their creating phase, David decided instead of making the group collage he would stay with the individual focus. He asked someone to discuss what they had created and its significance to them and a lively discussion followed.

David acknowledged that his strategy of going with the flow could have been problematic, however, he felt that the group had its own volition and he was prepared to go with them at that moment in time. He felt that he was skilled enough to work with the unfolding situation and support the members and the task.

David's supervisor asked if he would have chosen this course of action at the start of his placement? David considered his response; he felt possibly not but reflected that his experiences over the past weeks of being part of the group, and gradually taking more responsibility for leading the sessions had given him a level of confidence and a feel for the participants that supported his 'on the spot' decision.

The factual strand: This acts to set the scene; briefly it describes the context of the practice situation. Events are recalled in time order; what happened; how did you feel, think and *why*? Practitioners are asked to pinpoint any critical incidents that arose during the situation.

The retrospective strand: This considers what patterns are visible in the practice as a whole. It asks what aims were set, and were these achieved. It asks practitioners to see themselves in relation to the practice event.

The sub-stratum strand: This requires practitioners to review what customs, traditions, beliefs were brought into a situation or were already there? Furthermore, what assumptions, beliefs or values underpinned the actions they took and the decisions they made.

The connective strand: This brings it all together: what has been learnt from this practice experience and how will it relate to future practice? How might thoughts and actions specific to this situation be modified in light of experiences or further thought or reading? Finally, it considers the implications for future practice (Box 5.9).

Box 5.9

Illustrating strands of reflection – Michelle's school visit

The factual strand: Michelle recently took over a small number of children who were on the caseload of a practitioner who has left the service. Michelle has become involved with these specific children as they have outstanding areas of occupational performance to be assessed. Michelle visited one child (Fiona) in a mainstream school. Following a 30-minute session with Fiona that was conducted in the therapy room Michelle returned Fiona to the class as she wished to discuss her performance with the class teacher. It was just before lunchtime. Michelle waited till the class had gone and then fed back to the teacher on her session with Fiona. This took about 10 minutes. Michelle made suggestions to help Fiona in the classroom. The teacher listened, thanked her and then left for lunch. Michelle was surprised by what she perceived as a lack of interest from the teacher.

So let's unpack what happened here, **the retrospective strand**: Michelle went about her business as she always did when assessing children in school. She always reported back to the class teacher offering some suggestions if possible. She had aimed to assess the child and this was completed successfully. Michelle reflected that this was her usual approach. Why was the teacher uninterested in her input? **The substratum strand:** Michelle considered what beliefs and customs she brought to this situation or that were already there. As she thought through the exchange, she considered that although she had worked in her normal manner this was a new school to her and a teacher whom she had not worked with before. Michelle began to recognise that although she had positive relationships in the schools where she worked this was a new area for her and perhaps she needed to spend more time with the teachers: finding out what they already knew about occupational therapy, explaining how she hoped to work with the children and them. She began to consider that perhaps she should have done more preparatory work both for herself going into a new school with the school staff. She also realised that she had assumed that the previous therapist had worked in a similar manner to her, which may not have been the case. **The connective strand:** Michelle decided that to build collaborative relations with the teachers here and to learn how best to work with them to support the child in their classroom she would have to do some work with this school. This could involve Michelle doing some information sessions with the staff either in small groups or individually to explore how they could all best work together.

The strands of reflection model and the process undertaken by Michelle are described as the DATA method (Peter, 1991). DATA outlines the four stages of the process namely:

- **D**escribe   What you did and what occurred
- **A**nalyse   Why you choose this approach
- **T**heorize   What assumptions influenced your initial choices; do these give an accurate explanation to what occurred
- **A**ct   If not, act by revising the assumptions or the approach.

This provides a useful shorthand way to remember those reflective steps.

The final model discussed comes from nursing, Johns (1998, 2000, 2004) developed the 'model of structured reflection' (MSR) which like the strands of reflection model is composed of a series of questions, in a logical order to help the reflective practitioner tune

Box 5.10

Model for Structured reflection –14th Edition (Johns 2004)

Reflective cue	Way of knowing
Bring the mind home	Aesthetics
Focus on a description of an experience that seems significant in some way	
What particular issues seem significant to pay attention to?	Aesthetics
How were others feeling and what made them feel that way?	Aesthetics
How was I feeling and what made me feel that way?	Personal
What was I trying to achieve and did I respond effectively?	Aesthetics
What were the consequences of my action on the patient/client, others and myself?	Aesthetics
What factors influenced the way I was feeling, thinking or responding?	Personal
What knowledge did or might have informed me?	Empirics
To what extent did I act for the best and in tune with my values?	Ethics
How does this situation connect with previous experiences?	Reflexivity
How might I respond more effectively given this situation again?	Reflexivity
What would be the consequences of alternative actions for the patient/client, others and myself?	Reflexivity
How do I NOW feel about this experience	Reflexivity
Am I more able to support myself and others better as a consequence?	Reflexivity
Am I more able to realize desirable practice monitored using reflexivity	
Appropriate frameworks such as framing perspectives, Carper's fundamental ways of knowing, other maps?	

into an experience and to understand the different ways of knowing, e.g. personal, ethical, empiric; that inform their practice – when practitioners share their stories they describe their aesthetic response. The MSR is as Johns (1998) states a 'device to enable practitioners to penetrate the essence of reflection on experience' (p. 3). The model commences by focusing in on the self, which encourages the practitioner to pause amidst their busy practice and find a quiet space to focus on their thoughts and feelings. The main part of the MSR is 'looking out' which offers a series of reflective cues that focus the practitioner's attention on significant issues within their work-based experience (Box 5.10).

The 'model for structured reflection' is not meant to be used prescriptively (Johns 2004). Johns (2004) offers an illuminative discussion of the model's use in practice and those interested should read further.

Other methods for promoting reflection

The models discussed in this chapter are not meant to be taken as the only methods for reflecting, many other models exist, practitioners can choose the model that they find most useful. We each tune into different elements so diversity is required. Moving away from specific models of reflection it is worthwhile considering two other distinct methods that can assist in developing reflection further; story telling (see the work of Mattingly) and critical incidents (see the work of Brookfield) both these methods encourage sharing practice with others.

Telling stories

We all tell stories of our practice informally with our colleagues on a daily basis. Telling stories or narrative is proposed as the primary form by which human experience is made meaningful (Polkinghorne 1988). As personal meaning is offered through the individual's story, Mattingly (1991) considers stories are particularly useful for addressing experiences and are therefore a useful tool for reflection. Mattingly (1998) regards story telling as being 'event and experience-centred, which create experiences for the listener or audience' (p. 8). Therefore the sharing and discussion of stories can aid all participants' reflections. Stories hold our experiences together, allowing links to the past, present and crucially, to the future. Through our own practice stories we are trying to make sense or give coherence to our actions and experiences and importantly give coherence and meaning to our clients' stories (Mattingly 1998). Thus using stories to promote reflection is vital for practitioners to develop their practice. Stories can be written or verbal: they can be sketches/vignettes or portraits of practice in words (Fish 1998) that capture the essence of the story or can be developed to give detailed accounts of our practice, for example, writing reflective journals. Recalling our stories may be part of an individual's supervision session or a feature of team meetings. Living (1999) offers perspectives of a specific client from a range of different team members; each offering a slightly different view. Reflecting on our stories highlights the cognitive, affective and temporal aspects of experience (Johns and Freshwater 1998) sharing our practice stories illustrates our thinking, our practice and promotes reflection.

Exploring critical incidents

Critical incidents are not exactly what they sound like; they are not dramatic events such as life and death situations or crisis; indeed they are often small or indeed common events that are meaningful to an individual, often, because these incidents touch them at an emotional level. The critical incident's significance lies with the practitioner and what they do following the event (Brookfield 1990). The incident is described verbally or written, shared with others and the question asked – why was the incident critical? McAllister (2003) offers a guideline for the analysis of critical incidents to promote advance practice. These include:

- Identify the critical incident
- Crystallise the event – focus on the event and examine in depth, hone in on the specifics, the values and assumptions and your reactions, the context of the incident.
- Clarify the nature of the problem or the issue
- What are the lessons to be learnt here?
- Identify what you might do to address the problem or issue.

Critical incidents by their nature are unplanned, it is important that they are explored as such incidents can be a powerful learning tool for those involved.

When and how to reflect are questions often asked by practitioners. Reflection should take place when you are involved in something that is new or surprising, when faced with complex or difficult situations, and after CPD activities. What is important is that you take the time to reflect on such activities. Table 5.1 summarises a range of strategies for developing reflection both as an individual practitioner and as a shared task for peers and teams.

Table 5.1 Techniques for doing and being reflective

	Individual	Peers	Mentors	Multi-disciplinary teams	Further Reading
Pre-briefing & debriefing	✓	✓	✓		Boud et al (1985)
Story telling (written/oral)	✓	✓	✓	✓	Bolton (2001)
Exploration of attitudes and beliefs		✓	✓	✓	Fish et al (1991)
Reflective questions	✓		✓		Johns (2004)
Continuing Professional Development Portfolio	✓		✓	✓	Paschal et al (2002)
Reflective journal	✓				Ghaye and Lillyman (1997)
Wait time or Think time		✓	✓		Stahl (2007)
Critical incidents		✓	✓	✓	McAllister (2003)
Directing attention	✓	✓			Boud et al (1985)

Signs of reflections

This chapter has looked at various ways of 'doing and being' reflective. A question often asked is how do we know that we are reflecting? Reflective processes can be observed in several ways; for example, the intensity of a discussion may be evidence of reflection. Alternatively it may be the quality of silence, or it may be the nature of questions asked. For example:

- What was I/were we aiming for when we did that?
- What exactly did I/we do?
- Why did I/we choose that particular action?
- What was I/we trying to achieve?
- What criteria am I/are we using to judge success?
- How did the client feel about it?
- How do I/we know the client felt like that?

You can of course think of others in relation to your own or your team's practice. Changes in practice and reconstructing a different way forward may also be evidence of a reflective process in action. Such changes may of course be small and cumulative and as a result they may not be noticed immediately by others, so it is important that you note such changes and share them with your colleagues.

Outcomes of reflection

The above models, storytelling, critical incidents, and other strategies identified all must lead to action by the individual or by the team. It is imperative that action follows reflection, otherwise the reflective process becomes a closed activity. The actions that result from reflection may take a number of forms but they all have implications for practitioners and their practice.

- Practitioners/teams may gain new perspectives on an experience
- Practitioners/teams may seek further knowledge or related research
- Practitioners/teams may change their future behaviour in light of their reflections
- Practitioners/teams faced with a similar situation in the future, may have a readiness to apply different strategies or have a commitment to a specific course of action.

Reflection takes active involvement, time, structure and support from others. It is important that reflection leads to action – those actions have implications for your practice and ongoing continued professional development. Doing reflection is after all a professional imperative to being a reflective practitioner. To conclude the words of Drucker, an American educator, are fitting 'Follow effective action with quiet reflection. From the quiet reflection will come even more effective action'.

Summary

This chapter has reviewed reflection and reflective practice; it has considered the significance of reflective practice for the practitioner, both, at an individual and at a team level. Being a reflective practitioner is a key skill in today's health and social care environment. Reflection on practice and experience is necessary for continuing professional development. Key theorists have been included to trace the historical and recent development of reflective practice. A number of models and a range of methods for developing reflection in practice have been introduced and illustrated. Readers are encouraged to use the 'Promoting Reflection' activities in their work setting.

References

Alsop A, Ryan S 1996 Making the most of fieldwork education: a practical guide. Nelson Thornes, Cheltenham, UK

Bolton G 2001 Reflective practice: writing and professional development. Paul Chapman Publishing Ltd., London

Boud D 2006 Relocating reflection in the context of practice: Rehabilitation or rejection? Paper presented at Professional Lifelong Learning: Beyond Reflective practice. July 2006. http://www.leeds.ac.uk/medicine/meu/lifelong06/ 28 June 2007

Boud D, Knights S 1996 Course design for reflective practice. In Gould NG, Taylor I (eds) Reflective Learning for Social Work: Research, Theory and Practice, pp. 23–34. Arena, Aldershot, UK

Boud D, Walker D 1991 In the midst of experience: developing a model to aid learners and facilitators. Paper presented at the National Conference on Experiential Learning empowerment through experiential learning: explorations of good practice. University of Surrey, 16–18 July 1991

Boud D, Keogh R, Walker D 1985 Promoting reflection in learning: a model. In Boud D, Keogh R, Walker D (eds) Reflection: Turning Experience into Learning, London, Kogan Page

Boud D, Cohen R, Walker D 1993 Using Experience for Learning. Milton Keynes, UK, Open University Press

Brookfield S 1990 Using critical incidents to explore learners' assumptions. In: Mezirow J and associates (eds) Fostering Critical Reflection in Adulthood: A Guide to Transformative and Emancipatory Learning. San Francisco, CA, Jossey-Bass

Brown G, Ryan SE 2003 Enhancing reflective abilities: interweaving reflection into practice. In: Brown G, Esdaile SA, Ryan SE (eds) Becoming an Advanced Practitioner, pp. 118–144. Edinburgh, UK, Butterworth Heinemann

Cowan J 2006 On becoming an innovative university teacher: Reflection in action. Berkshire, Society for Research into Higher Education & Open University Press

Cressey P, Boud D 2006 The emergence of productive reflection. In: Boud D, Cressey P, Docherty P (eds) Productive Reflection at Work: Learning for Changing Organisations. Routledge, London

Denshire S 2005 'This is a hospital, not a circus': Reflecting on generative metaphors for a deeper understanding of professional practice. International Journal of Critical Psychology Issue 13: Critical Professional 13: 158–178

Dewey J 1910 How we Think. University of Chicago, Chicago

Drucker P 2007 http://www.brainyquote.com/quotes/authors/p/peter_f_drucker.html Accessed on 04/07/2007

Eraut M 1994 Developing Professional Knowledge and Competence. The Falmer Press, London

Eraut M 1995 Knowledge creation and knowledge use in professional contexts. Studies in Higher Education 10: 117–133.

Fade S 2007 Learning and assessing through reflection: a practical guide. Making practice-based work: www.practicebasedlearning.org accessed 24 February 2007.

Fish D 1998 Appreciating practice in the caring profession: Refocusing professional development and practitioner research. Butterworth Heinemann, Oxford

Fish D, Twinn S, Purr B 1989 How to Enable Learning Through Professional Practice. London, West London Press

Fish D, Twinn S, Purr B 1991 Promoting Reflection: Improving the Supervision of Practice in Health Visiting and Initial Teacher Training. London, West London Institute

Fraser SW, Greenhaugh T 2001 Coping with complexity: educating for capability. British Medical Journal 323: 799–803

Freire P 1972 Pedagogy of the Oppressed. London, Penguin

Fry H, Ketteridge S, Marshall S 2006 A handbook for teaching and learning in higher education. Enhancing academic practice. RoutledgeFalmer, London

Ghaye T, Lillyman S 1997 Learning journals and critical incidents: reflective practice for healthcare professionals. Dinton, Quay Books

Health Professions Council 2004 Standards of Proficiency: Occupational Therapists, London, Health Professions Council

Health Professions Council 2006 Your guide to our standards for continuing professional development. London, Health Professions Council

Johns C 1998 Opening the doors of perception. In: Johns C, Freshwater D (eds) Transforming nursing through reflective practice. Oxford, Blackwell Science

Johns C 2000 Becoming a Reflective Practitioner A Reflective and Holistic Approach to Clinical Nursing, Practice Development and Clinical Supervision. Oxford, Blackwell Science

Johns C 2004 Becoming a Reflective Practitioner. Oxford, Blackwell Science

Johns C, Freshwater D 1998 Transforming nursing through reflective practice. Oxford, Blackwell Science

Kember D 2000 Reflective teaching and learning in the health professions: action research in professional education. Oxford, Blackwell Science

Kinsella EA 2000 Professional development and reflective practice: Strategies for learning through professional experience – A workbook for practitioners. Ottawa, Ontario, CAOT Publications ACE

Kirkpatrick E M 1988 Chambers 20th Century Dictionary, Chambers, Edinburgh

Kolb DA 1984 Experiential learning; Experience as the source of learning and development, Englewood Cliffs, NJ, Prentice Hall

Kuit JA, Reay G, Freeman R 2001 Experiences of reflective teaching. Active Learning in Higher Education 2(2): 128–142

Living R 1999 The team's story of a client's experience of anorexia nervosa. In: Ryan SE, McKay EA (eds) Thinking and reasoning in therapy. Stanley Thornes, Cheltenham, UK

Mattingly C 1991 Narrative reflection on practical actions: Two learning experiments in reflective storytelling. In: Schön DA (ed.) The Reflective Turn. San Francisco, CA, Jossey Bass

Mattingly C 1998 Healing dramas and clinical plots. The narrative structure of experience. Cambridge, UK, Cambridge University Press

McAllister L 2003 Using adult education theories: facilitating others' learning in professional practice settings. In: Brown G, Esdaile SA, Ryan SE (eds) Becoming an advance healthcare practitioner. Butterworth Heinemann, Edinburgh, UK

McIntosh P, Webb C 2006 Creativity and reflection: An approach to reflexivity in practice. Paper presented at Professional Lifelong Learning: Beyond Reflective practice. July 2006. http://www.leeds.ac.uk/medicine/meu/lifelong06/ 28 June 2007

Murray R, McKay E, Thompson S et al 2000 Practising reflection: a medical humanities approach to occupational therapist education. Medical Teacher 22(3): 276–281

Osterman KF 1990 Reflective Practice: A new agenda for education. Education and Urban Society 22(2): 133–152

Paschal KA, Jensen GM, Mostrom E 2002 Building portfolios: a means for developing habits of reflective practice in physical therapy education. Journal of Physical Therapy Education 16(3): 38–53

Peters J 1991 'Strategies for reflective practice'. In: Brocket R (ed.) Professional development for educators of adult and continuing learning, No.51. San Francisco, CA, Jossey Bass

Polkinghorne D 1988 Narrative knowing and the human sciences. Albany, NY: State University of New York Press

Quality Assurance Agency for Higher Education 2001 Benchmark statement: Health care programmes phase 1, occupational therapy subject bench marking group. Quality Assurance Agency for Higher Education, Gloucester, UK

Schön D 1983 The Reflective Practitioner: how professionals think in action. New York, Basic Books

Schön D 1987 Educating the Reflective Practitioner. San Francisco, CA, Jossey Bass

Somerville D, Keeling J 2004 A practical approach to promote reflective practice within nursing. Nursing Times 100(12): 42–45

Stalh RJ 2007 Using think time and wait time skillfully in the classroom. Available at: http://atozteacherstuff.com/pages/1884.shtml accessed 6 July 2007

Winpenny K, Forsyth K, Jones C et al 2006 Group reflective supervision: Thinking with theory to develop practice. British Journal of Occupational Therapy 69(9): 423–428

Professional skills for practice

Assessment skills for practice

6

Susan Prior and
Edward A.S. Duncan

Highlight box

- Assessment is a term used to describe both a process and a tool.
- Assessments ensure that interventions meet the needs of clients, can measure change and reflect the unique contribution of occupational therapy to practice.
- 'Top-down approaches' to assessment, whilst lacking in objective evidence, have a strong theoretical rationale that supports their use in practice.
- There are a variety of different forms that assessments can take.
- Standardised and non-standardised assessments each have strengths and weaknesses in practice.

Overview

Accurate assessment is an essential component of occupational therapy. But what exactly is assessment and at what stage of therapy should it be carried out? And how do practitioners choose which assessments to use? These questions, amongst others, are discussed in this chapter. The chapter commences by examining why occupational therapists carry out assessments and considers why other stakeholders (such as the service manager or regularity body) feel strongly that assessment should be a core part of practice.

The chapter tackles head on the debate about whether or not conceptual models of practice should be selected prior to, or following (or not at all) the initial assessment process. Other factors that influence the selection of an assessment in occupational therapy are then described and discussed.

Assessments can be undertaken in various formats and these are each described in turn with key points highlighted for when they are appropriate to use. Finally the chapter concludes with discussion about the appropriateness of using standardised and non-standardised assessments in practice. Case vignettes are used throughout the chapter to illuminate relevant issues.

What is assessment and why assess?

Assessment is a term used to describe both a process and a tool. The process of assessment aims to develop practitioners' understanding of clients as occupational beings, recognising their strengths and difficulties. Assessment is the initial stage of the occupational therapy process and supports practitioners to appropriately carry out the second stage of the process: developing individualised intervention strategies tailored to client's needs. Without appropriate assessment therapy may not meet the requirements of clients (Laver Fawcett 2002, Cohn et al 2003). Assessments are used at the evaluation stage of the occupational therapy process, identifying changes from the initial assessment and determining the effectiveness of the interventions.

Assessments and the assessment process help to ensure that occupational therapy practice not only meets the needs of clients but also reflects the unique contribution that occupational therapy practitioners can make to the health and wellbeing of clients. McMillan (2006) suggests that assessments that reflect occupational therapy values should be the initial tools used by occupational therapists. These include assessments drawn from two conceptual models of practice: The Model of Human Occupation (Kielhofner 2007) and the Canadian Model of Occupational Performance and Engagement (Townsend et al 2007). This is known as a top-down approach to assessment (Mathiowetz 1993, Trombly 1995, Kramer et al 2003), where practitioners first consider clients' occupational roles, performance and skills. Without this understanding it will be much harder to understand what the consequences of specific problems will be on clients' lives. For example, the impact of limited grip strength will be different for a needlework artist and a manual labourer. Thereafter a practitioner may decide to further investigate specific performance components. And it is at this stage that measurement of grip strength (in this example) may or may not be appropriate.

It is often the case that practitioners will not discover anything new by conducting an assessment; the same information may have been gathered through informal conversation and observation. However by gathering information systematically through a standardised assessment a practitioner can be confident that a comprehensive review has been completed and this can then be used for comparison at a later stage of therapy.

An occupational therapy assessment may have considerable consequences for clients. It could indicate whether they are safe to be discharged from hospital or to continue living at home, or it may identify goals of getting back to work or entering education. These implications have considerable impact on clients' lives so it is each practitioner's professional responsibility to ensure that all assessments are conducted sensitively, thoroughly and reliably.

In addition to the direct clinical requirements of carrying out assessments, practitioners may be required to assess by service managers in order to demonstrate the service's clinical effectiveness. Professional or regulatory bodies also insist that practitioners use assessments in practice. For example, in the UK the Health Professions Council (2007) Standards of Proficiency for Occupational Therapists requires that registrants must be able to use assessment techniques, gather, analyse and evaluate information. Assessment, therefore, as both a process and a tool, is an essential component of the occupational therapy process.

Who benefits from assessment?

At times external influences and the drive for evidence-based practice led practitioners to consider the assessment strategies that they are using. But, whilst evaluating outcomes of intervention is important for occupational therapy services and helps demonstrate their effectiveness, it is vital not to lose sight of the value that this evaluation will have for individual clients and practitioners (Table 6.1).

Table 6.1 The value of evaluation

Client	Practitioner	Service	Profession (when outcomes are published)
To be listened to and understood by the practitioner Establishing a collaborative relationship	Better understanding of client initially and throughout therapy	To ensure that resources are being used in the most effective way	Developing an evidence base which other practitioners may draw on
Occupational therapy is tailored to individual needs	Time is spent focusing on clients needs and priorities	To evidence need for new resources to develop new services	To allow others to build on previous work
Provides evidence of change and allows reassessment of goals	Professional development providing material for reflective learning	To identify areas where intervention is ineffective and practice needs to be reviewed or redirected	
To identify when therapy is no longer required			

Assessment may occur throughout therapy, but assessments should only be carried out when necessary. So why would an occupational therapist decide to conduct an assessment? There are various reasons. For example:

- At the beginning of occupational therapy involvement:
    - To determine need for occupational therapy intervention
    - To understand a client's current strengths and needs in relation to their occupational performance
    - To gain an accurate picture of a client's occupational lifestyle prior to illness or injury
    - To determine current and predict future functional ability
    - To provide a baseline assessment prior to intervention
    - To assist in goal setting for intervention
- Throughout occupational therapy involvement:
    - To evaluate the effectiveness of an intervention programme
    - To review, adapt or redesign an intervention
    - To identify needs best met by other services leading to referral onto other agencies
- At the end of occupational therapy involvement:
    - To identify appropriate time for discharge from services
    - To determine on-going needs for support and make recommendations for further services.

Shared (or needs) assessments

Occupational therapists may work within clinical settings where they contribute to assessments where there is a multi-professional shared responsibility to gather information. This is likely to be an important aspect of their role with other team members relying on the occupational therapist to assess a client's independence in activities of daily living. However a therapist should consider if this shared assessment should be informed by a profession-specific assessment. Shared assessment tools tend to be global measures and are therefore useful for screening strengths and difficulties, however are insufficient to gain the detail an occupational therapist would require to plan an appropriate intervention. Supplementing the shared assessment with an occupational therapy tool will be vital as illustrated in Vignette 6.1.

Vignette 6.1

Mrs Jones attends the local day hospital, she has been suffering from depression since the death of her husband 6 months ago. She was first seen by a member of the local authority access team who conducted the locality's single shared assessment used by both health and local authority staff. The assessment identified that Mrs Jones had needs in terms of diet and meal making and subsequently 'Meals on Wheels' were provided. Mrs Jones regularly expresses her frustration reporting that she does not need this service and asks for it to be discontinued.

Before contacting the home care team the occupational therapist assessed Mrs Jones, by carrying out an OCAIRS (Forsyth et al 2005), and identified that Mrs Jones missed the routine that meal preparation tasks gave her, prior to the meals on wheels she sometimes skipped meals as she couldn't face going shopping. Before his death her husband had always driven her to the supermarket. An AMPS (Assessment of Motor and Process Skills assessment: an observational measure of activities of daily living which rates a clients effort, efficiency, safety, and independence in carrying out familiar tasks (Fisher 1999)) had demonstrated that Mrs Jones had necessary skills to prepare her meals. In discussion with the multi-professional team it was decided to arrange an alternative care package for Mrs Jones utilising a shopping service rather than Meals on Wheels. This service would collect a shopping list from Mrs Jones and then deliver her order.

How to select an assessment

There are numerous assessment tools that occupational therapists could use in practice, so how do practitioners know which to select? Practitioners use a wide variety of types of assessment the selection of which depends on the information they wish to gather. Frequently more than one type of assessment may be required in order to gain a comprehensive understanding of a situation, or client's functioning, etc. Various factors should be considered when deciding which type of assessment to use with a client.

Conceptual models and selecting assessments

Which comes first: the assessment or the choice of conceptual model? This occupational therapy alternative to the better known chicken and egg scenario has taxed the profession for a number of years, and continues to do so today. In essence it is the argument of whether or not to use the 'top-down' assessment approach previously discussed.

The top-down approach suggests that an occupation-focused conceptual model of practice is selected as the first stage of the occupational therapy process (ensuring, amongst other issues, that the assessment is occupationally focused) and from that point an initial or screening assessment can take place. Following this assessment it may then be necessary to conduct further, more specific, assessments depending on the initial assessment's findings. A good example of this way of practising and selecting assessments is outlined by Forsyth and Kielhofner (2006). These authors provide a flow chart that very clearly outlines the process of assessment selection based on the use of the Model of Human Occupation (MoHo) (Kielhofner 2008). Similarly, the Canadian Model of Occupational Performance and Engagement (CMOP-E) (Townsend et al 2007) is intrinsically linked to the Canadian Occupational Performance Measure (COPM) (Law et al 2005a). Law et al's (2005b) argument for using the COPM as an initial assessment is that, 'the tone of the therapeutic relationship, lets the client know you will be working as partners, and helps to focus your further assessment and intervention on the issues that the client feels are priorities'.

Both the MoHo and the CMOP-E have been developed within a generally Western societal context. Interestingly, the Western perspective of occupational therapy practice has been criticised for being excessively reductionistic, linear and scientific (Iwama 2006): But it is beyond the scope of the current chapter to consider whether the differences between Western and Eastern perspectives are truly significant in occupational therapy practice and if so what its effect on the assessment process would be.

It is important to highlight that using a top-down approach to practice does not restrict the practitioner to only using assessments that have been developed within the selected conceptual model; there may be times when an unstructured assessment is appropriate and an impromptu assessment opportunity may also occur when the practitioner has not had time to prepare a more structured assessment process. Furthermore a specific issue best understood from a specific frame of reference (for example mood and the cognitive-behavioural frame of reference) may also be appropriate after the initial conceptual model assessments are carried out. The use of a top-down approach to assessment, therefore, does not restrict practitioners to using assessments solely associated with that model.

An alternative approach to assessment is presented by Creek (2003), amongst others. In a document published by the College of Occupational Therapists, Creek presented 'the complex content of occupational therapy practice' (p. 7). Creek's (2003) account makes no mention of employing a conceptual model of practice at any stage. Instead, Creek (2003) lists a broad range of factors that should be considered when assessing a client. These include:

- information about self-maintenance, productivity and/or leisure
- examining functioning in the physical, intra- and interpersonal and cognitive domains
- considering a client's strengths and challenges
- examining the client's social and physical environments and the amount and duration of any assistance that may be required.

The dozen factors listed above are a summary of the fuller list recommended by Creek (2003). Students and practitioners rightly question which of these two differing approaches is more effective? Does it matter if a top-down approach to assessment is used or not? To date, there does not appear to be any research that has rigorously studied this question. However, at a theoretical level, an argument can be made that a top-down approach is least likely to leave practitioners vulnerable to making errors through peoples' known limitations; specifically in working memory capacity and personal biases in information gathering. In other words using a top-down approach may minimise the errors that practitioners make. Various issues leave practitioners vulnerable to making errors in assessing clients.

Given that the maximum number of pieces of information a person can hold in their working memory is 7 ± 2 (Miller 1956), it can be seen that listing an extensive range of factors that should be considered when assessing an individual (without placing them in the context of a well-developed structured assessment) is likely to lead to practitioners accidentally omitting some aspects of the assessment. Miller's research, therefore, lends weight to the idea that practitioners should consider using a top-down approach and intentionally use a conceptual model of practice when initially conducting an assessment.

It has also been clearly evidenced in a range of studies in differing contexts that individuals are not reliable information gatherers and are biased in the manner in which information gathered from assessments is analysed (Paley et al 2007). Assuming that occupational therapists are no different (and there is no reason to assume they are) it can be seen that if practitioners do not impose an assessment structure that has been thoroughly tested they leave themselves open to bias, focusing in on areas of particular interest to themselves, potentially not giving due weight to certain issues raised by their clients, and emphasising some issues more than others when reporting the findings of their assessment. Each of these dangers is lessened when a practitioner uses a structured scoping or initial assessment founded in a conceptual model of practice. Practitioners are in effect 'forced' to consider the range of aspects covered in the assessment thus lessening the potential for bias or omission. For example both the Model of Human Occupation Screening Tool (Parkinson et al 2006) and the Canadian Occupational Performance Measure (Law et al 2005) contain specific questions that cover each of the aspects that are included within their respective conceptual models. This assessment structure ensures that individual practitioners gather information about the whole range of occupational functioning (as conceived by each respective model) and are less likely to succumb to personal biases and shortcuts, or accidentally omit certain aspect of the assessment.

As with so many areas of practice, research into the superiority of differing assessment approaches is needed before it can be said with confidence whether or not it is more beneficial to use a top-down assessment approach. However, the well-established literature surrounding heuristics and biases (Gilovich et al 2002) and existing knowledge about human's limited working memory capacity (Miller 1956) lends strength to the theoretical arguments that support using a top-down assessment approach rather than a theoretical list of a multitude of factors such as those listed by Creek (2003) and others.

Work context

The area of practice an occupational therapist works in will also shape the assessment strategies they use. The priorities of the service and time available each influence the selection of appropriate assessments (see Vignette 6.2).

In a long-term setting there may be benefits in investing time in comprehensive assessments to ensure that an intervention programme is thorough, while there may not be the time available to conduct several assessments in acute settings where practitioners are required to make quick decisions based on rapid assessments. As in the case of Mr MacDonald this may result in referral onto another service where longer-term needs are suggested.

Decisions about assessments may also be influenced by the clinical specialism, some assessments are designed for particular areas of practice while others can be applied across most areas. Assessment manuals often provide guidance about when using it would be inappropriate; for example using a self-report assessment with a client who has limited insight. Occupational therapists also work in a variety of settings

Vignette 6.2

Mr MacDonald

The rapid response team has been asked to visit Mr MacDonald by his GP. He was found, having fallen this morning, by a neighbour. The GP visited and has decided not to admit Mr MacDonald as he has only sustained minor bruising. However the GP would like occupational therapy and physiotherapy to assess him and refers Mr MacDonald to the Rapid Response Service.

The Rapid Response Service is a busy service which responds to referrals within 24 h. Their priority is to ensure peoples' safety at home. They use a quick checklist to assess the home environment and individuals' functional abilities. They visit Mr MacDonald in the morning spending about 30 min with him. From the assessment the occupational therapist identifies that a toilet frame, bed rail and high-back chair would improve his safety and the physiotherapist recommends a walking frame. The team is able to deliver and fit these items the same day.

The occupational therapist is confident that the situation has improved but recognises there are longer-term issues her service is not able to deal with. She recommends that Mr Macdonald be seen by the community rehabilitation service who can offer a longer-term input aiming to increase Mr Macdonald's independence and safety. This team conducts a more thorough assessment through interview and observation over two home visits.

including hospitals, clinics and in clients' homes. There may be some practical limitations that restrict the available range of assessments for use, for example if the equipment is not easily portable.

Occasionally an occupational therapist may be asked to assess an individual only to provide a report, for example in a compensation claim. However, usually assessments are a means to an end: to begin, review or end a programme of intervention. It is therefore important that practitioners consider what to do with the information that they gather.

Standardised assessments provide a structure for organising information into a logical format, and may provide information for interpreting the findings. Practitioners may also have gathered information from one or several assessments. Taking time to formulate all the information gathered through the assessment process into a conceptualisation of the individual is an important step in the assessment process and vital to enable appropriate planning of an intervention. The conceptualisation, drawn from the information gathered, will provide a portrait of a client's occupational life and their needs. This information should be considered as a whole. In a collaborative therapeutic relationship the practitioner should then return to their client, share their understanding and confirm whether or not the client views the situation in a similar way (see Chapter 9 for further information as this issue is often much easier to suggest than to truly achieve). Sharing and confirming your understanding is an important step towards developing shared goals.

Report writing is a useful way of synthesising the findings of assessments, provides a document in the clinical records to demonstrate occupational therapy's intervention and can be used to compare future assessment findings (see Chapter 6). Some assessments provide a quantitative summary of findings (for example the Assessment of Motor and Process Skills (AMPS) (Fisher 1999), but a narrative interpretation of findings is also useful to describe what this means for the client.

The type of information required

The type of information required will also influence the type of assessment used. Practitioners wishing to gain a broad understanding of a client may decide to use a general screening tool. Alternatively, where more detailed information is desired about client's specific abilities, a structured observational measure may be more appropriate. Which assessment is ultimately selected depends on a variety of issues including client ability, timing and the form of assessment the practitioner wishes to undertake.

The ability of the client to participate in the assessment process

Clients who are non-verbal or have very low levels of concentration will be unable to participate in interviews; clients who are unable to read will not be able to complete self assessment forms without assistance, etc.

The timing of the assessment

An assessment at the start of therapy will initially be broad in nature: practitioners will frequently conduct a screening procedure or initial interview to ascertain whether or not a client requires occupational therapy, and if so broadly what the issues are. Towards the end of therapy assessments are likely to be much more focused to measure (whether narratively or numerically) what difference (if any) occupational therapy intervention has made.

Forms of assessment

Several different forms of assessment exist and have been mentioned within the chapter so far. Each method of assessment has its strengths and weaknesses.

Case note review

Frequently clients have already seen several health-care professionals before they meet an occupational therapist. Looking through multidisciplinary notes (where available) is an excellent way in which to gain some extra knowledge about a client before a practitioner sees them for the first time. Frequently case notes are interdisciplinary, and there may not be separate case notes held by each professional discipline. Either way there are often medical case notes that are held separately and these can contain additional valuable background information.

Some practitioners prefer not to look at case notes before they meet a client, and may suggest this to students. The rationale for this is that it is best to form your own initial impressions without having your assessment tainted by the clinical information and reasoning of others. However, there is no evidence to suggest that reading case notes before meeting a client significantly affects practitioners' opinion of them, and if a practitioner was aware of the potential of forming an unhelpful attitude towards clients they can consciously try to avoid doing so (Creek 2002). There are several other reasons why reviewing a client's notes before meeting them is very sensible:

- Clients may already have related their 'story', background and key clinical features to several clinicians before you get involved. Having to repeat this information can be intensely frustrating for a client and gives the impression that services do not communicate with each other.
- The client may have recently (or historically) undergone a traumatic life event which practitioners may inadvertently touch upon during an assessment if they were not aware of them. Examples of this include death of a family member or close friend, experiences of sexual abuse, etc.

- It may be necessary to conduct a risk assessment for meeting a client. Some clients may have histories of violent or sexually inappropriate behaviour. It cannot be guaranteed that such information would always be included in a referral. Not knowing this information before meeting a client could place the practitioner in danger.
- Case note reviewing can help a practitioner to understand a client's case and context in much greater detail than most referral forms allow. Reading case notes can assist in developing further areas of assessment such as interviews or observational assessments.

Observation

Observation is an essential assessment skill for every practitioner. Observational assessments can be either structured or unstructured. An excellent example of an unstructured observational assessment process, and the richness of information that can be gained through this process, is recounted in the book 'Dibs in search of self' (Axline 1964). This section outlines various forms of observational assessments commonly used in practice.

Whilst all forms of observation could be categorised as structured or non-structured, more detailed categorisations also exist and are useful ways of considering the various forms of observation. Creek (2002) outlines three types of observation: general observation, observation of specific performances and observation of set task performance. Using the theoretical framework of the Model of Human Occupation, observation can also be used to understand both the performance and participation levels of clients' occupational functioning.

An observation of performance skills could include assessing a client's dressing ability post stroke. Whilst an observation of occupational participation could include assessing a client with multiple sclerosis working in their office to see if any adaptations are required. As well as unstructured observations of a client's skill level, the practitioner may also wish to conduct a structured observation of a client's communication and interaction or motor and process skills. Two well-known assessments developed from the Model of Human Occupation enable practitioners to do this and provide extremely detailed information about clients actual abilities (Fisher 1999, Forsyth et al 1998) (see Vignette 6.3).

Vignette 6.3

Mrs Harris is a 78-year-old widow, she lives alone and has no local family. After a recent home visit, the district nurse has referred Mrs Harris to the community rehabilitation team. The district nurse was concerned that Mrs Harris is not looking after herself and her home environment is deteriorating. The occupational therapist in the team is asked to visit to carry out a functional assessment.

During the visit it quickly becomes apparent that Mrs Harris is a poor historian and has limited insight into the difficulties she is experiencing, she does not know why the district nurse has asked for this assessment. When discussing her daily routine Mrs Harris reports going to the shops every morning, coming home to do some housework before cooking her own lunch. There is only out-of-date food in the fridge and no signs of recent cooking even though it is early afternoon. The occupational therapist decides that in order to get an objective assessment of Mrs Harris' abilities she should carry out an AMPS assessment (Fisher 1999). This is suggested to Mrs Harris, who agrees.

The environmental location of both participation and performance skills are highly dependent on the environment in which they occur: how a client completes an activity can significantly differ between an occupational therapy department and a client's home for example. This differentiation in skill level may be due to environmental differences (for example the kitchen in the occupational therapy department is at a more suitable height for the client than their own kitchen at home), but it can also be due to volitional differences.

Volition is most easily understood as the thoughts and feelings that a person has about what they have done, are doing, and will be doing in the future (Kielhofner 2008). Volitional deficits can have a significant effect on a clients' functioning. Some clients may be able to accurately articulate these issues, others (such as people with severe mental illness or learning difficulties) will find this harder. In these cases it is useful to carry out an observational assessment.

Whilst it can therefore be very important to observe a client in the environment in which the activity will normally take place, it can also be useful, depending on the reason for the assessment, to observe a client in a variety of settings. This variation in environment can be used to good effect to demonstrate a client's occupational potential. The Volitional Questionnaire (de les Haras et al 2007) (a structured assessment developed from the Model of Human Occupation) provides an excellent method of measuring volition through observation. This assessment can be used to good effect when a practitioner wishes to understand in greater depth why a client performs better in one environment than another, or to demonstrate the significance of this altered behaviour to other members of the clinical team.

Interviews

At their most basic level interviews are where a practitioner asks questions from a client in order to gain a better picture of their occupational performance. Like observation, interviews can generally be categorised as unstructured or structured.

Unstructured interviews. Unstructured interviews are those where the practitioner is not following a standardised interview assessment or formal information-gathering schedule.

Unstructured interviews may vary in their formality and presentation. At their most informal a practitioner may conduct an unstructured interview whilst participating in another task. An example of this is the 'interview' that occurs when a client and practitioner are jointly preparing a meal, doing the dishes, or driving somewhere in a car. Participating in such activities can make information sharing for some clients much easier and often a practitioner is able to elicit more information from a client whilst participating in such tasks than they would ever manage to gain if they had formally sat down in a room together with the specific aim of talking!

Of course it will often be appropriate and feasible to sit down together to interview a client. In these situations, even when the interview is unstructured, it is important to consider factors that will improve the interview process. These factors can be broadly categorised as expectations (of both practitioner and client) and environment (where the interview will take place), and are equally relevant and worthy of consideration when carrying out structured assessments.

Clients should be informed in advance of the reason for an interview, the time and location that it will take place, and the length of time a client should expect it to take (Creek 2002). Practitioners should also have gained the client's agreement to be interviewed.

The physical and social environment where an interview is to take place should be closely considered. Interviews should be carried out in a peaceful setting, free from distractions and interruptions. Let other people know that an interview is taking place so that unnecessary interruptions are avoided. Consideration should be given to the seating arrangements of both parties: a 90° angle of seats that are comfortable and allow the feet of both client and participant to be flat on the floor is ideal (see Figure 6.1). Seats should be the same height so neither party is looking up or down on the other. It is important that clients are as relaxed as possible during interviews, so practitioners need to employ all their skills in the therapeutic use of self (see Chapter 9).

Structured interviews Structured assessments have a relatively fixed format. They may form the basis of an initial assessment developed by a department or service which contains a list of questions that are asked of all clients who enter the service. Alternatively a practitioner may wish to gather particular information about occupational functioning and may use a structured assessment from a conceptual model of practice. One such example is the Occupational Circumstances Interview and Rating Scale (Forsyth et al 2005) which is developed from the Model of Human Occupation and now has specific formats and guiding questions for physical, general mental health and forensic settings (see Vignette 6.5). It is important to read the instructions for all structured assessments carefully: some require the use of precise words in questions, whilst others (including the majority of those associated with the Model of Human Occupation) provide examples of questions to use, but have specific guidelines for scoring the assessment. Familiarity with structured interview assessments is essential to enable the interview to flow smoothly. They can feel awkward to use at first, due to a lack of experience, but frequent use helps practitioners to feel more comfortable with them, which in turn helps the interview to flow more like a good conversation.

Self-report questionnaires and checklists

Self-report questionnaires and checklists are commonly used in practice. They can be generic (such as measures of depression (e.g. Kroenke and Spitzer 2002) or anxiety (Beck and Steer 1990)) or occupation specific (such as measures of client's self assessment of occupational interests (Kielhofner and Neville 1983) or time use (Smith et al 1986)). Whilst questionnaires and checklists do not provide a depth of information about a client, they can be very useful methods of gathering specific information.

When deciding whether or not to use a self-report method of assessment consideration should be given to the client's eyesight quality, as well as reading, comprehension and concentration levels.

Assessments that combine information-gathering methods

Some assessment measures do not 'fit' nicely into either observation, interview or self-report categories, as they use a combination of methods to gather information. Two examples of such measures are the Model of Human Occupation Screening Tool (MOHOST) (Parkinson 2006) and the Canadian Occupational Performance Measure (Law et al 2005).

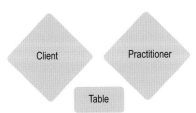

Figure 6.1 Seating plan for one to one interviews

Vignette 6.4

James is a long-term client of the mental health services, he lives independently in the community supported by his keyworker (a community psychiatric nurse). The key-worker is concerned that he is isolated and has no social network. She has discussed her concerns with the occupational therapist (Beth); they plan a joint visit for James' next appointment.

However on introducing James to Beth he immediately refuses to work with her, James explains that he has seen occupational therapists in the past and they always wanted him to join sports and art groups, he tells her he has no interest in these activities. Beth asks him about what he does enjoy, he tells her about his interest in computers. Beth explains that if he were to agree to work with her she would initially interview him using the OCAIRS (Occupational Circumstances Assessment Interview and Rating Scale) (Forsyth et al 2005). Beth explained that this would help her to fully understand what is important to him and what, if any, difficulties he was having. Beth told James she would then share her assessment with him and then they would be able to discuss what they could work on together. She guaranteed that as James was not interested in sports or art group she would not ask him to attend these. Beth recognized that by using this interview as an initial assessment her intervention could be tailored to James' specific needs and they could work in collaboration to set meaningful goals.

The MOHOST was developed by a group of clinicians in the United Kingdom who worked with clients who were very low functioning. The practitioners wished to use a broad screening assessment to gather information about clients' general occupational functioning difficulties, but found the interview structure of assessments such as the OCAIRS (Forsyth et al 2005) too intense and challenging for this client population. Over time and in collaboration with academic colleagues they developed the MOHOST. Whilst primarily an observational measure, information can also be gathered through case note

Vignette 6.5

Potter House is a new residential rehabilitation unit built in the community as an intermediary step between hospital and independent tenancy as part of the neuro-rehabilitation service. The multi-professional team has been asked to consider appropriate assessments to be used at monthly intervals during a client's stay in the unit. It is planned that residents will be in the unit for between 3 and 12 months.

The practitioner considers that it will be important to gain a comprehensive picture of a client's occupations in self care, work and leisure pursuits; she wants to be able to identify areas of need and priorities for the client. She is particularly aware that while in hospital clients tend to follow the routine of the busy ward and priorities tend to be set by the clinical team. This has led to clients finding it difficult on discharge as they feel overwhelmed with the responsibility of planning for the future. The occupational therapist decides to utilise the COPM (Canadian Occupational Performance Measure) (Law et al 2005b). She recognises that this assessment gathers information about a client's self perception of their occupational performance and facilitates clients' setting their own priorities for rehabilitation. She anticipates that through supporting clients in setting their own goals the transition to independence may be assisted.

review, interview and even third-party information gathering from relatives or other care staff to inform the scoring of the MOHOST.

The Canadian Occupational Performance Measure (Law et al 2005) combines an interview format with a self report rating of satisfaction and importance. This assessment is closely linked with the Canadian Occupational Performance Model and Engagement and addresses the three occupational performance areas covered by the model: self-care, productivity and leisure (see Vignette 6.5).

Standardised or non-standardised assessments?

Standardised assessments

Assessments can be standardised in two main ways: in terms of their process, materials and scoring instructions, and by normative standardisation (that is by providing statistics that outline what healthy 'normal' individuals could expect to score on the assessment) (de Clive Lowe 1996). De Clive Lowe (1996) outlined the importance of standardised assessments for occupational therapists. Standardised assessments can provide objective information about the health status or occupational functioning of a client. Such objectivity is important as it provides a very useful outcome measurement of a client's progress and can form the basis of decision making that is more defensible than a practitioner's judgement alone (Stewart 1999). Further, and as previously discussed, human memory is very fallible (Schacter 1999) and self reporting is recognised to be a very subjective process, with tenuous reliability and open to numerous biases. All of these reasons provide a sound rationale for using standardised assessments. Taking these factors into account Laver Fawcett (2002) rightly concluded that, 'Inadequate, and even inaccurate, decisions may be made from non-standardised assessments and can have negative consequences both for the care of an individual and, where the effectiveness of occupational therapy intervention cannot be reliably demonstrated, for service provision as a whole' (p. 135). Given this, why do non-standardised assessments continue to be used in practice?

Non-standardised assessments

Non-standardised assessments continue to form a part of practitioners' assessment toolkit for a variety of reasons, some of which are more defensible than others! These include:

- Flexibility (Laver Fawcett 2002)
- Lack of training or confidence in using standardised assessments
- Assessment of the qualitative aspects of performance and dynamics between key individuals (Chia 1996)
- Standardisation of assessment process being perceived as a lack of flexibility (Laver Fawcett 2002)
- Unhelpful culture of the therapeutic environment (for example 'Standardised assessments! We don't use those here!')
- Lack of accountability (practitioners are still too rarely called to account for the differences they do/or do not make in clients' lives)
- Lack of an existing structured (standardised) assessment (Kielhofner 2008)
- Client resistance to completing a standardised assessment (Kielhofner 2008)
- Lack of time (Kielhofner 2008)

- An opportunity presents itself to gather information and the practitioner is unable to use a standardised measure (Kielhofner 2008).

Non-standardised assessments lend themselves to those serendipitous moments in therapy when a client shares some information during the course of intervention that helps the practitioner to understand the client's occupational performance in a new or more profound manner. Further, there is no standardised measure that can help a practitioner to understand what it means to a client to be affected by the illness or disability they themselves are experiencing. However, this does not mean that due care and attention should not be made to the process of gathering this sort of information. Kielhofner (2008) outlines three strategies that support the dependability of the information gathered by unstructured means: evaluating context, triangulation and validity checks.

Evaluating context

The circumstances in which a client shares information often influences the degree of confidence a practitioner has in the information received: Information shared by a child who is refusing to go to school may be interpreted quite differently if given in the presence of their school teacher than in a one-to-one interview scenario.

Triangulation

Information that is yielded in a non-structured assessment should be checked, using an alternative source, for accuracy: This can be achieved by observing the client do the activity they discussed or by asking another person who knows them well (e.g. nurse or spouse) for their perspective of the situation.

Validity checks

It is important that practitioners ensure that their understanding of information shared is accurate. This can be done by:

- reflecting on the information and asking if it 'fits' with what is already known about the client
- continuing to collect information through a variety of assessment methods to either confirm or refute the information already gathered
- checking with the client to see if they agree with the practitioner's interpretation.

Thus, whilst Laver Fawcett's (2002) argument that lack of use of standardised assessments, where they are already developed, could place practitioners and clients at risk is true; sound reasons to use non-standardised assessments also exist (Kielhofner 2008). The challenge for the discerning practitioner is to have the skill to know when to use each to their best effect.

Summary

This chapter has described what, why, where and when practitioners should consider undertaking assessments in practice. Basic information about the various types of assessments and the appropriate stages at which assessments could be carried out were presented. More contemporary issues, such as whether or not a top-down approach to conducting assessments is appropriate, were also discussed. It was suggested that, whilst objective evidence of the superiority of a top-down assessment approach over a more traditional assessment strategy is still lacking, there are well-grounded theoretical arguments that support the use of an assessment strategy that commences with the selection of an occupation-focused conceptual model of practice and initially uses assessments drawn from the model.

References

Axline VM (1964) Dibs in Search of Self. Ballantyne Books, Toronto, Canada

Beck AT, Steer RS 1990 Beck Anxiety Inventory. The Psychological Incorporation, Oxford, UK

Chia 1996 The use of non standardised assessments in occupational therapy with children who have disabilities: a perspective. The British Journal of Occupational Therapy 59(8): 363–364

Cohn ES, Schell BAB, Neistadt ME 2003 Overview of Evaluation. In: Crepeau EB, Cohn ES, Schell BAB (eds) Willard and Spackman's Occupational Therapy, 10th ed. Lippincott Williams and Wilkins, Philadelphia, PA

Creek J 2002 Assessment. In: J Creek (ed) Occupational Therapy and Mental Health, pp. 93–118. Churchill Livingstone, Edinburgh, UK

Creek J 2003 Occupational Therapy Defined as a Complex Intervention. College of Occupational Therapists, London

de Clive-Lowe S 1996 Outcome measurement, cost effectiveness and clinical audit: the importance of standardised assessments to occupational therapists in meeting these new demands. British Journal of Occupational Therapy 59(8): 357–362

de las Heras C, Geist R, Kielhofner G et al 2007 The Volitional Questionnaire (VQ) (V.4.1) The Model of Human Occupation. Clearing House, Chicago, IL

Fisher AG 1999 Assessment of Motor and Process Skills, 3rd edn. Three Star Press, Fort Collins

Forsyth K, Kielhofner G 2006 The model of human occupation: integrating theory into practice and practice into theory. In: EAS Duncan (ed) Foundations for Practice in Occupational Therapy, 4th edn. Churchill Livingstone, Edinburgh: 69–107

Forsyth K, Salamy M, Simon S et al 1998 A users guide to the Assessment of Communication and Interaction Skills (ACIS). Model of Human Occupation. Clearinghouse, Department of Occupational Therapy, College of Applied Health Sciences, University of Illinois at Chicago, Chicago

Forsyth K, Deshpande S, Kielhofner G et al 2005 The Occupational Circumstances Assessment Interview and Rating Scale (OCAIRS) Version 4.0, The Model of Human Occupation. Clearing House, Chicago, IL

Gilovich T, Griffin D, Kahneman D 2002 (eds) Heuristics and Biases: The Psychology of Intuitive Judgment. Cambridge University Press, Cambridge, UK

Health Professions Council 2007 Standards of Proficiency: Occupational Therapists

Iwama M 2006 The Kawa Model. Culturally Relevant Occupational Therapy. Churchill Livingstone/Elsevier, London

Kielhofner G 2008 A model of human occupation: theory and application, 3rd ed. Lippincott, Williams & Wilkins, Philadelphia, PA

Kielhofner G, Neville A 1983 The Modified Interest Checklist. Available at http://www.moho.uic.edu/images/Modified%20Interest%20Checklist.pdf Accessed on 2 November 2007

Kramer P, Hinojosa J, Royeen CB 2003 Perspectives in Human Occupation: Participation in Life. Lippincott Williams & Wilkins, Philadelphia, PA

Kroenke K, Spitzer RL 2002 The PHQ-9: A new depression and diagnostic severity measure. Psychiatric Annals 32: 509–521

Laver Fawcett A 2002 Assessment. In: Turner A, Foster M, Johnson SE (eds) Occupational Therapy and Physical Dysfunction, 5th edn., pp. 107–144. Churchill Livingstone, Edinburgh

Law M, Baptiste S, Carswell A et al 2005a Canadian Occupational Performance Measure. Canadian Association of Occupational Therapists

Law M, Baptiste S, Carswell A et al 2005b Canadian Occupational Performance Measure. Questions and Answers. http://www.caot.ca/copm/questions.html#1. Accessed on 4 November 2007

McMillan I 2006 Assumptions underpinning a biomechanical frame of reference in occupational therapy. In: Duncan EAS (ed) Foundations for Practice in Occupational Therapy, 4th edn. Elsevier, Edinburgh, UK

Mathiowetz V 1993 Role of physical performance component evaluations in occupational therapy functional assessment. American Journal of Occupational Therapy 47(3): 225–230

Miller G 1956 The magical number seven, plus or minus two. The Psychological Review 63: 81–97

Paley J, Cheyne H, Dalgleish L et al 2007 Nursing's ways of knowing and dual process theories of cognition. Journal of Advanced Nursing 60(6): 692–701

Parkinson S, Forsyth K, Kielhofner G 2006 The Model of Human Occupation Screening Tool (MOHOST) Version 4.0, The Model of Human Occupation. Clearing House, Chicago, IL

Schacter DL 1999 The seven sins of memory: Insights from psychology and cognitive neuroscience. American Psychology 54: 182–203

Smith N, Kielhofner G, Watts J 1986 The relationship between volition, activity pattern and life satisfaction in the elderly. American Journal of Occupational Therapy 40: 278–283

Stewart S 1999 The use of standardised and non-standardised assessments in a social service setting: implications for practice. The British Journal of Occupational Therapy. 62(9): 410–423

Townsend E, Polatjko HJK 2007 Enabling Occupation II: Advancing an Occupational Therapy Vision for Health, Well-being, & Justice through Occupation. Canadian Association of Occupational Therapists, Ottawa

Trombly CA 1995 Occupation: purposefulness and meaningfulness as therapeutic mechanisms. American Journal of Occupational Therapy 49(11): 960–972

Activity analysis

Gary Kielhofner and
Kirsty Forsyth

Highlight box

- Activity analysis is the process for finding and/or adjusting an occupation to achieve some therapeutic benefit or allow a person to engage in a former or new occupational role.
- The demands of an occupation can only be identified in relation to the client or client group who is receiving occupational therapy.
- Analysis that is based on theory provides the additional benefits of the explanatory power of theory to identify the activity characteristics and how they influence a client.
- This chapter presents a theory-driven approach to activity analysis consisting of four steps.

Overview

Activity analysis is a process for finding and/or adjusting an occupation to achieve some therapeutic benefit or allow a person to engage in a former or new occupational role. Its aim is to find a fit between the characteristics and needs of a client or client group and an occupation. While there are a number of approaches to activity analysis, basing it on theory both provides a structure for the analysis and brings the explanatory power of theory to help identify activity characteristics and how they influence a client or group.

This chapter presents a theory-driven approach to activity analysis. It begins by identifying key principles underlying activity analysis. Then the chapter presents and discusses four key steps in theory-driven activity analysis. The application of these steps is illustrated through the following case examples.

Selma is an occupational therapist providing service to Elsie a 72-year-old who has osteoarthritis as well as a fracture in her right dominant hand, and is having challenges bathing. Elsie has been referred to occupational therapy. The therapist needs to complete an analysis of the bathing challenges for Elsie in order to support her re-engage with this activity.

Vincent is an occupational therapist providing services to children with special needs in a primary school classroom. He typically works with pupils (students) who have cerebral palsy and are integrated into regular classrooms. A common task Vincent must address is how to enable these pupils to engage in typical classroom activities such as taking notes and completing exams.

Gwen works as an occupational therapist in a residential home. The director of the residential home has approached her and asked if she could initiate some group activities designed to reduce the social isolation observed among many residents with limited cognitive function. Gwen is concerned to identify group activities she can implement that provide opportunities for engaging in meaningful activities, which will not be too difficult for these residents. Additionally, she recognises that since all groups are voluntary, she will need to find activities that will be motivating to entice residents to participate.

Philip is an occupational therapist working in an industrial setting. His responsibilities typically include making recommendations for how clients with a variety of impairments can complete work tasks efficiently and without sustaining further injury.

While each of the practitioners described above face quite different tasks, each will have to engage in a process that is ordinarily referred to in occupational therapy as activity analysis. The aim of this chapter is to provide a practical approach to activity analysis in the context of contemporary practice, which emphasises the importance of theory and evidence.

Overview of activity analysis

Activity analysis is one of the oldest occupational therapy processes. It emerged out of occupational therapists' need to find and/or adjust an occupation to achieve some therapeutic benefit or allow a person to engage in a former or new occupational role. Basically, the core of all activity analysis is to find a fit between the characteristics and needs of a client or client group and an occupation. The analysis of occupations and their use within therapy are the unique skills of the occupational therapist (Hagedorn 2001). Despite being an essential skill for any occupational therapist, there is not a single definition or set of agreed-upon procedures for activity analysis in the field. In fact, a variety of different discussions can be found on the topic (Fidler and Fidler 1963, Mosey 1986, Lamport et al 2001, Foster and Pratt 2002, Creek 2002, Crepeau 2003).

Discussions of activity analysis do agree that the core of the analysis involves asking questions about the occupation. These questions are designed to help the practitioner understand what doing the occupation involves and what therapeutic potential the activity might have. The following are examples of the types of questions one might ask about an occupation. Is it a simple or complex occupation? Where does the occupation take place? What are the stages or sequences of the occupation? Does the occupation require more than one performer? Sometimes the questions that are asked are based on the type of client or client group that the therapist has in mind when doing the activity analysis? So, for instance, if the client has an impairment that affects movement, the practitioner may focus on asking questions about the kinds of movements required for doing the occupation.

Some authors offer a structure for doing activity analysis. In some instances these structures try to include all things that need to be considered in order to determine what capacities are needed for doing an occupation. This approach to activity analysis will seek to describe physical, sensory, cognitive, social, emotional and cultural demands of the occupation. Box 7.1 shows an example of such a structured approach to activity analysis.

Box 7.1

Having identified the purpose, sequence, and duration of the performance of the activity and the spaces, tools and materials required. It may be necessary to ask any of the following questions and to identify how, when and where within the activity or tasks any particular skills or changes in demands and requirements are needed.

Physical skills

Position
What is the starting position when carrying out the activity – sitting, standing, lying?
Any changes that occur during the sequence of performance of the activity?

Movements
Which joints are involved and what movements are required?
Which muscle groups are involved at specific stages?
What ranges of specific movements are required at each joint?
Is the action unilateral or bilateral?
Is the movement required: active, static, or passive? Repetitive assisted or resisted?
Fast, slow, smooth or irregular?

Strength
Does the activity require a high moderate or low level of muscle strength
Is the effort continuous or intermittent?
Does the activity require high, medium, or low levels of stamina and endurance?

Coordination
Does the activity require gross or fine motor coordination?
Is the coordination unilateral or bilateral?
Where does the coordination take place? – hand/hand, hand/eye, lower limbs?
Hand function:
Does the activity require grip – cylinder, ball, hook, plate, pincer, tripod grip?
What levels of manipulative or dexterous movements are needed?
Are any precise actions needed?
Are both hands required equally?

Sensory & perceptual skills

Does the activity require vision – short and/or long distance, colour recognition?
Auditory – is hearing necessary to identify particular sounds, tones or volume?
Gustatory – does the activity involve the ability to identify or discriminate between tastes?
Olfactory – is the ability to identify or discrimate between smells necessary?
Touch–does the activity require gross or fine sensation?
Is the ability to distinguish shapes, textures or temperatures necessary?
Are stereognosis, proprioceptive or vestibular skills required?

Cognitive skills

Is the level of thinking concrete or abstract?
What level of concentration does the activity require – is it constant or changing?
Is short term, long term or procedural memory required?
Are organisational skills needed – logical thinking, planning, decision making, problem solving?
Is specific level of numeracy or literacy required?
Does the activity involve time recognition and time management skills?
What levels of responsibility and control does the activity involve?
Are there any opportunities for use of imagination, creativity or improvisation?

(Continued)

> **Box 7.1—Cont'd**
>
> ### Social interaction skills
> Is the activity carried out with others?
> Is the interaction formal or informal, cooperative, competitive, in parallel or compliant?
> What forms of communication are involved?: receptive (listening and interpreting) expressive (verbal, written, technological), non verbal, touch?
> Does the activity involve attention to others through debate or negotiation?
>
> ### Emotional skills
> Does the activity require insight or ability for else expression?
> Are attitudes and values inherent in the activity?
> Is the activity likely to demand conflict, handling feelings, testing reality, or role identity?
> Does the activity require patience managing impulses or self control?
>
> ### Cultural demands
> Is the activity specific to certain cultural groups in terms of gender, ethnicity, class or age?
> What is the sociocultural symbolic meaning of the activity?
> Does the activity require particular cultural values, approaches or techniques?

More recently, authors have advocated using occupational theories as a framework for activity analysis (Katz 1985, Foster and Pratt 2002, Crepeau 2003). Crepeau (2003) outlines theory-focused activity analysis. This approach to activity analysis examines the properties of an activity from the perspective of a particular practice theory. She notes that this approach is most appropriate when analysing an occupation in terms of its appropriateness for a particular client or a particular group of clients who share a common impairment or challenge.

This chapter takes the position that activity analysis should always be theory driven. An analysis that is based on theory provides the additional benefits of the explanatory power of theory. Using an occupational therapy theory as the structure for activity analysis serves not only to provide a structure or a framework for the analysis but also an explanation of how the elements identified operate together to support or prevent a person engaging with occupation. Traditional structured approaches to activity analysis that provides 'lists' of issues to consider (or lists of questions) offer the first part of what a theory offers (i.e., a structure) but they cannot provide the explanation that enriches the activity analysis making it more comprehensive.

Towards a definition of theory-driven activity analysis

Before discussing the process of theory-driven activity analysis, some key principles that should guide the process are outlined.

Principle 1: Theory-driven activity analysis should reflect the occupation-centred approach that characterises the field's contemporary perspective

Contemporary occupational therapy emphasises that practice should be occupation-focused (Clark 1993, Trombly 1993, 1995, Polatajko 1994, Fisher 1998, Wood 1998, Christiansen 1999). Along with this is the theme that, while underlying performance components are recognised as necessary to occupational performance, they must always be viewed in the larger context of the client's occupational life. This top-down approach (Trombly 1993) means that thinking in occupational therapy always begins with asking what a client wants and needs to do in their occupational lives and then proceeds to consideration of personal and environmental barriers and supports to performance.

Principle 2: Theory-driven activity analysis should be part of the therapeutic reasoning process whereby practitioners plan a course of action for a particular client or a group of clients

Analysis is most useful when it is employed as a step in the therapeutic reasoning that guides practice with a given client or client group. As noted at the beginning of this chapter, analysis is undertaken to make specific decisions about selecting and adapting an occupation in order to meet the needs of a specific client or group. Thus, the analysis occurs and relational questions arise about how the characteristics of an occupation compare with the characteristics of a client or group. Analysis, therefore, should always be done to determine how the occupation can be used as part of therapy or modified to allow the clients to engage in occupation part of their overall occupational participation. Analysis is always undertaken with reference to a particular individual or group. To illustrate this point it is helpful to return to the examples with which this chapter began. In these instances analysis would be undertaken to:

- Determine how to change the environment to support Elsie engage in bathing
- Determine how typical classroom occupations can be adapted so as to allow pupils with cerebral palsy to do them
- Identify occupations appropriate for implementation with a group of adults with cognitive impairments
- Recommend strategies for clients with impairments to complete work occupations efficiently and safely.

Principle 3: Theory driven-activity analysis should be both theoretical and empirical

The most efficient way to do analysis that is theoretical and empirical is to base it on conceptual practice models. Conceptual practice models are bodies of knowledge in occupational therapy that provide explanations of some phenomena of practical concern in the field, while providing a rationale and methods for therapy (Kielhofner 2004). Since conceptual practice models include both theoretical concepts and empirical testing of those concepts and their application in therapy, using them allows a practitioner to be both theoretically and empirically based when doing analysis. Practice-based theories have the added advantage of providing an understanding of how different elements of analysis relate to each other and provides an insight into the change process (Creek 2002).

Each model of practice addresses different phenomena. Most of the traditional models (biomechanical, sensory integration, cognitive disabilities, cognitive-perceptual, motor control) address some aspect of the underlying capacity for performing occupation. In contrast, the model of human occupation (Kielhofner 2007) addresses the motivation for occupation, the lifestyle or pattern of occupation in a person's life, the environmental context. This model also offers a unique view of skills (Kielhofner 2007) which have been recommended as an important dimension of task/activity analysis (Crepeau 2003, Watson and Wilson 2003).

Let us briefly consider how these principles would frame analysis by returning to one of the examples at the start of this chapter. Consider Vincent who typically works with children who have cerebral palsy in a mainstream school. Vincent will routinely use analysis to determine what gaps exist between the physical, interpersonal, cognitive and socio-cultural demands of the various activities required for being a student and the characteristics of the students he serves. His use of analysis will help him recommend ways that the student can be better integrated into the daily activity stream of a classroom. His analysis will lead him to a series of solutions that enable children to engage in the occupational role of student. In order to undertake analysis Vincent can use the model of human occupation as a broad framework for considering the interpersonal, social and cultural aspects of the analysis as well as the skills involved in classroom activities. He can also employ the motor control model that addresses issues of movement that these children face. To the extent that his clients may have cognitive or sensory problems he might also employ other models that address these concerns as well. Because his analysis is guided by these conceptual practice models, he would go beyond a simple taxonomy of elements to consider and instead, be able to create a more in-depth explanation of the gaps between necessary activities and his pupils' characteristics which will guide him in seeking ways to close those gaps. Vincent would also have the reassurance that the conceptual practice models that he uses have an identifiable evidence base.

The process of theory-driven activity analysis

This section presents a process of theory-driven activity analysis consisting of four steps. These steps are as follows:

- Identify the appropriate practice model(s) to guide the analysis
- Select the occupation to be analysed
- Generate questions to guide the analysis
- Identify ways the occupation(s) can be adapted and/or graded.

The section below discusses the four steps of analysis in detail. The process of activity analysis will be illustrated with one of the cases presented at the start of this chapter: Selma is a practitioner who is supporting Elsie with bathing challenges.

Step 1. Identify the appropriate practice model(s) to guide the analysis

Before selecting the models one should reflect on the person or group for which the analysis is being done. It is the characteristics of the person or group for which the analysis is being done that should influence the choice of conceptual practice models to be used for the activity analysis.

The conceptual practice model(s) chosen to guide the analysis should reflect:

- the occupational and client-centred focus of contemporary practice and
- the unique impairment status of the client.

The model of human occupation (MOHO) provides a comprehensive view of key aspects of occupation and client-centredness (Kielhofner 2007). MOHO also has a substantial evidence base (Kramer and Kielhofner 2007). Moreover, it is designed to be used in combination with models that address performance components and, therefore, easily dovetails with such models.

In addition to MOHO, one should select additional models that address the impairment(s) experienced by the client or client group. If the client has a cognitive impairment, one should choose an appropriate cognitive model, if the client has muscle weakness, one should choose the biomechanical model. If the client has problems controlling motion, one should choose the motor control model. Moreover, if the client has problems with all the above, one should include all the relevant models (see Figure 7.1).

Illustration of step one: selecting models for an analysis of bathing for Elsie

Elsie is a 72-year-old Scottish woman who has osteoarthritis and is having difficulty bathing. As described above, MOHO would be appropriate to understand the broader occupational issues Elsie faces in relation to bathing. MOHO provides an analysis structure for considering such factors as the value of bathing for Elsie, the usual routine within which the bathing occupation happens, the responsibilities Elsie holds that are reliant on bathing, the sense of efficacy Elsie feels towards bathing. MOHO will also call attention to the physical and social environment and how it may impact on Elsie's bathing. In short, MOHO provides an analysis framework that views bathing in the context of Elsie's occupational participation. Additionally MOHO will provide a detailed framework for examining what skills Elsie will need to employ in order to complete bathing.

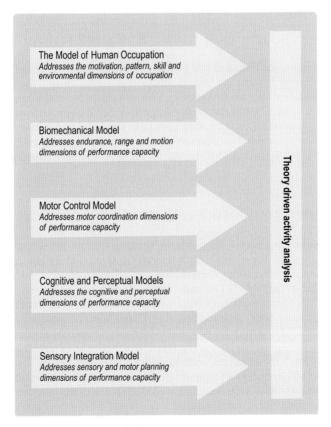

Figure 7.1 Theory-driven activity analysis

Other models of practice will also be important for this analysis. Because Elsie has osteoarthritis, has fractured her right dominant hand and has orthopaedic limitations, the biomechanical model would provide a structure for considering whether Elsie has the strength and range of motion to get in and out of the bath and whether she has enough endurance to complete bathing safely.

On review of medical notes and feedback from the multidisciplinary team it would be noted that Elsie did not have any cognitive challenges and, therefore, cognitive models are not necessary for this analysis. Similarly because Elsie did not have any sensory or motor control impairments, no additional models were required to provide a comprehensive analysis of her bathing.

Step 2: Select the occupation to be analysed

Selection of the occupation(s) to be analysed should be guided by a top-down approach. That is, the occupation selection should always begin by examining the relevance of the occupation to the volition, habituation and environment of the client or group. If an occupation has no relevance to the person's/group's interests, values and sense of competence and if it is not relevant to the client's/group's roles or lifestyle, it is hardly worth considering for occupational engagement or participation. Without such relevance, it has no meaning for the client/group. Behind these first considerations, a practitioner will then begin to ask whether the occupation involves at least some skills that the client/group possess and whether the capacities required (e.g., strength, movement, coordination, perception and cognition) overlap with those of the client/group. If not, then the occupation is not a reasonable candidate for the client/group.

An illustration of step 2: Elsie

Bathing has meaning for Elsie and is a part of her longstanding routine. Elsie has high standards of personal hygiene for herself. She previously attended a social club twice a week and this was her only leisure activity. She also reads to local schoolchildren as a volunteer once a week. She has not been doing either occupation because she feels conscious of her body odour. This is causing Elsie to feel isolated and is lowering her mood. Bathing, therefore, is a valued occupation in Elsie's life and is significantly impacting on her occupational participation. It is, therefore, an appropriate occupation to select for analysis.

Step 3: Generate questions to guide the analysis

Once an occupation is selected for analysis, the practitioner must begin to carefully examine it in light of the client's characteristics as guided by the model(s) being used for analysis. At this stage the practitioner moves from the more broad kinds of questions shown in Table 7.1 to much more detailed elaborations of those questions in Table 7.2. The aim is to generate a detailed inspection of the occupation and its relationship to the client's characteristics. Thus, how the analysis is undertaken, depends on the client or group for which it is being done and the needs that are being addressed.

Since activity analysis is done with reference to a particular individual, not all concepts from each model will be necessary to generate necessary questions. Communication and interaction skills questions were not generated since bathing was a solitary activity and process skills questions were not generated because she did not have any cognitive challenges that may impact her processing skills.

Table 7.1 Examples of broad questions to guide analysis

MOHO-based questions

What is Elsie's sense of efficacy with bathing?

Does Elsie value bathing? If so, why?

Does Elsie find bathing enjoyable?

What is Elsie's routine of bathing?

When in the day does Elsie bathe?

Does Elsie have full responsibility of bathing?

What of Elsie's responsibilities are dependent on bathing?

What physical and/or mental capacities are affecting her bathing?

What physical environment does Elsie bathe in?

What social supports does Elsie have to support bathing?

Biomechanical-based questions

What range of motion does Elsie have at her knee joints?

What muscle strength does Elsie have in her limbs?

Do Elsie's physical capacities allow Elsie to transfer in and out of the bath?

Does Elsie have reduced strength in her right dominant hand following her fracture?

Does Elsie have enough physical endurance to complete the full bathing occupation?

Does Elsie have pain anywhere that restricts movement?

Does Elsie have enough physical flexibility to be able to reach her toes and her back while bathing?

Does Elsie have contractures that may be restricting range of motion or strength?

Table 7.2 Examples of detailed MOHO questions to guide analysis

MOTOR SKILLS

♦ **Posture: Can Elsie stabilise and align her body while moving and in relation to bathing objects?**

Can Elsie steady her body and maintain trunk control and balance while sitting, standing, walking, reaching, or while moving, lifting or pulling objects while bathing?
Can Elsie maintain the vertical alignment of the body over the base of support while bathing?
Can Elsie place her arms and body in relation to bathing objects in a manner that promotes efficient arm movements.

♦ **Mobility: Can Elsie move her entire body or a body part in space when bathing?**

Can Elsie ambulate on level surfaces, including turning around and changing direction while bathing?
Can Elsie stretch or extend her arm and, when appropriate, her trunk to grasp or place bathing objects that are out of reach.
Can Elsie actively flex, rotate, or twist her body in a manner and direction appropriate to bathing?

(Continued)

Table 7.2 Examples of detailed MOHO questions to guide analysis—Cont'd

♦ **Coordination: Can Elsie move body parts in relationship to each other and to the bathing environment?**

Can Elsie use different parts of her body together to support or stabilise bathing objects during bilateral motor tasks?
Can Elsie use dexterous grasp and release, as well as coordinated in-hand manipulation patterns while bathing?
Can Elsie use smooth, fluid, continuous, uninterrupted arm and hand movements while bathing?

♦ **Strength and Effort: Can Elsie generate muscle force appropriate to actions needed in bathing?**

Can Elsie push, shove, pull, or drag bathing objects along a supporting surface or about a weight bearing axis?
Can Elsie carry bathing objects while ambulating or moving from one place to another?
Can Elsie raise or hoist bathing objects off of a supporting surface?
Can Elsie regulate or grade the force, speed, and extent of movements?
Can Elsie pinch or grasp in order to securely hold handles or other bathing objects?

♦ **Energy: Can Elsie have enough physical exertion and sustained effort over time while bathing?**

Can Elsie persist and complete an activity without evidence of fatigue, pausing to rest, or stopping to "catch her breath"?
Can Elsie maintain a rate or tempo of performance across an entire bathing occupation?

PROCESS DOMAINS AND SKILLS

♦ **Energy: Can Elsie sustain and appropriately allocate mental energy while bathing?**

Can Elsie maintain a rate or tempo of performance across an entire bathing experience?
Can Elsie maintain attention focused on bathing?

♦ **Using Knowledge: Can Elsie seek and use knowledge while bathing?**

Can Elsie select appropriate tools and materials for bathing?

Can Elsie employ tools and materials according to their intended purposes while bathing?
Can Elsie support, stabilise, and hold tools and materials in an appropriate manner while bathing?
Can Elsie use goal-directed task performance that is focused toward the completion of bathing?
Can Elsie seek appropriate verbal/written information by asking questions or reading directions.

♦ **Temporal Organisation: Can Elsie initiate, logically order, continue, and complete the steps and action sequences required when bathing?**

Can Elsie start or begin doing an action or step without hesitation while bathing?
Can Elsie perform an action sequence of a step without unnecessary interruption and as an unbroken, smooth progression?
Can Elsie perform steps in an effective or logical order for efficient use of time and energy while bathing?
Can Elsie finish or bring to completion single actions or steps without perseveration, inappropriate persistence, or premature cessation while bathing?

Table 7.2 Examples of detailed MOHO questions to guide analysis—Cont'd

♦ **Organising Space and Objects: Can Elsie organise bathing space and objects?**

Can Elsie look for and locate tools and materials through the process of logical searching while bathing?

Can Elsie collect together needed or misplaced bathing tools and materials?

Can Elsie logically position or spatially arrange bathing tools and materials in an orderly fashion while bathing?

Can Elsie return/put away bathing tools and materials, and restore her immediate space to original condition.

Can Elsie modify the movement of the arm, body, or wheelchair to avoid or manoeuvre around existing obstacles that are encountered in the course of moving the arm, body, or wheelchair through space while bathing?

♦ **Adaptation: Can Elsie relate to the ability to anticipate, correct for, and benefit by learning from the consequences of errors that arise in bathing?**

Can Elsie respond appropriately to nonverbal environmental/perceptual cues that provide feedback regarding bathing progression?

Can Elsie modify her action or locate objects within the bathing area in anticipation of or in response to circumstances/problems that might arise in the course of bathing or to avoid undesirable outcomes?

Can Elsie change environmental conditions in anticipation of or in response to circumstances/problems that arise in the course of bathing or to avoid undesirable outcomes?

Can Elsie anticipate and prevent undesirable circumstances/problems from recurring or persisting while bathing?

Step 4: Identify and test ways occupation(s) can be adapted and/or graded based on identified gaps between the activity and the person

Occupations can be adapted and/or graded, for example:

- Providing adaptive equipment
- Modifying how the occupation is done
- Providing assistance/encouragement
- Making environmental alterations.

Since step four involves coming up with possible strategies to address identified gaps between the activity and the person or group, it is important that these strategies be tested to see whether they work.

An illustration of step 4: adapting Elsie's bathing

Links between the theory base and Elsie's case example are highlighted in parentheses. Elsie had previously been provided with a bath board and tap spray (MOHO – physical object) in 2003 and had been using this equipment independently until about 4 weeks ago. She reported she is no longer bathing for a variety of reasons including:

- she was physically having more difficulty due to osteoarthritis stiffening in her knees (biomechanical – range of motion)

- she has decreased confidence (MOHO – personal causation) due to lack of power in her dominant hand following a fracture (biomechanical – strength) which she feels reduces her ability to grip (MOHO – skill) the side of the bath and
- water goes on the floor and she is anxious (MOHO – personal causation) she will slip on the lino floor (MOHO – physical environment) when she gets out. She has fallen in the house recently and so has a legitimate fear.

Not bathing is affecting other occupations. Her only leisure activity is going to the social club twice a week (MOHO – role) and she reads to local schoolchildren as a volunteer once a week (MOHO – role). She has not been doing either activity in the last 2 weeks because she feels conscious of her body odour. This is causing Elsie to feel isolated (MOHO – disengaged from roles).

The practitioner originally decided on the strategy of using a bath hoist since this was the least costly and involved a kind of adaptation that could be made. In order to assess the suitability of a bath hoist (MOHO – physical object) it was tried out with Elsie. During the assessment Elsie physically struggled to get her legs over the side of the bath tub due to restricted range of motion at her knee joints (biomechanical – range of motion) and required physical assistance (MOHO – social environment). This kind of physical effort against resistance is contraindicated by her high blood pressure and irregular heart beat. Moreover, when she was trying to transfer off the bath hoist her foot caught on the leg of the wash hand basin and she required physical assistance (MOHO – social environment) to move it. Elsie was visibly fearful during the assessment (MOHO – personal causation) which exacerbated her chronic obstructive airways disease (MOHO – performance capacity). In order to manage a bath hoist Elsie would need physical help (MOHO – social environment) due to physical restrictions (biomechanical), anxiety (MOHO – personal causation) and medial conditions (MOHO – performance capacity). Elsie, however, lives alone and does not have physical support available (MOHO – social environment). Thus it was determined that a bath hoist was not an adequate solution for closing the gap between the demands of bathing and Elsie's characteristics. As a result, the practitioner determined that the only option for bathing would be to have a walk-in shower with non-slip flooring (MOHO – physical environment) which she could manage independently and would allow her to feel she can return to her volunteer responsibility and her social club (MOHO – roles).

Summary

This chapter presented an approach to theory-driven activity analysis. We argue that the demands of an occupation can only be identified in relation to the client or client group who is receiving occupational therapy. We also argue that an analysis that is based on theory provides the additional benefits of the explanatory power of theory to identify the activity characteristics and how they influence a client. That is, theory-driven occupational analysis provides a framework that not only identifies areas of analysis but also provides a theory that supports an explanation of how the identified elements operate together to support or prevent a person engaging in an occupation.

References

Christiansen C 1999 Defining lives: Occupation as identity: An essay on competence, coherence, and the creation of meaning: Eleanor Clark Slagle Lecture. American Journal of Occupational Therapy 53: 547–558

Clark FA 1993 Occupational embedded in a real life: Interweaving occupation science and occupational therapy. American Journal of Occupational Therapy 47: 1067–1077

Crepeau EB 2003 Analyzing occupation and activity: a way of thinking about occupational performance. In: EB Crepeau, ES Cohn, BA Boyt Schell (eds) Willard and Spackman's Occupational Therapy, 10th edn. Lippincott, Williams & Wilkins, Philadelphia, PA

Creek J, 3rd 2002 The knowledge base of occupational therapy In: J Creek (ed) Occupational therapy and mental health, pp. 29–49. Churchill Livingstone, Edinburgh, UK

Fidler G, Fidler J 1963 Occupational therapy: a communication process in psychiatry. Macmillian, New York

Fisher AG 1998 Uniting practice and theory in an occupational framework. American Journal of Occupational Therapy 54(7): 509–521

Foster M, Pratt J 2002 Activity analysis In: A Turner, M Foster, SE Johnston (eds) Occupational Therapy and Physical Dysfunction: Principles, Skills and Practice, pp. 145–163. Churchill Livingstone, Edinburgh, UK

Hagedorn R 2001 Foundations for Practice in Occupational Therapy, 3rd edn. Churchill Livingstone, Edinburgh, UK

Katz N (ed.) 2005 Cognition and occupation across the life span: Models for Interventions in Occupational Therapy, 2nd edn. AOTA Press, Bethesda, MD

Kielhofner G 2004 Conceptual Foundations of Occupational Therapy, 3rd edn. FA Davis, Philadelphia, PA

Kielhofner G 2007 A Model of Human Occupation: Theory and Application, 4th edn. Lippincott, Williams and Wilkins, Baltimore, MD

Kramer J, Kielhofner, G 2007 Evidence for practice from the model of human occupation In: G Kielhofner (ed.) A Model of Human Occupation: Theory and Application, 4th edn. Lippincott, Williams and Wilkins, Baltimore, MD

Lamport N, Coffey M, Hersch G 2001 Activity analysis and application building blocks of treatment. SLACK Incorporated, Thorofare

Mosey A 1986 Psychosocial Components of Occupational Therapy. Raven Press, New York

Polatajko HJ 1994 Dreams, dilemmas, and decisions for occupational therapy practice in a new millennium: A Canadian perspective. American Journal of Occupational therapy 48(7): 590–594

Trombly C 1993 The issue is – Anticipating the future: Assessment of occupational functioning. American Journal of Occupational Therapy 47(3): 253–257

Trombly C 1995 Occupation: purposefulness and meaningfulness as therapeutic mechanisms: Eleanor Clark Slagle Lecture. American Journal of Occupational Therapy 49(10): 960–972

Watson DE, Wilson 2003 Task Analysis: An Individual and Population Approach, 2nd edn. American Occupational Therapy Association, Bethesda, MD

Wood W 1998 It is jump time for occupational therapy. American Journal of Occupational Therapy 52(6): 403–411

Goal setting in occupational therapy: a client-centred perspective

8

Steve Park

Highlight box

- Client-centred goal setting focuses on the daily life activities of concern to clients.
- Goal setting evaluates significant progress from the client's viewpoint.
- Enacting client-centred goal setting is a challenging prospect for practitioners.
- Time is required to identify client priorities and negotiate meaningful goals.
- Occupational therapy intervention should be guided by client-centred goals.

Overview

This chapter focuses on implementing *client-centred goal setting*, illustrating the process for occupational therapy services. The current standing of goal setting in occupational therapy is presented, underscoring the challenges practitioners face to enact client-centred practice during goal setting. Using as a guide the three phrases of goal setting, (1) identifying client concerns, (2) formulating client-centred goals, and (3) evaluating goal achievement, the knowledge and skills to enact client-centred goal setting are presented, with particular attention to documentation.

Goals and goal setting

> 'Humans yearn for the "unattainable" and pursue practical goals; they marshal all possible resources against great odds to reach the most grand, and sometimes the most simple, objectives.' (Crabtree 2000: 122)

Occupational therapists focus on facilitating a client's engagement in daily life activities that possess meaning to the client. Essential to the process is client-centred practice, a collaborative approach that respects each client's perspective, particularly when negotiating goals that become the focus for assessment, intervention and evaluation (Law et al 1995, Sumsion 2000). During negotiation, practitioners and clients explore all daily life activities of concern because even the most mundane and commonplace activities possess the potential for clients to make and express meaning in daily life (Crabtree 2000). Subsequently, goals are identified that express the future state clients hope to experience in regard to their daily life activities.

Although goal setting is common in practice, overwhelming evidence indicates practitioners require additional skill to negotiate and document goals that are client-centred and reflect engagement in daily life activities (Neistadt 1995, Northen et al 1995, Nelson and Payton 1997, Andrew et al 1999, Lund et al 2001, Barclay 2002, Hanna and Rodger 2002, Palmadottir 2003, Eschenfelder 2005). For example, documented goals sometimes reflect the practitioner's plan, such as *Conduct home evaluation & recommend adaptive equipment* or *Refer to social services for meal programme*. Other times, practitioners use the SMART acronym, attempting to ensure goals are *Specific, Measurable, Achievable, Realistic* and *Timely* (SMART). Often, though, goals are unclear and not client-centred. How then should practitioners frame goals for intervention?

What are goals?

Most persons think about what they hope to accomplish, whether relatively straightforward tasks, such as tidying the living room, scheduling a dentist appointment, or paying the monthly bills, or more complex activities in which they desire to participate in the future, such as playing the guitar, driving a car, or operating a construction crane. Hopes may focus further in the future, centring on desired roles, such as a partner, parent or employee. Hopes also may reflect a person's dreams, such as scoring the winning goal during the World Cup or touring the world as a rock star. All of these hopes, though, are often referred to as goals, making little distinction between 'things to get done today' and 'wishful dreams for the future'. These 'goals' comprise a continuum, from simple tasks to global aims (Geen 1995) (Figure 8.1). What then along this continuum would be considered a goal during occupational therapy intervention?

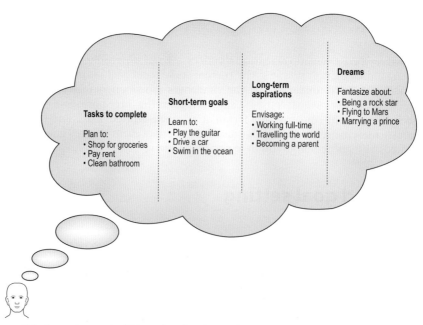

Figure 8.1 A continuum and hierarchy of tasks, goals, aspirations and dreams. From Park 2006, with permission

For intervention, a goal is an end-state (an *outcome*) that expresses what a person hopes to accomplish, is considered attainable, and requires some degree of effort by the client to attain (Schut and Stam 1994, Geen 1995, Quinn and Gordon 2003). Thus, a goal reflects a *short-term* (but significant) accomplishment rather than a task that is relatively easy to complete or a dream that is unrealistic to attain. Moreover, a goal signifies something in the near future to be accomplished by the person that he or she cannot accomplish now (Quinn and Gordon 2003) and that reflects the attainment of a standard of proficiency within a designated time frame (Locke and Latham 2002).

Benefits of setting goals with clients

Why should practitioners use goal setting? First, they have a professional responsibility to provide individualised services, focusing on the client's daily life activities of importance (Wallen and Doyle 1996, College of Occupational Therapists 2000, Creek 2003). Client-centred practice is a cornerstone of occupational therapy intervention and as Rebeiro (2000) stated '[If] occupational therapy strives to be client-centred, the profession must allow practice to be guided by "client visions"' (p. 13). Second, focusing on client goals promotes effective use of time and resources (Welch and Foster 2003, Wressle and Samuelsson 2004). Third, actively involving clients during goal setting helps them to understand the focus of intervention (Welch and Foster 2003) and provides a specific direction to intervention (Conneeley 2004). Finally, goals that evolve from client concerns provide a means to identify small changes that are meaningful to clients (Wallen and Doyle 1996) and facilitate the evaluation of outcomes (Wressle et al 2003).

Whilst limited in scope and based in physical rehabilitation, research evidence supports the premise that clients who set goals achieve better outcomes than those who do not (Ponte-Allan and Giles 1999, Wressle et al 2002a). From his review of published research, Wade (1998) concluded reasonable evidence exists that: (a) more behavioural change occurs when goal setting is used; (b) change is more likely to occur when goal setting is reinforced with specific interventions intended to facilitate the desired change; and (c) setting goals may improve long-term effectiveness. Locke and Latham (2002), from their summary of evidence regarding goal setting in the business field, identified the following characteristics:

- Setting goals focuses a person's attention and directs his or her effort to those activities most relevant to goal attainment.
- Establishing challenging (yet realistic) goals leads to greater effort and persistence.
- Identifying specific, challenging goals leads to higher performance versus just encouraging persons to do their best.
- Setting goals facilitates the use of goal-relevant knowledge and strategies, prompting persons to apply their current skills to achieve the goal.
- Effective goal achievement requires on-going feedback that reflects the person's progress toward the goal.

Although successful implementation of goal setting has occurred within occupational therapy services (Rosa and Hasselkus 2005, Sumsion 2005), most research indicates that practitioners need to involve clients more during the goal-setting process and further develop their skills to negotiate and formulate client-centred goals (Northen et al 1995, Neistadt 1995a, Nelson and Payton 1997, Andrew et al 1999, Lund et al 2001, Barclay 2002, Hanna and Rodger 2002, Palmadottir 2003, Eschenfelder 2005). Indeed, the top three barriers to client-centred practice identified by occupational therapists all centred around goals: (a) practitioners and clients identify different goals; (b) practitioners cannot accept clients' goals due to practitioners' values and beliefs; and

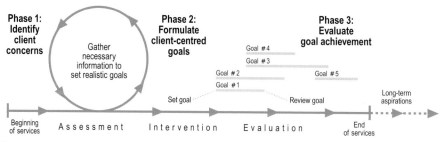

Figure 8.2 The three phases of client-centred goal setting. From Park 2006, with permission

(c) practitioners are uncomfortable allowing clients to choose goals (Sumsion and Smyth 2000). Rosa and Hasselkus (2005) pointedly concluded: '[In] spite of the recent professional emphasis on collaborative therapeutic relations…these ideals may continue to elude occupational therapists, perhaps much of the time.' (p. 206). Given this, how can practitioners successfully implement client-centred goal setting? To address this challenge, this chapter illustrates the process in three phases: (a) identifying client concerns; (b) formulating client-centred goals and (c) evaluating goal achievement (Figure 8.2).

Collaborating with clients: the goal-setting process

'[T]here [are] two different types of goals: those that were negotiated with the [client] and those that were not.' (Playford et al 2000: 494)

Client-centred practice and goal setting

Occupational therapists should acknowledge that clients are experts about their lives, capable of indicating what is of importance and concern (Gage 1994, Blackmer 2000, Guidetti and Tham 2002). Everyday, people seek specialists to help resolve problems that they identified as important, for example, enlisting the services of a builder, accountant or lawyer (Sumsion 2006a). This is comparable to a client receiving occupational therapy services – he or she identifies 'problems' for which the practitioner can provide specialist advice. Furthermore, the client identifies the problem and the practitioner provides the expertise, similar to the person who identifies (and prioritises) a leaky kitchen tap and hires a plumber to fix it. As Sumsion (2006a) clearly stated: 'If a therapist cannot accept a person's right to be a client and all that this right entails then he or she cannot be a client-centred therapist.' (p. 41).

Practitioners should recognise that clients might identify goals that place them at risk for failure or injury (Law et al 1995). As long as clients are competent to understand the risk or chance for failure and practitioners are not acting in a manner that places clients in perilous circumstances, practitioners should recognise that undertaking such a risk is often a valuable learning experience for clients. Clients' preferences should be respected as long as realistic concerns do not exist (Blackmer 2000, College of Occupational Therapists 2000).

Practitioners also should consider that client participation during goal setting exists along a continuum – not all clients want to participate equally during the process (Lund et al 2001, Wilkins et al 2001, Palmadottir 2003). Some clients are comfortable sharing their concerns and making decisions whilst others are challenged to make simple choices (Wilkins et al 2001). From research conducted in physical rehabilitation settings, Lund and colleagues (2001) discovered three categories of clients: (a) *participants* – those who participate in shared decision-making to an extent that meets their need; (b) *occasional participants* – those who occasionally participate but tend to allow practitioners to make the primary decisions; and (c) *relinquishers* – those who are not interested in participating and readily accept practitioners' decisions. Lund and colleagues further discovered that practitioners were inclined to use the same approach for each client, encouraging all clients to participate regardless of a client's preference. Sumsion (2005), during her review of client-centred practice, revealed further characteristics associated with goal setting: Persons more likely to participate in shared decision-making tend to be younger, more educated, and from a higher social class whilst persons less likely to participate are those with acute and severe illnesses or whose cultural practices sanction decision making by family consensus or the family patriarch.

Phase 1: Identifying client concerns

'Eliciting and incorporating [clients'] views and setting goals are demanding and potentially time-consuming activities.' (Parry 2004: 679)

As the practitioner establishes rapport and gathers information about and shares information with the client during the initial assessment, the discussion should evolve to identify what is of concern and important to the client regarding his or her engagement in daily life activities (Park 2006). This process should clearly establish the client's concerns and priorities; these may not be in agreement, however, with the practitioner, the client's family, or the reason for the referral (Sumsion 2006b). The objective is to understand the client's (and others') perspective. To do so, the practitioner should listen carefully to the client and help the client to identify and clarify his or her concerns.

When identifying concerns, all areas of a client's engagement in daily life activities, as appropriate, should be explored, including personal care, domestic, productive, play/leisure, and social activities (Park 2006). The client and practitioner work together to identify *specific* daily life activities of concern to the client and establish which are priorities. Often, these are the activities considered a challenge by the client and for which a change is desired (Park 2006). Whilst some practitioners have raised concerns about focusing on client 'problems' (Halladay 2001, Parry 2004), the intent is *not* to identify what is wrong; rather, the intent is to listen and solicit areas of concern from the client's perspective. The practitioner should help the client to identify immediate, realistic concerns with daily life activities. Clients benefit far more if intervention is based in the 'here and now' of daily life and targets issues that could be more 'immediately' resolved (Park 2006). Questions such as the following can help clients identify specific concerns about their engagement in daily life activities.

- Which activities in your daily life are important to you?
- Which daily life activities are of concern at home? Outside your home? At work?
- What are your specific concerns with your morning activities? Weekend activities? Domestic activities? Getting around? Leisure? Work? Social?
- Which activities concern you the most and would like to see a change?
- What are your priorities about how you currently spend your time?

Some clients may state their concerns as 'to go home' or 'taking care of myself'. Practitioners should not be satisfied with such general statements and should explore these further (Neistadt 1995). For example, a parent (also considered a client) shares her concern that her child is not performing successfully in school. The practitioner needs to assist the parent to identify specific school activities, such as 'My daughter doesn't play with any friends during the break (recess)' and 'She takes too much time answering written questions – her handwriting is so laborious'.

Evidence exists that informal means of eliciting clients' concerns (and goals) are more common than methods based on structured assessments (Neistadt 1995, Wressle et al 2002b, Palmadottir 2003). Although informal discussion is important when establishing therapeutic rapport, practitioners vary in their interview skills and styles; this can affect the quality and extent of information gathered (Neistadt 1995). Because formal interview methods identify a broader range of concerns and lead to more distinct goals (Pollock and Stewart 1998, Bodium 1999, McColl et al 2000, Wressle et al 2002b, 2003, Donnelly et al 2004), practitioners should consider adopting formal methods to elicit client concerns.

Although various methods exist and the choice depends on each situation, the Canadian Occupational Performance Measure (COPM) (Law et al 2005) is a standardised assessment designed to elicit the client's perspective of problems and priorities with specific daily life activities. The COPM has been used successfully with a variety of clients, including children (and their parents and teachers), adolescents and adults with physical, cognitive and psychosocial health conditions (Carswell et al 2004). Because setting goals requires identifying current 'problems' and the COPM prompts clients to consider framing their 'problems' in terms of daily life activities, the COPM is well suited to identify client concerns.

During initial discussions with clients, goals should *not* be the primary focus. Before goals are formulated, the client and practitioner need to possess all necessary information on which to base realistic goals (Law et al 1995, Sumsion 2006b). Moreover, clients (and practitioners) need to appreciate the realities and limitations of existing resources (Sumsion 2006b) and some clients may need to experience their current 'problems' in daily life activities before they can identify realistic goals (Chan and Lee 1997, Spencer and Davidson 1998, Bodium 1999, Playford et al 2000, Guidetti and Tham 2002). As Sumsion (2006b) cogently stated: 'The client-centred approach requires that time and energy be dedicated to the analysis and understanding of the assessment information before the goals are set.' (p. 26). Therefore, beginning the assessment process by asking a client 'What do you hope to achieve during occupational therapy?' or 'What are your goals for therapy?' is *not* recommended (Park 2006). These questions can be difficult to answer, particularly if the client is experiencing the onset of a new health condition, and are more appropriate after the client and practitioner possess a clearer picture of the client's health condition and potential for change, its effect on the client's engagement in daily life activities, and the available support and resources.

Sometimes, clients may not be able to participate in a discussion or readily indicate their concerns. Practitioners should make every effort to solicit the viewpoints of principal persons in the client's life in order to identify potential concerns (and goals) that are in the client's best interest. Further, every effort should be made to help the client understand the identified concerns and provide an opportunity to agree (or not).

Differences in priorities

Differences of opinion regarding concerns (and goals) will exist amongst practitioners, clients, family members and others; these need to be acknowledged and negotiated (Hanna and Rodger 2002). Although goal setting is client-focused, this does not mean practitioners will always agree with the client's priorities – at times, the practitioner will need to inform the client that he or she is unable to support the client's priority. As Parry (2004) stated: 'Accounting for why it is not...relevant whilst avoiding outright dismissal of a [client's] stated preference may involve considerable interactional time and effort.' (p. 675).

Vignette 8.1

Gerard

Gerard experienced a severe TBI 3 months ago and currently receives community services. When asked about his concerns, Gerard insists he wants to drive again. His practitioner empathises with him but also recognises that Gerard's concern does not readily convert to a realistic goal that could be achieved over the next 4 months (the anticipated course of intervention). She skilfully shares this perspective with Gerard (without dismissing his long-term aspiration to drive) and continues to collaborate with Gerard to identify concerns that are realistic and potentially achievable over the next 4 months.

Clients and family members may differ in their priorities for intervention. For example, when asked to select which activities should be the focus of intervention, parents tended to prioritise academic tasks such as printing and drawing whereas their children's preferences leaned more toward self-care and leisure activities (Missiuna and Pollock 2000). When clients and family members do not agree, practitioners need to negotiate an equitable solution before goals can be set, particularly when they propose fostering a client's ability to engage in desired daily life activities and the client's family may be more interested in protecting the client from harm, real or imagined (Foye et al 2002).

Phase 2: Formulate client-centred goals

Once a client's concerns and priorities are identified and sufficient information has been gathered, the practitioner and client work together to identify realistic goals that could be achieved over the course of intervention (Park 2006). To ensure that a goal is client-centred, it should describe a client's future experience in a specific daily life activity that is

Vignette 8.2

Moira

Moira, a 34-year-old with learning difficulties, lives with her mother who plans to work an evening shift. Moira remarked that she wants to prepare hot meals when her mother is away. Her mother (whose interests must also be considered) believes that Moira could stay by herself but she does not want her to use the electrical or gas appliances; instead, she wants hot meals to be delivered. The practitioner agrees that Moira could stay by herself but she also believes that Moira has the potential to safely use appliances. If Moira's mother agrees to Moira preparing hot meals, a goal could be set, such as 'Moira to safely prepare hot meals at home without supervision'. If Moira's mother does not agree and arranges for hot meals to be delivered, no goal could be set as no significant change will occur with Moira's engagement in a daily life activity, particularly as the delivery of hot meals represents a service Moira will receive, not a goal she will achieve. In this case, further negotiation must occur between all three to identify and agree to a client-centred goal for intervention.

relevant and meaningful to the client (Park 2006). Goals should reflect specific daily life activities in which clients need or want to engage, such as safely preparing evening meals, getting dressed in the morning on their own, playing with friends after school at the local park, successfully completing homework on time, engaging in fun social activities at the local leisure centre, or managing their own medications throughout the week. Asking the question, 'So what difference does performing this activity mean to the person?' (Randall and McEwen 2000: 1202) can help identify if a goal is client-centred.

Framing goals from the client's perspective also helps ensure that goals are client-centred. The practitioner should work with the client to 'match' the goal to the client's description of the problem (Parry 2004), and use phrases that reflect common, everyday language. Thus, a goal might state 'Louvain to sit comfortably in her wheelchair throughout the day with no significant red areas developing on her bottom' rather than 'Louvain to prevent development of decubiti whilst in wheelchair'. In this case, the phrase 'sitting comfortably throughout the day' is Louvain's personal perspective of the 'problem' and the practitioner 'translated' the importance of preventing decubiti into the phrase 'no significant red areas developing'. Concerns do exist that goals framed from the client's perspective are not 'objective' or 'measurable' (Parry 2004). On the contrary, client-centred goals, in addition to being more relevant to clients, are intrinsically more 'testable' than conventional goals created using a formula (Quinn and Gordon 2003).

Specific elements of goals

Because client-centred outcomes for intervention focus on persons engaging in daily life activities within various environments (Figure 8.3), goals should reflect this premise. Thus, documented goals should contain three elements: the person, a daily life activity, and a context (Table 8.1).

Person The person for whom the goal is set and for whom a change is anticipated should always be identified in the goal. Although this most often is the person with a health condition (i.e., the client, service user or patient), the person may be a family member, carer or another person involved in the client's daily life and with whom the practitioner is working (Park 2006). In many instances, the goal focuses on a carer's or parent's ability to care for and interact with the client, such as 'Mother to safely and with confidence bathe her child each day on her own' or 'Carer to help client in and out of bath at home without undue effort and only providing help as necessary'.

Daily life activity The goal should specify the anticipated 'level' of engagement in a specific daily life activity and describe the expected *quality* of the client's experience, focusing on the manner in which the client engages in the activity and, as appropriate, the client's feelings about engaging in the activity. The anticipated activity should be of sufficient challenge given the client's abilities (Williams et al 1999, Quinn and Gordon 2003)

Vignette 8.3

Nisha

Nisha, a 32-year-old woman who experienced the onset of Guillain-Barre syndrome 6 months ago, is unhappy with how she applies her make-up. When asked to elaborate, Nisha shares that she frequently drops items, smears her make-up, gets frustrated with the amount of effort for disappointing results, and often asks for help. Rather than suggest a more conventional goal, such as 'Nisha to independently apply make-up', the practitioner collaborates with Nisha, formulating a goal from Nisha's perspective: 'Nisha to apply make-up by herself and be pleased with the effort and result'.

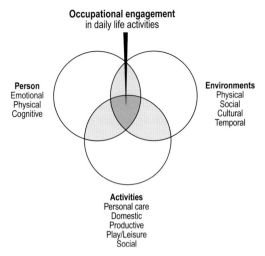

Figure 8.3 Occupational engagement is the interaction between a person, activities and environments. From Park 2006, with permission

and clearly identify the next 'level' of engagement the client might achieve. Practitioners might imagine a client starting on a step (as described later, this reflects the client's *current status*) (Figure 8.4). The client and practitioner decide where, on the steps ahead, the client hopes to be in the future – this step represents the goal. In deciding which step ahead is the goal, the magnitude of change is specified – an essential feature of goal setting. To credibly evaluate client outcomes, clients and practitioners need to identify exactly which 'step' represents the goal, such as 'Client to arrive safely on the second step from the top' or 'Client to climb steadily halfway up the steps'. One exception does exist – goals may reflect maintenance of a client's engagement in daily life activities. When improvement is not expected, particularly in the presence of degenerative conditions, goals may focus on maintaining a client's current status (Cott and Finch 1991, Wallen and Doyle 1996).

Context The environmental conditions under which the person will engage in the activity should be described. Aspects such as where, with whom, when, or how long may be included, particularly as qualitative differences with a person's engagement in daily life activities may occur that directly reflect the environment in which the person engages (Park 2006). For example, Aiden, who experiences schizophrenia, will shop for items at

113

Table 8.1 Components and characteristics of client-centred goals

Components of client-centred goals		Characteristics of goals
A PERSON engaging in a specific DAILY LIFE ACTIVITY within a specific CONTEXT	*Client to consistently check for oncoming traffic and wait for traffic lights when crossing road to corner shop throughout the week.*	• Be relevant and motivating • Express what clients hope to accomplish • Be positively defined • Be put in behavioural terms • Be explicit and commonly understandable • Be attainable • Enable measurement (After Schut & Stam 1994)

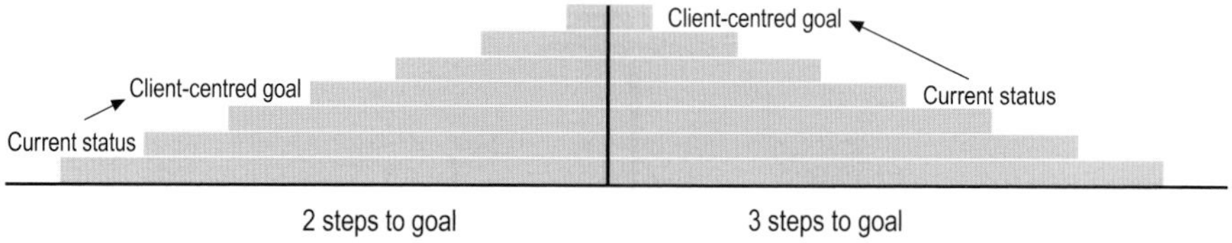

Figure 8.4 When setting goals, exactly how 'far' a client hopes to 'go' (in relation to the starting point) must be explicitly identified. From Park 2006, with permission

the corner shop but is apprehensive about shopping at the nearby superstore and declines to shop there (although he would like to). The goal, 'Aiden to shop for groceries at super store over the course of a month and feel pleased with accomplishment', reflects the next level of challenge for Aiden – shopping within a different environment and over a specified time period. Although including contextual information may require additional words, their inclusion enables practitioners to more precisely determine if a goal is achieved (Randall and McEwen 2000).

Identifying current status to assist with goal formation

'A well-defined problem converted into a goal guides the [intervention] plan and the interventions in a direction that is essential for the [client].' (Wressle et al 2002a: 34)

When formulating goals with clients, practitioners should identify (and document) the client's current status in relation to the goal (Table 8.2). Current status is the starting point, a brief description of the 'problem' the client is experiencing with the specific daily life activity and that the client and practitioner agree is amendable through

Table 8.2 Examples of current status and client-centred goals. After Park 2006, with permission

Current status	Client-centred goal
Client repeatedly washes the same item until prompted to stop and start washing another item, taking an inordinate amount of time to finish washing up	Client to wash up all items on the bench within a reasonable amount of time and without prompting
Client is bullied by other ward patients for cigarettes and readily gives them away without protest	When on the ward, client, in an assertive yet considerate manner, to decline to share cigarettes when he does not want to
At day care, child often wets himself without indicating he needs to toilet	Throughout the morning, child to consistently indicate (without prompting) need to use toilet before wetting himself
Spouse says he is nervous using the hoist at home to move client in/out of bed and declines to use it unless someone else is present	Spouse to safely use hoist to move client in/out of bed and feel confident doing so on his own

intervention (Park 2006). Identifying current status helps to: (a) identify the qualitative features of a client's experience in daily life activities that will become a target for intervention; (b) 'quantify' the expected magnitude of change during intervention; and, (c) determine if the goal was achieved when evaluating the outcome.

Most often, current status describes the client's occupational performance, that is, the manner in which the client currently engages in a daily life activity. Essentially, if the client was videotaped participating in the activity, current status would reflect important highlights of the client's performance that were challenging and which are expected to change during intervention – that is, the occupational 'problem' the client is experiencing. Note: This is *not* the same as the cause of the problem. Current status reflects the client's experience engaging in a daily life activity, not the reason why he or she is encountering the problem. Moreover, current status may also identify the feelings the client experiences whilst engaging in the activity.

Additional considerations when setting goals

Whilst a client's performance of specific daily activities is often the primary focus of intervention, the fact a client can perform an activity may not be the only desired outcome. Often, a client's feelings regarding his or her experience in specific activities are an important outcome to consider and include in the goal. This does not mean, however, the goal reflects a change in the client's general feelings or mood, such as sadness, happiness, discouragement or joy. Rather, the client's feelings about his or her experience in a specific daily life activity (termed 'occupational disposition') are the focus. For example, Dorothea currently declines to ride the bus to the town centre and conveys she doesn't feel confident to do so on her own. If the goal were to solely focus on Dorothea's performance, such as 'Dorothea to ride the bus independently into town', an important concern is ignored. Moreover, Dorothea might well ride the bus into the city centre on her own, effectively achieving the stated goal, but feel miserable whilst doing so. Such an outcome would not be acceptable to Dorothea (or the practitioner). Thus, Dorothea's feelings about her confidence are essential to target during intervention and include in the goal, such as 'Dorothea to ride the bus into town centre on her own and feel confidence doing so'. If a client's occupational disposition is neither likely to change over the course of intervention nor of primary concern to the client, a description of the client's feelings is *not* required.

Because occupational disposition is difficult to quantify, how can these goals be reliably evaluated? If the goal is formulated such that the client can respond with a simple 'yes' or 'no' response, the goal can be evaluated (Table 8.3). For example, Oliver experiences extreme anxiety whilst attending community outings and often declines to go (his current status). If the goal was 'Oliver to be less anxious during community outings', two concerns exist: (1) The goal does not specify the magnitude of expected change, an essential requirement for goals; and (2) Intervention may well help Oliver experience less anxiety but is this lesser degree acceptable to him? To address these concerns, a goal could be set 'Whilst attending community outings to the local leisure centre, Oliver to enjoy the outings with a manageable degree of anxiety'. When the goal is reviewed, Oliver can respond with a definitive 'yes' or 'no' when asked if he enjoyed the outings and if he experienced a manageable degree of anxiety.

If safety whilst engaging in a daily life activity will be a target of intervention, the client's risk for personal injury or damage to the environment should be described. For example, when Fiona prepares hot meals in her kitchen, she frequently does not attend to what she is doing, spilling and dropping hot materials and sharp objects. The goal in this case could be 'Fiona to consistently prepare hot meals with an acceptable degree of risk to her and her partner'. Note: When the goal is evaluated, Fiona and her partner would identify if any safety concerns existed and if these are acceptable.

Table 8.3 Examples of terms to distinguish the difference in a client's feelings about experiencing a daily life activity between 'now' and in the 'future'. From Park 2006, with permission.

Occupational disposition	
Current status	**Client-centred goal**
painful	significant reduction in pain
not satisfied	satisfied, to client's satisfaction
very anxious, unacceptable anxiety	acceptable degree of anxiety
unmanageable anxiety	manageable level of anxiety
unreasonable amount of time	reasonable amount of time
not confident	confident, reasonably confident
intolerable, not tolerable	tolerable
not enjoyable, not fun	enjoyable, fun
embarrassed	not embarrassed

Practitioners are accustomed to setting goals that focus on amount of assistance, such as 'Client will be able to dress with minimal assistance'. Is independence the most important factor to the client (Cederfeldt et al 2003)? Or does the notion of independence serve the professional's need to evaluate progress (Crabtree 2000)? Other factors of equal or greater importance may exist for clients, such as amount of effort, timeliness, efficiency, or the quality of the process or outcome (Park 2006). Setting goals that focus exclusively on independence may not illustrate the meaning of the activity to the client nor indicate important and beneficial qualities that could change during intervention.

Goals may also focus on engaging in a routine of daily life activities as clients may be quite capable of performing an activity but the challenge is sustaining participation over time. For example, Jackson will prepare nutritious meals for a few days in a row but then reverts to his previous habit of eating non-nutritious food. The goal could focus on sustaining a routine of meal preparation, such as 'Jackson to consistently prepare nutritious and satisfying meals throughout the month'. Table 8.4 provides additional considerations when documenting goals.

Time frame for realistic goals

As clients and practitioners formulate goals, the time frame of intervention must be considered. To effectively monitor change, goals should reflect accomplishments that clients could realistically achieve whilst receiving intervention; this contrasts with aspirations to be achieved after discharge. To distinguish the difference, *short-term goals* reflect what might be achieved over the course of intervention and *long-term aspirations* focus on the client's life after intervention. When initially discussing goals, clients frequently focus on long-term aspirations. Practitioners should help clients identify 'smaller' short-term goals for intervention that subsequently lead to the achievement of long-term aspirations (McClain 2005).

Each short-term goal should reflect an accomplishment that could be potentially achieved within 6 months or less. As such, a review date should be designated, at which time it will be determined if the goal was achieved. Two to five short-term goals may be in 'play' at any one time and as goals are achieved, additional ones may be identified. Moreover, short-term goals are not set in stone – some goals may be modified or even abandoned (Hass 1993, Blackmer 2000, Quinn and Gordon 2003, Eschenfelder 2005). As clients gain an understanding of their capacities or re-evaluate the meaningfulness of specific daily life activities, the goal-setting process should accommodate their shifting perspectives.

Table 8.4 In order to evaluate goals, attention to detail is required whilst documenting.

Additional Considerations When Documenting Goals

(based on Park 2006, with additional references as noted)

"Word selection is also important in describing change and the measurement of change."
(Sames 2005, p. 92)

Use the word TO or *will*; avoid the phrase *will be able to*

The phrase *will be able to* is not essential and implies the person can do the activity but might choose not to (Quinn and Gordon 2003, Randall and McEwen 2000)

Current Status	Client-Centred Goal
When shopping for groceries on his own at the local corner store, client usually returns with 3–4 non-essential items; essential items are frequently not included.	NO: *Client will be able to shop on his own.* YES: *Over the course of a month, client to shop on his own, consistently returning with essential items and only occasionally 1–2 non-essential items.*

Ensure goals are clearly understood; avoid professional language

Goals should be stated so that clients understand them.

Current Status	Client-Centred Goal
When attempting to write her name on lined paper, child holds her pencil with a fisted grasp; her signature is illegible.	NO: *Child to display age-appropriate tripod grasp.* YES: *Child to neatly write her name on lined paper, using a three-point grasp to hold her pencil.*

Identify specific goals; avoid goals that are broad

Broad goals do not provide information about specific needs or how to guide intervention most relevant to the client (Forker et al 1999)

Current Status	Client-Centred Goal
Client has never been employed and is unaware of process to search for and obtain a job.	NO: *Client will obtain a job* YES: *When applying onsite for a job, client to legibly, thoroughly & accurately complete application by himself.*

Focus on one activity per goal; avoid including multiple activities

Focusing on one activity makes it easier to monitor change over time.

Current Status	Client-Centred Goal
Client receives help of one person to get in/out of bed and does so in an unsafe manner. *Client receives help of two people to transfer to/from toilet at home.* *Client receives help of two people to get him in/out of bathtub in a safe manner.*	NO: *Client will be able to safely transfer with assistance of one person on/off bed & toilet and in/out of chair & bathtub.* YES: *Client to receive help of one person to get safely in/out of bed.* YES: *Client to safely transfer with help of one person on/off toilet.* YES: *Client to safely transfer with help of one person in/out of bathtub.*

(Continued)

117

Additional Considerations When Documenting Goals—Cont'd

Focus on client achievements; do *not* include the intervention plan

Including information about the intervention plan invalidates the goal setting process. Note: Adaptive equipment is *not* considered an intervention plan; rather, it specifies the manner in which the client will perform the activity.

Current Status	**Client-Centred Goal**
Carer doesn't know how to use bathlift safely with client.	NO: *Carer to be educated to safely use bathlift.* YES: *Carer, by herself, to safely & confidently use bathlift with client at home.*

Focus on what clients will do; avoid focusing on a reduction in behaviour

Goals should specify what a client will do, not what he won't do (Schut & Stam 1994).

Current Status	**Client-Centred Goal**
Client frequently hits out at peers and occasionally spits when playing together on the playground.	NO: *Client will not spit whilst playing with peers on the playground.* YES: *Client to play cooperatively in a socially suitable manner with his peers on the playground.*

Focus on activity engagement; avoid including information about underlying capacities

Information about a client's physical, cognitive, or emotional capacity should not be included—a change in capacity is only a means to goal achievement, not an end (Moorhead & Kannenberg 1998).

Current Status	**Client-Centred Goal**
Client frequently misses appointments throughout the week and, on occasion, has shown up on the wrong day.	NO: *Client will increase memory to complete appointment diary.* YES: Client to arrive to all appointments on time over the course of a month.

Vignette 8.4

Raji

When asked about his priorities, Raji, a 19-year-old in-patient rehabilitation client with an incomplete C-6 spinal cord injury, identifies one priority is to complete a vocational course and receive a First Diploma in Sport. Because this priority cannot be achieved before discharge, it does not make sense to set a goal that states 'Client will successfully complete vocational course'. The practitioner, however, acknowledges Raji's long-term aspiration and together they review the daily life activities required to attend college, such as writing papers, giving presentations and using public transportation. They decide that using a computer to write papers and riding public transportation to college would be meaningful and significant challenges to address. Together, they formulate two goals: 'Using a computer, Raji to accurately type a 2-page paper within a reasonable time' and 'Raji to successfully negotiate the bus from hospital to college, arriving on time and satisfied with effort required'.

Phase 3: Evaluating goal achievement

'When the client's need or desired behavior is successfully identified in the [goal], the task of selecting suitable intervention is straightforward' (McLeod & Robnett 1998: 29).

Table 8.5 An example of documentation based on client-centred goal setting. After Park 2006, with permission

Background: Irisa, a retired 72-year-old shopkeeper, lives with her husband of 47 years. Irisa has an extensive history of major depression (her last hospitalisation occurred 2 months ago) and she is currently receiving community services. Her husband is concerned about her favoured activities of preparing meals, attending music group, and taking care of their dog; Irisa expresses hopelessness that she can reclaim her life but identifies it would be nice to help out more around the house and to enjoy life once again.

Documentation

Current status	Client-centred goals	Client outcomes
Client requires much encouragement from husband to assist with preparing evening meals. She often declines to help, stating she just can't do it	*Irisa to help with preparing evening meals throughout the week with only a bit of encouragement from her husband*	*Irisa reports she helped prepare evening meals with her husband's occasional encouragement. Irisa's husband concurs and says he is pleased with the progress*
01.02.00	01.03.00	01.03.00
Irisa's husband prepares lunch for his wife as she will not prepare any food when he is away at work. Irisa says she feels overwhelmed with the prospect of preparing anything to eat	*For Monday through Friday, Irisa to consistently prepare a satisfying and nutritional lunch*	*Irisa and husband report she prepared four nutritious lunches that she liked. Irisa said she now feels she will continue to make lunch but that occasionally she might not feel like eating*
01.02.00	01.04.00	01.04.00
Irisa stays at home during the day and will not attend the twice-weekly music group in which she previously participated	*Irisa to consistently attend music group twice a week for 2 weeks and enjoy herself*	*Irisa reports she attended 4 music groups over the past 2 weeks and felt good about going*
01.02.00	01.05.00	01.05.00
Irisa does not feel able to look after the family dog. The dog is currently living nearby at her daughter's house	*Irisa to take care of her dog at her home over the course of a month and feel confident in doing so*	*Although Irisa says she is still apprehensive, she did assume all care for their dog during the past month and would like to continue keeping the dog at home*
01.05.00	01.08.00	01.08.00

119

Although each goal is reviewed at a specified date, to guide and monitor intervention, goals should be referred to regularly during intervention (Cott and Finch 1991, Quinn and Gordon 2003). At the review date, the client and practitioner together should determine if the goal was achieved. All available information can be used to evaluate the outcome, including client self-report, and family members, partners, carers, or other persons can provide relevant information. As well, the practitioner may observe the client in the specified activity, gathering information with which to determine if the goal was achieved. No matter the means, evaluating goal achievement is a collaborative effort between the client and practitioner. It is then the practitioner's responsibility to document the outcome, providing a complete description such that any reader could compare the outcome to the current status and goal, and conclude if the goal was achieved. Additional information to substantiate why the outcome is important may also be included. Table 8.5 outlines how a client's current status, goals and outcomes are documented when using client-centred goal setting.

Conclusion

As Welch and Foster (2003) discovered, time and support are needed to assist occupational therapists to incorporate client-centred goal setting into traditional health-care services (and likely others). Goal setting is not just asking clients to identify their goals – it requires practitioners to interlace therapeutic rapport with professional skills to enable clients to find meaning in everyday life activities and to support client efforts to achieve the most ordinary desire and grandest dream. Giving voice to clients through goal setting allows them to experience a key benefit of occupational therapy – engagement in meaningful daily activities to support their health and well-being in everyday life.

References

Andrew E, McDermott S, Vitzakovitch S et al 1999 Therapist and patient perceptions of the occupational therapy goal-setting process: A pilot study. Physical & Occupational Therapy in Geriatrics 17(1): 55–63

Barclay L 2002 Exploring the factors that influence the goal setting process for occupational therapy intervention with an individual with spinal cord injury. Australian Occupational Therapy Journal 49: 3–13

Blackmer J 2000 Ethical issues in rehabilitation medicine. Scandinavian Journal of Rehabilitation Medicine 32: 51–55

Bodium C 1999 The use of the Canadian Occupational Performance Measure for the assessment of outcome on a neurorehabilitation unit. British Journal of Occupational Therapy 62(3): 123–126

Carswell A, McColl MA, Baptiste S et al 2004 The Canadian Occupational Performance Measure: A research and clinical review. Canadian Journal of Occupational Therapy 71(4): 210–222

Cederfeldt M, Lundgren Pieree B, Sadlo G 2003 Occupational status as documented in records

for stroke inpatients in Sweden. Scandinavian Journal of Occupational Therapy 10: 81–87

Chan CH, Lee TMC 1997 Validity of the Canadian Occupational Performance Measure. Occupational Therapy International 4(3): 229–247

College of Occupational Therapists (COT) 2000 Code of ethics and professional conduct for occupational therapists. COT, London

Conneeley AL 2004 Interdisciplinary collaborative goal planning in a post-acute neurological setting: A qualitative study. British Journal of Occupational Therapy 67(6): 248–255

Cott C, Finch C 1991 Goal-setting in physical therapy practice. Physiotherapy Canada 43(1): 19–22

Crabtree J 2000 What is a worthy goal of occupational therapy? Occupational Therapy in Health Care 12(2/3): 111–126

Creek J 2003 Occupational therapy defined as a complex intervention. College of Occupational Therapists, London

Donnelly C, Eng JJ, Hall J et al 2004 Client-centred assessment and the identification of meaningful treatment goals for individuals with a spinal cord injury. Spinal Cord 42(5): 302–307

Eschenfelder VG 2005 Shaping the goal setting process in OT: The role of meaningful occupation. Physical & Occupational Therapy in Geriatrics 23(4): 67–81

Forker JE, Gallagher B, Lewis A 1999 Care planning for the homebound elderly client. Home Health Care Management & Practice 11(6): 42–48

Foye SJ, Kirschner KL, Wagner LCB et al 2002 Ethical issues in rehabilitation: A qualitative analysis of dilemmas identified by occupational therapists. Topics in Stroke Rehabilitation 9(3): 89–101

Gage M 1994 The patient-driven interdisciplinary care plan. Journal of Nursing Administration 24(4): 26–35

Geen R G 1995 Human motivation: A social psychological approach. Brooks/Cole, Pacific Grove, CA

Guidetti S, Tham K 2002 Therapeutic strategies used by occupational therapists in self-care training: A qualitative study. Occupational Therapy International 9(4): 257–276

Halladay K 2001 Measuring the occupational performance of mental health clients – How hard should we try? OT News 21

Hanna K, Rodger S 2002 Towards family-centred practice in paediatric occupational therapy: A review of the literature on parent–therapist collaboration. Australian Occupational Therapy Journal 49: 14–24

Law M, Baptiste S, Mills J 1995 Client-centred practice: What does it mean and does it make a difference? Canadian Journal of Occupational Therapy 62(5): 250–257

Law M, Baptiste S, Carswell A et al 2005 Canadian Occupational Performance Measure, 4th edn. Canadian Association of Occupational Therapists, Ottawa, Ontario

Locke EA, Latham GP 2002 Building a practically useful theory of goal setting and task motivation. American Psychologist 57(9): 705–717

Lund ML, Tamm M, Bränholm IB 2001 Patients' perceptions of their participation in rehabilitation planning and professionals' views of their strategies to encourage it. Occupational Therapy International 8(3): 151–167

McClain C 2005 Collaborative rehabilitation goal setting. Topics in Stroke Rehabilitation 12(4): 56–60

McColl MA, Paterson M, Davies D et al 2000 Validity and community utility of the Canadian Occupational Performance Measure. Canadian Journal of Occupational Therapy 67(1): 22–30

McLeod K, Robnett R 1998 Psychosocial documentation: Are your objectives functional, measurable and reimbursable? Occupational Therapy in Mental Health 14(3): 21–31

Missiuna C, Pollock N 2000 Perceived efficacy and goal setting in young children. Canadian Journal of Occupational Therapy 67(2): 101–109

Moorhead P, Kannenberg K 1998 Writing functional goals. In: Acquaviva JD (ed) Effective documentation for occupational therapy, 2nd edn., pp. 75–82. Rockville, MD, American Occupational Therapy Association

Neistadt ME 1995 Methods of assessing clients' priorities: A survey of adult physical dysfunction settings. American Journal of Occupational Therapy 49(5) 428–436

Nelson CE, Payton OD 1997 The planning process in occupational therapy: Perceptions of adult rehabilitation patients. American Journal of Occupational Therapy 51(7): 576–583

Northen JG, Rust DM, Nelson CE et al 1995 Involvement of adult rehabilitation patients in setting occupational therapy goals. American Journal of Occupational Therapy 49(3): 214–220

Palmadottir G 2003 Client perspectives on occupational therapy services. Scandinavian Journal of Occupational Therapy 10: 157–166

Park SW 2006 Client-centred, goal-oriented outcome evaluation in occupational therapy [course manual]. Harrison Associates, London

Parry RH 2004 Communication during goal-setting in physiotherapy treatment sessions. Clinical Rehabilitation 18: 668–682

Playford ED, Dawson L, Limbert V et al 2000 Goal setting in rehabilitation: Report of a workshop to explore professionals' perceptions of goal setting. Clinical Rehabilitation 14: 491–496

Pollock N, Stewart D 1998 Occupational performance needs of school-aged children with physical disabilities in the community. Physical & Occupational Therapy in Pediatrics 18(1): 55–68

Ponte-Allan M, Giles GM 1999 Goal setting and functional outcomes in rehabilitation. American Journal of Occupational Therapy 53(6): 646–649

Quinn L, Gordon J 2003 Functional outcomes documentation for rehabilitation. Saunders, St Louis, MO

Randall KE, McEwen IR 2000 Writing patient-centered functional goals. Physical Therapy 80(12): 1197–1203

Rebeiro KL 2000 Client perspectives on occupational therapy practice: Are we truly client-centred? Canadian Journal of Occupational Therapy 67(1): 7–14

Rosa SA, Hasselkus BR 2005 Finding common ground with patients: The centrality of compatibility. American Journal of Occupational Therapy 59(2): 198–208

Sames KM 2005 Documenting occupational therapy practice. Pearson Prentice Hall, Upper Saddle River, New Jersey

Schut HA, Stam HJ 1994 Goals in rehabilitation teamwork. Disability and Rehabilitation 16(4): 223–226

Spencer JC, Davidson HA 1998 The Community Adaptive Planning Assessment: A clinical tool for documenting future planning with clients. American Journal of Occupational Therapy 52(1): 19–30

Sumsion T 2000 A revised occupational therapy definition of client-centred practice. British Journal of Occupational Therapy 63(7): 304–309

Sumsion T 2005 Facilitating client-centred practice: Insights from clients. Canadian Journal of Occupational Therapy 72(1): 13–20

Sumsion T 2006a Implementation issues. In: Sumsion T (ed) Client-centred practice in occupational therapy: A guide to implementation, pp. 39–53. Elsevier, Edinburgh, UK

Sumsion T 2006b The client-centred approach. In: Sumsion T (ed) Client-centred practice in occupational therapy: A guide to implementation, pp. 19–28. Elsevier, Edinburgh, UK

Sumsion T, Smyth G 2000 Barriers to client-centredness and their resolution. Canadian Journal of Occupational Therapy 67(1): 15–21

Wade DT 1998 Editorial. Evidence related to goal planning in rehabilitation. Clinical Rehabilitation 12: 273–275

Wallen M, Doyle S 1996 Performance indicators in paediatrics: The role of standardized assessments and goal setting. Australian Occupational Therapy Journal 43: 172–177

Welch A, Forster S 2003 A clinical audit of the outcome of occupational therapy assessment and negotiated patient goals in the acute setting. British Journal of Occupational Therapy 66(8): 363–368

Wilkins S, Pollock N, Rochon S et al 2001 Implementing client-centred practice: Why is it so difficult to do? Canadian Journal of Occupational Therapy 68(2): 70–79

Williams WH, Evans JJ, Wilson BA 1999 Outcome measures for survivors of acquired brain injury in day and outpatient neurorehabilitation programmes. Neuropsychological Rehabilitation 9(3/4): 421–436

Wressle E, Samuelsson K 2004 Barriers and bridges to client-centred occupational therapy in Sweden. Scandinavian Journal of Occupational Therapy 11: 12–16

Wressle E, Eeg-Olofsson A, Marcusson J et al 2002a Improved client participation in the rehabilitation process using a client-centred goal formulation structure. Journal of Rehabilitation Medicine 34: 5–11

Wressle E, Marcusson J, Henriksson C 2002b Clinical utility of the Canadian Occupational Performance Measure – Swedish version. Canadian Journal of Occupational Therapy 69(1): 40–48

Wressle E, Lindstrand J, Neher M et al 2003 The Canadian Occupational Performance Measure as an outcome measure and team tool in a day treatment programme. Disability and Rehabilitation 25(10): 497–506

Therapeutic use of self: a model of the intentional relationship

9

Renee R. Taylor and
Jane Melton

Highlight box

- Though significant progress has been made in knowledge development regarding use of self in occupational therapy, research suggests that an increased focus is needed
- There is still a lack of clarity regarding the exact definition, use and relevance of therapeutic use of self in occupational therapy.
- Clients possess a number of interpersonal characteristics that, when discovered, can guide therapists' decision making within the relationship.
- An interpersonal event is a naturally occurring communication, reaction, process, task or general circumstance that occurs during therapy and that has the potential to detract from or strengthen the therapeutic relationship.
- The Intentional Relationship Model provides a means of mapping, interpreting and responding to client characteristics and to the challenging interpersonal events of therapy by incorporating a variety of perspectives, skills and approaches.

Introduction

A recent survey of practising occupational therapists within the United States revealed that more than 80% of therapists consider therapeutic use of self to be the most important variable in successful therapy outcomes (Taylor et al in press). In a similar study in the UK 83% of respondents placed a significant amount of importance upon therapeutic use of self and 72% felt it is a key determinant of therapy (Forsyth et al submitted). At the same time, fewer than half of US therapists and just half of UK therapists felt they were adequately trained in this area upon graduation. Additionally, about two-thirds of both cohorts of therapists felt that there was sufficient knowledge about use of self in occupational therapy (Forsyth et al submitted, Taylor et al in press).

These therapists' perceptions of the importance of therapeutic use of self are supported by other research studies; a growing number of which indicate that the client–therapist relationship is a key determinant of whether occupational therapy has been successful or not (Ayres-Rosa and Hasselkus 1996, Cole and McLean 2003). In this chapter, we provide an overview of the historical foundations and literature on use of self within the field of occupational therapy. This is followed by a rationale for the introduction of a new conceptual model of use of self and an explanation of the research that has been conducted thus far to support the development of this model. The model and its four components and functions are then described. Ultimately, a case example is presented that illustrates a clinician's use of this model in a practice situation.

Historical overview

The topic of therapeutic use of self has been addressed throughout occupational therapy's history. Recommendations about how therapists should interact with clients have changed as our thinking about practice has evolved over time. An historical account has identified three distinct eras in occupational therapy (Kielhofner 2004). Each of these eras offers a unique perspective and emphasis on the role of the client–therapist relationship in the therapy process.

The earliest occupational era reflected ideals embraced by the field's founders (Kielhofner 2004). Initial descriptions of therapeutic use of self came from Europe in the late 1700s during the time of moral treatment (Bockoven 1971, Bing 1981). Moral treatment emphasised the facilitation of self-determination through engagement in everyday activities such as arts and crafts, sports and other pursuits. When more formalised approaches to occupational therapy emerged in the early 1900s, the humanistic approaches of moral treatment were emphasised. Supporters of moral treatment argued that all activity prescriptions should be based on an in-depth understanding of the patient's personality, preferences and interests (Bing 1981). Consideration and kindness were put forward as essential interpersonal values. During this era, the therapeutic relationship was viewed as existing solely as a means for encouraging the client to engage in occupation. In creating this relationship, the therapist's role was to serve as an:

- expert
- guide
- role model
- motivator through persuasion
- emulator of the joy of occupation
- instiller of confidence
- creator of a positive physical and social milieu.

In the mid-20th century, the early occupational era was replaced by a more analytical era labelled the era of inner mechanisms (Kielhofner 2004). In this era, concern for addressing a client's underlying impairment became the focus. Rooted in the medical establishment, the role of the occupational therapist during this era was to understand the nuances of and correct internal failures of body and mind. The client–therapist relationship was viewed as the central mechanism for change and understanding of this relationship was largely based on principles borrowed from literature influenced by the psychoanalytic perspective. Often, the relationship was viewed as a means by which to understand a client's unconscious motives, desires and behaviour toward others and toward occupations. Within the relationship, the therapist's role was to:

- behave in a competent and professional manner
- assume an impersonal and objective attitude toward the client

- instil hope
- be tactful
- exert self-control
- exercise good judgement
- privately identify with and use emotional reactions to patients in planning how to respond.

Within mental health settings, which then comprised a significant amount of occupational therapy practice, it was common to expect that the client would achieve catharsis by acting out unconscious motives and desires within the therapeutic relationship. The therapist then assisted the client in achieving insight into any issues that were viewed to be at the core of the client's pathological feelings and behaviours. By the 1970s, some believed that occupation had lost its place as the key dynamic of therapy (Yerxa 1967, Shannon 1977, Schwartz 2003 , Kielhofner 2007).

In the latter part of the 20th century a new, contemporary era was born, which returned the field to its initial focus on occupation. This era was labelled the return to occupation (Kielhofner 2004). In part, this new era represented a reaction to what was perceived as an over-emphasis on the role of the therapeutic relationship during the era of inner mechanisms. In this contemporary era, the strong focus on the therapeutic relationship has been set aside in favour of a renewed emphasis on occupational engagement as the true mechanism for change and positive outcomes in occupational therapy (Yerxa 1967, Kielhofner and Burke 1977, Shannon 1977, Schwartz 2003). Similar to the early occupational era, the role of the relationship in the contemporary era is more uni-dimensional in its focus, which is strictly to facilitate the client's engagement in occupation. The therapist's role is to use a variety of interpersonal strategies to make occupations appealing.

Within this contemporary era, there have been three central movements with which the client–therapist relationship has been associated:

- collaborative and client-centred approaches
- emphasis on caring and empathy
- use of narrative and clinical reasoning.

Collaborative and client-centred approaches (e.g. Mosey 1970, Townsend 2003, Duncan 2006) have focused on re-adjusting power imbalances within the therapeutic relationship and on facilitating client control over decision-making and problem-solving. Generally, these approaches emphasise open communication, orientation toward the client's perspective, recognition of the client's strengths, shared goals and priorities, and a collaborative partnership. There has also been an emphasis on therapist self-awareness. Therapists are encouraged to recognise, control and correct non-therapeutic reactions, incorporate their own life experiences into an understanding of their client's perspectives, and to draw upon their personal reactions to clients to guide their clinical reasoning.

In conjunction with collaborative and client-centred approaches, the contemporary era has also been characterised by an emphasis on empathy and caring within the therapeutic relationship. This can be summarised as an emphasis on the emotional exchange that occurs between client and therapist, on goal-directed activity, and on activities that promote personal growth (Baum 1980, Gilfoyle 1980, King 1980, Yerxa 1980, Devereaux 1984, Peloquin (1989a, 1989b, 1990, 1993, 1995, 2002, 2003). Caring was put forth as a much-needed value and it was defined as follows (Baum 1980, Gilfoyle 1980, King 1980, Yerxa 1980, Devereaux 1984):

- intimate knowing
- communicating effectively

- eliminating the focus on impairment
- flexibility in adapting to environmental and situational demands
- harnessing the will of each client
- believing in the innate potential of the individual
- using humour
- connecting at an emotional level
- using touch to connect, and
- restoring personal control through activity.

More recently, empathy has been written about extensively and defined as a communication of partnership:

- a turning of the soul toward the client
- a recognition of how one is similar to the client and how the client is unique
- an entry into the client's experience
- a connection with the feelings of the client
- the power to recover from that connection and maintain strength to continue therapeutic work.

Peloquin (1989b, 1990, 1993) emphasised the roles of art, literature, imagination and self-reflection. She further argued that the fundamental characteristics required to develop one's therapeutic use of self are well conveyed through reading literature and viewing and doing art (Peloquin 1989b). She believed that providing therapists with both fictional and non-fictional poems and stories that illustrate empathy and the depersonalising consequences of neglectful attitudes and failed communication could be a powerful motivator for the development of caring (Peloquin 1990, 1993, 1995).

Clinical reasoning and narrative approaches comprise the final general category of contemporary scholarship that includes the client–therapist relationship as a focal point (Rogers 1983, Crepeau 1991, Mattingly 1991, 1994, Clark 1993, Schell and Cervero 1993, Fleming 1994, Mattingly and Fleming 1994, Kielhofner 1997, Jonsson et al 2001, Lyons and Crepeau 2001, Schwartzberg 2002, Schell 2003, Schwartz 2003). These approaches emphasise the role of therapist understanding and reflection about the unique way in which clients think about and summarise key events in their lives (Kielhofner 2004). Clinical reasoning approaches incorporate thinking about the relationship as a component of one's overall approach to making sense of assessment findings and developing a treatment plan (Mattingly and Fleming 1994). This element has been referred to as interactive reasoning (Mattingly and Fleming 1994) and it has been described as an 'underground practice' in occupational therapy (Fleming 1991) because relatively little is known about the mechanisms that underlie it. One exception involves work by Mattingly and Gillette (1991), which resulted in six relationship-building strategies pertinent to clinical reasoning. These included:

- providing clients with choices
- individualising treatment
- structuring therapy activities to maximise the potential for success
- going outside of the formal therapeutic role and doing special favours or acts of kindness for clients
- sharing one's personal stories with clients, and
- joint problem solving.

Narrative approaches (e.g., narrative reasoning) were developed in tandem with clinical reasoning approaches (Mattingly 1994, Kielhofner 1997). Narrative approaches seek to organise and make sense of information from clients by encouraging them to present information about themselves through storytelling, poetry or metaphor. Thinking in story form is thought to allow both the client and the therapist to discover the meaning of the impairment experience according to the client's unique perspective. Therapeutic approaches are then focused toward reconstructing more hopeful narratives to re-shape one's life story.

Rationale for a model of use of self

We have seen that occupational therapy's view of the therapeutic relationship has changed and developed throughout history. Early perspectives of the field's first era emphasised the centrality of occupation and the therapist's role in promoting occupational engagement. The second era redefined the therapeutic relationship as a psychodynamic process that, according to some perspectives, replaced occupation as the central dynamic of therapy. With some exception (e.g., Blair and Daniels 2006) this idea was, in large part, rejected in favour of the contemporary, renewed focus on occupation.

During our contemporary era of heightened occupational focus, the three major themes related to the therapeutic relationship described in the prior section have been introduced: (1) collaborative and client-centred approaches; (2) an emphasis on caring and empathy; and (3) clinical reasoning and use of narrative. These are important themes that offer broad and useful principles related to the therapeutic use of self.

Despite the fact that these approaches coexist with the field's returned emphasis on occupational engagement, they do not directly address the question of how therapeutic use of self can be used specifically to promote both occupational engagement and positive therapy outcomes. Their relationship to an occupationally focused practice is assumed, but not made explicit.

In addition, some implicitly assume that, when therapists achieve a reflective, appreciative, and emotionally connected state with clients, a positive therapeutic process will simply emerge. This assumption is a large one that appears to be contradicted in the experience of most practising therapists. Despite the existence of a fairly extensive contemporary literature on collaboration, client-centred practice, caring, empathy, clinical reasoning and narrative, the vast majority of practising therapists that we surveyed, believe occupational therapy does not have sufficient knowledge to support the therapeutic use of self (Forsyth et al submitted, Taylor et al in press). Their perspectives suggest that something is still missing.

To date, there has been no effort to integrate all of the contemporary interpersonal approaches in occupational therapy into a coherent explanation of the therapeutic relationship. Moreover, beyond broad principles, there are few details about how the therapeutic relationship should be approached and managed in light of the central focus on the client's engagement in occupation. Consequently, there is still a lack of clarity regarding the exact definition, use and relevance of therapeutic use of self in occupational therapy.

These observations were the impetus for developing the conceptual practice model presented in this chapter, the Intentional Relationship Model. The model was developed in an attempt to clarify and provide more detailed guidance of how to enact the therapeutic use of self in occupational therapy. Therapeutic use of self involves a highly personal, individualised and subjective decision-making process. For some therapists, the process is driven by emotional reactions to clients and a perceived reliance on an innate or nurtured intuitive capacity. Others perceive the process as largely rational and grounded in the disciplined application of a set of interpersonal guidelines. Irrespective of such viewpoints, therapeutic use of self is, in large part, a product of the extent to which one possesses a knowledge base and interpersonal skills that can be applied thoughtfully to common interpersonal events in practice. Accordingly, therapeutic use of self is an occupational therapy skill that must be developed, reinforced, monitored and refined.

The Intentional Relationship Model explains therapeutic use of self and its relationship with occupational engagement. Additionally, it provides a means of mapping, interpreting and responding to the unique and everyday interpersonal events of therapy by incorporating a variety of perspectives, skills and approaches. The model provides educators, supervisors, students, clinicians with a common vocabulary with which to discuss and describe the interpersonal phenomena that have an ongoing impact on everyday practice.

The Intentional Relationship Model

The Intentional Relationship Model is an empirically based model that was developed over a 3-year period. In part, its concepts were based on practitioner responses to a large-scale ($n = 1000$, response rate 64%) nationwide survey of occupational therapists' knowledge, attitudes and interpersonal behaviours related to use of self (Taylor et al in press). In addition, 12 occupational therapy practitioners from various regions of the world were observed and interviewed using a semi-structured interview measure developed by the first author. In each region, these therapists were nominated by their local peers as having exceptional talent in terms of their ability to form successful therapeutic relationships with a wide range of clients. They also participated in an initial introductory interview with the first author to determine their suitability for participation in the formal interview and observation. The insights that emerged from the observation of these expert therapists were critical to the development of this model. The second author is one of the therapists who was selected and studied for her expertise and her approach to the therapeutic use of self will be used later in this chapter to illustrate some aspects of this model.

Many of the concepts for the intentional relationship model have their origins in theory underlying psychotherapy practice models. However, the intentional relationship model recognises a fundamental difference between occupational therapy and traditional psychotherapy. Figure 9.1 portrays the traditional psychotherapy process. In psychotherapy, interpersonal relating between client and therapist is the central focus. The verbal communication between client and therapist is lengthy, intense, highly complex, nuanced and derived from detailed conceptual models of how psychological change is intended to occur. Interpersonal communication is typically the only activity that occurs during psychotherapy.

In occupational therapy the client–therapist relationship does not and should not pretend to emulate the intensity, duration and complexity of a traditional psychotherapy relationship.

By contrast, the central focus of occupational therapy is occupational engagement. A diagram of the unique role that the therapeutic relationship plays in occupational therapy is presented in Figure 9.2.

As it shows the occupational therapist employs a number of therapeutic strategies, usually rooted in existing models of practice, to facilitate the client's engagement in occupation. Depending on the occupational needs, capacities and diagnosis of the client, any number of occupational therapy practice models might be employed alone or in combination to promote occupational engagement. However this main task of promoting occupational engagement through employing the specific methods and strategies of occupational therapy does not exist in isolation of a larger process of relating that occurs between client and therapist.

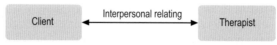

Figure 9.1 The client–therapist relationship in traditional psychotherapy

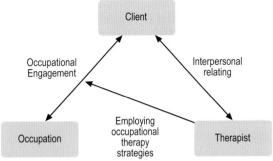

Figure 9.2 The unique relationship between client, therapist and occupation in occupational therapy (fix arrows)

The intentional relationship model explains the relationship between client and therapist that is part of the overall process of occupational therapy. Accordingly, the intentional relationship model is intended to complement existing occupational therapy conceptual practice models rather than replace any single model. It explains the detailed and overarching aspects of the client–therapist relationship, an important aspect of occupational therapy not addressed extensively by other conceptual practice models. Figure 9.3 shows how the intentional relationship is designed to supplement the use of other occupational therapy conceptual practice models.

As shown, the intentional relationship model should complement the usual concepts and strategies of occupational therapy that are directly aimed at facilitating occupational engagement. The model's utility for occupational therapy lies in addressing the otherwise unarticulated aspects of the interpersonal relationship that occur during the therapy process and that influences both occupational engagement and therapy outcomes. The next section defines the elements of this model and provides an explanation of how the elements interact to optimise the circumstances for a successful client–therapist relationship in occupational therapy.

To reiterate, the intentional relationship model is not a free-standing model of practice for occupational therapy. If a therapist only utilised this model, the essential work of occupational therapy would not occur. The model was designed to fill a gap in our practical

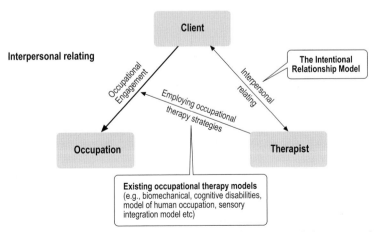

Figure 9.3 The intentional relationship model as a complement to existing occupational therapy models

knowledge about how to manage the interpersonal aspects of therapy – particularly the more challenging ones. This model should complement the field's existing methods and models by making the process of establishing a successful relationship with clients easier, clearer and more straightforward.

Elements of the Intentional Relationship Model

This chapter provides only a basic overview of the Intentional Relationship Model (IRM). Those who are interested in a more thorough treatment should consult *The Intentional Relationship: Therapeutic Use of Self in Occupational therapy* (Taylor 2008). The IRM views the therapeutic relationship as being comprised of four central elements:

1. The client
2. The interpersonal events that occur during therapy
3. The therapist
4. The occupation.

A summary diagram of the model is presented in Figure 9.4.

The model explains the requirements for a functional client–therapist relationship and it incorporates guidelines for responding to common interpersonal events that frequently occur in therapy. In the following section, the relevant aspects of each element of the model and their relationships with one another are described.

The client

According to the IRM, the client is the focal point. It is the therapist's responsibility to work to develop a positive relationship with the client and to respond appropriately when interpersonal events occur. In order to develop this relationship and respond appropriately to the client, a therapist must work to understand the client from an interpersonal perspective. This involves getting to know the client's interpersonal characteristics.

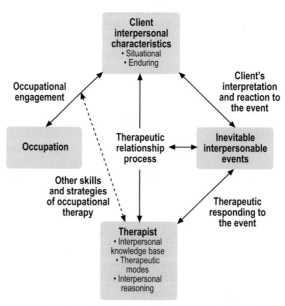

Figure 9.4 A model of the intentional relationship in occupational therapy

According to IRM, a client's interpersonal characteristics can be understood according to two dimensions:

- Situational characteristics
- Enduring characteristics.

Situational characteristics are interpersonal characteristics that are inconsistent with how a client typically and consistently behaves when interacting with others. Instead, they reflect a client's acute emotional reaction to a specific situation. Typically, a client's situational characteristics attract our attention when he or she is encountering a situation that is somehow painful, frustrating or stressful. For most of us, stressful situations result in some negative emotional state that makes it temporarily difficult for us to engage in occupations as planned. Thus, a client's situational characteristics are likely to surface when they interfere with the client's ability to engage in the activities of therapy as planned.

A client's situational characteristics are most likely to reveal themselves in therapy when the client is facing a situation where some immediate aspect of the impairment and/or the environment is experienced as stressful. Impairments, particularly when they are new or when there is a medical crisis or exacerbation in severity that disrupts one's usual relationship with the environment, often cause people to experience stress. Therapists are encouraged to assume, on some level, that a client's impairment situation and/or the client's interaction with an unaccommodating or difficult environment will cause the client to be more vulnerable to experiencing a variety of emotional reactions, many of which may be perceived as negative or at least atypical for that individual. For example, feelings of loss are common among newly disabled individuals and they may manifest in terms of sadness, irritability, anxiety, insecurity or anger. A therapist's interpersonal behaviour, if perceived as insensitive, judgemental or uncaring, may also serve as a source of stress and cause the client to interact in a manner that is generally inconsistent with his or her personality. It is important for newer therapists to recognise that these and other acute emotional reactions are normative. In fact they are givens in many health-care situations. They bear no reflection on the client's character or personality. However, they do have the potential to play out within the therapy relationship, and the way in which a therapist chooses to respond to them is often vital to the future of that relationship.

By contrast, *enduring characteristics* are more stable and consistent aspects of the client's interpersonal behaviour. They are not necessarily related to the situation of acquiring an impairment or to the environment's reaction or lack of accommodation to that impairment. Instead, they comprise an interpersonal profile that is idiosyncratic to the client. Enduring interpersonal characteristics include such things as a client's preferred style of communicating, capacity for trust, need for control, general orientation to relating and usual way of responding to change, challenge or frustration.

Because they coexist in each client, situational and enduring characteristics are mutually informative. Behaviour that reflects one's acute emotional reaction to a stressful event may temporarily attenuate, alter or intensify one's interpersonal behaviour in what are usually more stable categories. For example, a client that normally responds to a challenging situation adaptively may become irritated when the therapist recommends a more challenging activity if, earlier in that day, the client underwent a painful biopsy and then discovered that she did not have the funds to pay for transportation after leaving the physician's office. The rationale for distinguishing the two categories of interpersonal characteristics is to help inform therapists' understanding of the client in stressful and non-stressful situations so that therapeutic responses can be appropriately tailored and modulated.

The interpersonal events of therapy

An *interpersonal event* is a naturally occurring communication, reaction, process, task or general circumstance that occurs during therapy and that has the potential to detract from or strengthen the therapeutic relationship. In therapy, these events may be precipitated by the following kinds of circumstances:

- client resistance (e.g., a client refuses or feels unable to participate in some activity)
- therapist behaviour (e.g., the therapist asks a question that the client perceives as intrusive, or emotionally difficult to face)
- client display of strong emotions in therapy (e.g. an elderly client begins crying during transfer training or a child client runs up to the therapist and hugs her in the midst of a sensory motor activity)
- a difficult circumstance of therapy (e.g., a client is embarrassed because of losing bladder control, or becomes frustrated or fearful in the midst of an activity)
- a rift or conflict between client and therapist (e.g., the client is offended by a comment made by the therapist)
- differences concerning the aim of therapy (e.g., a client insists on a goal that the therapist believes is not attainable, or the therapist recommends a goal that the client rejects)
- client requests that test the boundaries or limits of the therapeutic relationship (e.g. the client invites the therapist to attend her wedding).

These, of course, are only a few of the myriad of possible interpersonal events that occur in the course of occupational therapy.

When interpersonal events of therapy occur, their interpretation by the client is a product of the client's unique set of interpersonal characteristics. Sometimes the event may have a significant effect upon the client and other times a client will be unaffected or minimally affected. When such events occur, what is important is that the therapist be aware that the event has occurred and take responsibility for responding appropriately.

Interpersonal events are:

- inevitable during the course of therapy, and
- ripe with both threat and opportunity.

Interpersonal events are part of the constant give and take that occurs in a therapy process. They are distinguished from other events or processes in that they are charged with the potential for an emotional response either when they occur or later upon reflection. Consequently, if they are ignored or responded to less than optimally, these events can threaten both the therapeutic relationship and the client's occupational engagement. When optimally responded to, these events can provide opportunities for positive client learning or change and for solidifying the therapeutic relationship. Because they are unavoidable in any therapeutic interaction, one of the primary tasks of a therapist practising according to the IRM is to respond to these inevitable events in a way that leads to repair and strengthening of the therapeutic relationship.

The therapist

Within the IRM, the therapist is responsible for making every reasonable effort to make the relationship work. Specifically, the therapist is responsible for bringing three main interpersonal capacities into the relationship:

- An interpersonal skill base
- Therapeutic modes (or interpersonal styles)
- Capacity for interpersonal reasoning.

This section provides a brief description of each of these interpersonal capacities. The first capacity involves development and application of a wide-ranging fount of knowledge about how to manage the various aspects of one's relationships with other people. The therapist's *interpersonal skill base* is comprised of a continuum of skills that are judiciously applied by the therapist to build a functional working relationship with the client. The perspective of the model is that, depending on the unique experiences, knowledge and innate capacities of the therapist, some of these skills will come more naturally while others will require significant effort and practice to develop.

These interpersonal skills are summarised in terms of nine categories:

- therapeutic communication
- interviewing skills and strategic questioning
- establishing relationships with clients
- families, social systems and groups
- working effectively with supervisors, employers and other professionals
- understanding and managing difficult interpersonal behaviour
- empathic breaks and conflicts
- professional behaviour, values and ethics
- therapist self-care and professional development.

The first category, therapeutic communication, involves activities such as verbal and nonverbal communication skills, therapeutic listening, assertiveness, providing clients with direction and feedback, and seeking and responding to client feedback. Interviewing skills is another skill set that involves being watchful and intentional about the way in which one approaches the process of asking a client questions. Socratic questioning is a specific approach to questioning born out of cognitive psychology (e.g., Beck 1995). It involves asking questions in a way that guides the respondent to think more broadly or differently. Establishing relationships with clients includes rapport building, matching one's therapeutic style to the interpersonal demands of the client, managing a client's strong emotion, judicious use of touch, and cultural competence.

Because many clients have caregivers, family members or other individuals with whom they have regular contact, understanding and working with families, social systems and groups is an essential aspect of occupational therapy practice. It includes using guiding principles of IRM, in combination with prominent systems theories, to gain the collaboration of partners, parents, other family and friends to serve the goals of therapy. It also involves understanding the structure, process and interpersonal dynamics of group therapy.

Another fundamental skill involves knowing how to work collaboratively with supervisors, employers and other professionals. It involves knowing how to communicate with other professionals about clients both in the presence and in the absence of those clients. Additionally, it requires understanding the power dynamics and value systems that underlie supervisor/student and employer/employee relationships. Understanding and managing clients' difficult behaviour is another category of necessary interpersonal skills required in many practice situations. It involves knowing how to respond effectively to behaviours that involve manipulation, excessive dependency, symptom focusing, resistance, emotional disengagement, denial, difficulty with rapport and trust, and hostility. Responding effectively will help limit the extent to which this behaviour disrupts the goal and process of therapy.

Knowing how to resolve conflicts and empathic breaks (or rifts in understanding between client and therapist) is another fundamental skill set that can salvage a failing relationship or repair minor threats to an otherwise functional relationship. Professional behaviour and ethics encompasses knowledge of how one's own values are consistent or inconsistent with the occupational therapy core values, ethical behaviour and decision making, behavioural self-awareness around clients, being reliable and dependable, upholding confidentiality, and setting and managing professional boundaries. Therapist self care incorporates knowing and managing one's own emotional reactions to clients and being accountable to those reactions, a general capacity for self-reflection, an ability to manage one's personal life and seek support when necessary, and the capacity to maintain perspective regarding client outcomes. More information about all of these skills, which comprise a therapist's interpersonal skill base, is provided in Taylor (2008).

The second interpersonal capacity that a therapist brings to the client–therapist relationship is her or his primary therapeutic mode or modes. A *therapeutic mode* is a specific way of relating to a client. The IRM identifies six therapeutic modes:

* advocating
* collaborating
* empathising
* encouraging
* instructing
* problem-solving.

A brief definition of each mode and an example of how the second author used the mode in practice is provided in Table 9.1.

Therapists naturally use therapeutic modes that are consistent with their fundamental personality characteristics. For example, a therapist who tends to be more of a listener than a talker and believes in the importance of understanding another person's perspective before making a suggestion would likely use empathising as a primary therapeutic mode in therapy. Therapists vary widely in terms of the range and flexibility with which they use modes in relating to clients. Some therapists relate to clients in one or two primary ways, while others draw upon multiple therapeutic modes depending upon the interpersonal characteristics of the client and the situation, or inevitable interpersonal events, at hand. One of the goals in using the intentional relationship model is to become increasingly comfortable utilising any of the six modes flexibly and interchangeably depending upon the client's needs. A therapeutic mode or set of modes define the therapist's general *interpersonal style* when interacting with a client. Therapists able to utilise all six of the modes flexibly and comfortably and to match those modes to the client and the situation are described as having a *multi-modal* interpersonal style.

According to the IRM, a therapist's choice and application of a particular therapeutic mode or set of modes should depend largely on the enduring interpersonal characteristics of the client. In addition, certain events or interpersonal events in therapy may call for a mode shift. A *mode shift* is a conscious change in one's way of relating to a client. Mode shifts are frequently required in response to interpersonal events in therapy. For example, if a client perceives a therapist's attempts at problem-solving to be insensitive or off the mark, a therapist would be wise to switch from the problem-solving mode to an empathising mode so that she can get a better understanding of the client's reaction and the root of the dilemma. An interpersonal reasoning process, described in the following paragraph, can be utilised to guide the therapist in deciding when a mode shift might be required and determining which alternative mode to select. Because the interpersonal aspects of occupational therapy practice are complex and require a therapist to possess a highly adaptive therapeutic personality, the IRM recommends that therapists learn to draw upon all six of the therapeutic modes in a flexible manner according to the different interpersonal needs of each client and the unique demands of each clinical situation.

The third therapist interpersonal competency involves the capacity to engage in an *interpersonal reasoning* process when an interpersonal dilemma presents itself in therapy. Interpersonal reasoning is a step-wise process by which a therapist decides what to say, do or express in reaction to the occurrence of an interpersonal dilemma in therapy.

Table 9.1 The six therapeutic modes in practice

Mode	Definition	Example
Advocating	Ensuring that the client's rights are enforced and resources are secured. May require the therapist to serve as a mediator, facilitator, negotiator, enforcer, or other type of advocate with external persons and agencies	Lobbying to secure adequate resources for the provision of ongoing support and environmental adaptation. This enabled a man with learning disabilities to participate safely in self care and domestic activities within his own home environment
Collaborating	Expecting the client to be an active and equal participant in therapy. Ensuring choice, freedom, and autonomy to the greatest extent possible	Setting recovery oriented occupational goals with a man who had been through an inpatient detoxification program for alcohol misuse. The service user reported that the structured routine for healthy activity choices coupled with feedback to the therapist helped to build him a sense of personal responsibility for achieving the goals
Empathising	Ongoing striving to understand the client's thoughts, feelings, and behaviours while suspending any judgement. Ensuring that the client verifies and experiences the therapist's understanding as truthful and validating	Taking care to fully appreciate the occupational requests and sensitivities of a woman experiencing psychotic symptoms. This approach enabled her to reclaim her values of being a vegan and being very environmentally conscious throughout her therapeutic recovery experience
Encouraging	Seizing the opportunity to instill hope in a client. Celebrating a client's thinking or behaviour through positive reinforcement. Conveying an attitude of joyfulness, playfulness and confidence	Spontaneously responding to a woman attending an occupational therapy group session who, inspired by some background music started to dance. Therapeutic connection was enhanced by this small gesture to join with her joy of the activity
Instructing	Carefully structuring therapy activities and being explicit with clients about the plan, sequence, and events of therapy. Providing clear instruction and feedback about performance. Setting limits on a client's requests or behaviour	Enabling a withdrawn woman with little belief in her own abilities to undertake self care activities. This was achieved by talking the woman through the task, all the while reinforcing verbally the support available with the task if required
Problem-solving	Facilitating pragmatic thinking and solving dilemmas by outlining choices, posing strategic questions, and providing opportunities for comparative or analytical thinking	Allowing a young man with Aspergers syndrome to undertake the activities of value to him that also supported his well-being. This involved analysing options and negotiating with his family, who were concerned about his extraordinary choices of some occupations and his neglect of others

It includes developing a mental vigilance toward the interpersonal aspects of therapy in anticipation that a dilemma might occur, and a means of reviewing and evaluating options for responding. The six steps of interpersonal reasoning include:

1. Anticipate
2. Identify and cope
3. Determine if a mode shift is required
4. Choose a response mode or mode sequence
5. Draw upon any relevant interpersonal skills associated with the mode(s)
6. Gather feedback.

An extensive description and discussion of these steps can be found in Taylor (2008).

The desired occupation

Occupational therapy is unique in that the crux of the therapy process is the client's occupational engagement. The final component of the IRM is the desired occupation. The ***desired occupation*** is the task or activity that the therapist and the client have selected for therapy. These desired occupations may include a wide range of tasks and activities such as dressing oneself, driving, shopping, gross motor play, participating in a goal setting group, completing a craft activity or engaging in a simulated or modified work task. The selection of the occupation and support for occupational engagement will be primarily informed by other occupational therapy conceptual practice models such as the biomechanical model, the sensory integration model, or the model of human occupation (Kielhofner 2004)

The primary function of the IRM is to enable the therapist to manage the interpersonal dynamic between the client and the therapist that also occurs as part of the therapy process. This interpersonal dynamic influences the occupational engagement and also serves as an arena in which the emotional reactions that stem from or influence occupational engagement can be positively managed. Thus, according to the model the therapeutic relationship functions both as:

* a support to occupational engagement and
* a place where the emotions and coping process associated with the client's impairment and its implications for occupational participation can be addressed.

Relationships within the model

According to the IRM, the client and therapist relationship can be viewed at two different levels or scales:

* the usual therapeutic relationship process that consists of the ongoing rapport and patterns of interaction between client and therapist. This relationship is enduring and it occurs outside of any unusual circumstances or stressors (macro-level)
* the therapeutic relationship process that is influenced by interpersonal events of therapy, or the stressors or highlights that have the potential to challenge or enrich the relationship depending upon how they are responded to and resolved (micro-level).

The ***therapeutic relationship*** is a socially defined and personally interpreted interactive process between the client and therapist. It is socially defined in that the therapist and the client are engaged in an interaction within publicly understood roles. The therapist is recognised as bringing a certain kind of expertise, ethical guidelines and values into a relationship. The client is recognised as a person receiving service in order to address a particular need. The relationship is understood to exist for the sole purpose of achieving an improvement in the client's situation. These parameters are given and provide an important definition of the relationship. Therapist and client are in a particular relationship that can be differentiated from other kinds of relationships such as friendships. At the same time, this relationship has a personal side. The client and therapist are human beings who encounter each other with the same potential range of thoughts and emotions that occur when any two people interact.

Consequently, the therapist's responsibility is to ensure that:

- the appropriate definitions and boundaries of the therapeutic relationship are sustained, and
- positive interpersonal relating such as trust, mutual respect and honesty characterise the relationship.

Sustaining the therapeutic relationship is an ongoing task that does not focus solely on interpersonal events. The everyday therapeutic relationship process that occurs outside of any specific interpersonal events is the macro dimension of the interpersonal process of therapy.

Responding to the immediate events that occur during therapy is the micro dimension. Responding to these interpersonal events of therapy requires that therapists detect the occurrence of an event, read the client's reaction to the event, and decide upon an appropriate way to address the event with the client.

Both the micro and macro scales of therapeutic interaction play a critical role in the overall process of occupational therapy. Moreover, they are interrelated. That is, the nature of the therapeutic relationship will have an influence on how the client interprets and how the therapist responds to interpersonal events and, in turn, interpersonal events and their resolution will either enhance or detract from the therapeutic relationship.

In some cases, the two scales of interaction are difficult to differentiate. For example, some therapy relationships only last for one or two sessions. In these cases, a therapist must work to respond to a client and to interpersonal events with much more vigilance and self-control because a more stable underlying therapeutic relationship does not yet exist. Moreover, the interpersonal events and their resolution during the therapy sessions will be the major determinants of the therapeutic relationship.

However, in most cases, therapy continues over a period of weeks or months, allowing for the development of some kind of predictable pattern or usual way of interacting within the therapeutic relationship. That therapeutic relationship will infuse and be shaped by interpersonal events that occur in the moment-by-moment therapy process. It will also be influenced by characteristics and behaviours that the client and therapist bring to the relationship, as well as by the circumstances surrounding the relationship. These circumstances include such factors as the nature and unfolding of the client's impairment and the context (e.g., school, rehabilitation setting, home, work) in which therapy takes place.

It is the therapist's responsibility to manage and continually strive to fortify the therapeutic relationship and to seek optimal resolutions to interpersonal events in therapy. The stability and success of a therapeutic relationship cannot be assumed. Rather, it begins early in treatment with attempts by the therapist to build rapport, followed by other efforts to develop a relationship that meets the client's immediate interpersonal needs and is appropriate in terms of the circumstances of therapy and the demands of the treatment setting. Recognising and sustaining a successful therapeutic relationship might include such things as:

- sharing certain interpersonal rituals that facilitate bonding (e.g., paying a visit to a garden or other favourite locale within the client's setting each time before the ending of therapy)
- witnessing the client enjoying or benefitting from therapy

- sharing mutual feelings of respect, admiration or appreciation
- feeling interested and engaged in the therapy process
- being open and comfortable digressing during therapy for discussion, venting or advice-seeking about events in his or her personal life (without interfering with progress toward goals)
- being able to discuss and overcome the interpersonal events that might otherwise challenge the relationship
- having a long-standing private joke with a client
- sharing a certain intensity of eye-contact that communicates mutual trust or
- noticing a certain way a client laughs that conveys her appreciation of the therapist.

These are only a few examples of myriad factors that might contribute to a successful therapeutic relationship. It is the responsibility of the therapist to be vigilant to explore, identify and sustain those factors that contribute to a relationship that supports positive therapy outcomes.

This is not to say that the client will not make positive contributions to the therapeutic relationship. In most instances, clients will bring important or essential characteristics and behaviours into the therapeutic relationship. However, the fundamental difference is that it is the therapist who must assume the ultimate responsibility for assuring that the relationship is positive. By assuming this responsibility the therapist creates a space in the relationship wherein a client can be vulnerable, distressed, frustrated or angry without fearing that the relationship will be ruptured. Moreover, this does not mean that the therapist assumes an expert or authoritative stance in the relationship. Rather, it means that the therapist must assume responsibility for the caring within the relationship.

The enduring aspects of the therapeutic relationship are systematically built and fortified as a result of naturally occurring variables in relationship (similar personality styles or interpersonal chemistry or other optimal circumstances and timing) and as a result of the therapist's consistent efforts to build the relationship in the face of the inevitable interpersonal events and challenges that occur. If the therapist's efforts to build a relationship are successful and the client is not particularly sensitive, untrusting or otherwise vulnerable, the therapeutic relationship becomes stronger over time and is more likely to withstand interpersonal events that would otherwise challenge or strain the relationship.

For any number of reasons, however, the therapeutic relationship may not develop adequately enough to endure threats caused by the interpersonal events that routinely emerge during therapy. Signs that there is difficulty within the therapeutic relationship may include, but are not limited to:

- change in affect, attitude or interpersonal behaviour
- becoming disengaged from therapy
- appearing/feeling impatient, irritable or angry
- therapy is experienced as 'boring'
- the utility of therapy becomes questionable
- questioning or criticism feels excessive
- taking therapy 'home'
- dreading or becoming apprehensive about the next appointment
- having a desire to refer or terminate prematurely
- conflict with the client
- client's attendance pattern changes or declines.

There are a number of potential reasons why difficulty may emerge within the therapeutic relationship. For example, a client may bring a particular interpersonal history into the treatment relationship that makes it difficult for the therapist to establish rapport in ways that usually work. Conversely, the client may be mistrustful of the therapist because of the circumstances under which he is being seen. For example, a client may have been mandated by an insurance company to receive an evaluation for work potential and the client perceives that the therapist has tremendous power to influence his life (i.e., whether he continues to receive disability support). Alternatively, a therapist may have a negative reaction to a client because the client reminds the therapist of someone with whom the therapist has had a difficult relationship in the past. General sources of difficulty within the relationship may include, but are not limited to:

- Client brings a difficult interpersonal history into the relationship or has an Axis II (DSM-TR 2000) diagnosis such as avoidant or antisocial personality disorder
- Circumstances under which the client is being seen are threatening or pressured (i.e., an evaluation is being conducted for the purpose of verifying disability to an insurance company)
- Poor match between client and therapist's interpersonal styles
- Inability to overcome challenges caused by differences in culture, values or worldview
- Client or therapist remind each other of someone with whom they have had a negative experience
- Client or therapist disappoint or fail to meet expectations
- Client or therapist inadvertently say or do something that is perceived as injurious and the situation is not processed and resolved.

These and other kinds of obstacles to a more stable enduring relationship with a client are only intensified by inevitable interpersonal events. Examples of events that are likely to further stress an already-vulnerable therapy relationship include such things as a therapist's unanticipated absence for a period of time, a common misunderstanding that occurs between client and therapist, a comment or question that is perceived by the client as insensitive or inappropriate, or an unexpected personal crisis that causes the client to regress or temporarily relinquish treatment goals. While these are normal and inevitable examples of difficult aspects of therapy, the way in which the therapist responds to them is a powerful mediator of the final outcome.

Irrespective of the extent to which the therapeutic relationship process is stable and strong, the process of therapeutic responding to interpersonal events is essential to good therapy. If a therapist does not respond adequately to interpersonal events or challenges to the relationship, the process of occupational engagement may suffer and the therapeutic relationship process will quickly erode.

Thus, for the duration of the therapy process, the therapist must engage in a process of interpersonal reasoning. **Interpersonal reasoning** is the process by which a therapist consciously and reflectively monitors both the therapeutic relationship and the interpersonal events of therapy in order to decide upon and enact appropriate interpersonal strategies. The six steps of this process were presented earlier in this chapter. A full description of the steps of interpersonal reasoning and examples of its application in practice are provided in Taylor (2008).

Case example

In the following section, a case example of how aspects of the IRM can be used in practice is provided by the second author, a practising occupational therapist for the Gloucestershire Partnership National Health Service Trust in Gloucestershire, England, United Kingdom. Jane has been practising for 20 years and her primary areas of expertise include inpatient and community interventions for adults with severe mental illness and for adults with learning disabilities. Jane also uses the model of human occupation (Kielhofner 2007) to underpin the formulation of her client's abilities and challenges with regard to their engagement in occupations.

Jane's interpersonal challenge: Resolving power struggles with Cecile

Cecile is a woman in her 40s who is divorced and lives alone. In the past, Cecile worked in a department store but was fired from her job, which she describes as one of many significant losses in her life. Cecile was referred for occupational therapy during a stay at an inpatient psychiatric unit. Her diagnosis has been difficult to determine, but Cecile has a long history of depression and anxiety with features of both borderline and narcissistic personality disorder.

Before she was referred to occupational therapy, Cecile had been using the psychiatric inpatient unit repeatedly during the previous 3 years. Cecile's behaviour was also characterised by a tendency to lose favour with her health-care workers. She often made strong and repeated demands for support and assistance but then became dismissive of any attempts to meet these demands. At times she has been known to become rejecting or subtly hostile towards care workers. Her non-verbal messages matched her verbal communication conveying that she was defensive, hopeless or angry. She often twisted facts about her care and distorted or ignored attempts at support from family, friends and caregivers. Her communication was redundant with statements like, 'I can not carry on like this' or 'You are not helping me' or 'This is not making me better'. In therapy, Cecile lacked curiosity and explored new environments only hesitantly. Though she was a highly capable person, she did not take pride in any current achievement nor seek out challenges. She was reluctant to show preferences, engage with others, complete activity, sustain focus or show that any activity was significant to her. This was particularly true when she was aware that staff were observing her, but were not prompting, instructing or encouraging her. Because of her attitude and behaviours, many health-care workers have become weary of providing support and some have refused to work with her.

The interpersonal response

Quickly I realized that issues of power were dominating our interactions and I began to specifically look for interpersonal events that presented power dilemmas. At once Cecile would say something that indicated a desire to change (e.g., 'I want to be myself again') and shortly thereafter she would tell me my approach was not working. Because this dynamic occurred repeatedly despite my many efforts to change my approach or incorporate her feedback, I interpreted this pattern's true meaning as 'I can say your intervention is not making me better and therefore I am powerful over you – even though I tell you that I want to change'. This played out in other ways. For example, we once shared a joke when visiting a local café and Cecile smiled. Because she rarely smiled, I pointed out that I enjoyed seeing her smile. She immediately returned to a mask-like expression. On another occasion I was gently questioning Cecile about her interests and achievements and she quickly became tearful and insisted we stop the conversation.

One of the central tasks of our work together involved understanding this power dynamic as an indication of Cecile's high need for control, which is one of her more consistent and enduring interpersonal characteristics. Knowing this, I then had to work with this dynamic to maximise Cecile's feelings of control so that she could develop other aspects of volition. On some occasions, this meant occasionally giving in to the dynamic and sometimes becoming vulnerable in her eyes. For example, I might use some self-disclosure about how her behaviour affects me. I did this with the hope of stimulating her self-reflection about our conversation and raising her awareness of how her use of power in this way affects other people.

On other occasions, I have worked with the power dynamic by standing my ground and providing a rationale for why my approach might assist her. I often validate Cecile's desire for me to see that she is deeply troubled, but I also remind her that if and when she is ready to build strength I will be there to assist her. On some occasions, we have also agreed to take short, planned breaks from our work together. The reason for these breaks is to give her space from the therapy process, to allow her time to reflect upon the responsibility that she holds within the therapy relationship, and to enable me to reform with ideas and energy to maintain the relationship. Aside from working with the power dynamic in these ways, an overarching aspect of my approach has been to not take any of Cecile's behaviours or comments personally.

The outcome

Cecile was discharged after an 8-month stay in the hospital. A structured and sophisticated support network was designed and implemented including regular occupational therapy appointments. Activities were set up and undertaken with the aim of engaging Cecile in making choices, taking control over her activities, regaining interest in past activities, and formulating a pattern within her occupations. Cecile's motivation for doing did not develop any further than what she needed to maintain independent functioning. Importantly, however, it was maintained at the same level and now after many months since her last hospitalisation Cecile has not yet felt the need to return to the hospital.

Jane is a very circumspect therapist who has mastered the delicate art of walking on eggshells without breaking them. Her judgement about what people need, particularly when they are feeling vulnerable or threatened, is very precise and a quality that any therapist would admire. The story above illustrates that Jane's level of sophistication in managing more difficult interpersonal issues within therapeutic relationships is highly developed. She utilised interpersonal reasoning to recognise inevitable power dilemmas within the relationship and she responded to them appropriately by shifting between the empathising and instructing modes to achieve a balance between acceptance-oriented strategies and change-oriented approaches. She was careful to select and time these modes carefully to accommodate Cecile's high need for control within the relationship in a way that allowed her to feel more empowered without feeling the need to dominate or manipulate the relationship.

Summary

In occupational therapy, therapeutic use of self is a fundamental aspect of practice that has significant implications in terms of the course and ultimate outcomes of therapy. In this chapter, we learned that initiating and maintaining a relationship that supports occupational engagement is a complex and dynamic process that must be intentional in order to be maximally responsive to a client's developing interpersonal needs in therapy. The chapter began with a historical overview of prior conceptualisations and approaches to therapeutic use of self throughout the history of our field. A rationale for the need for a conceptual model of practice that uniquely addresses the interpersonal aspects of occupational therapy and does not interfere with other models and approaches to practice was provided. A model that responds to that need, the IRM was presented. The primary components of the model and their relationships were described. A successful therapeutic relationship was defined according to the model's principles. Finally, a case example was provided by the second author to illustrate application of specific aspects of the model in a practice situation.

References

American Psychiatric Association 2000 Diagnostic and Statistical Manual of Mental Disorders – Text Revision IV. American Psychiatric Association

Ayres-Rosa S, Hasselkus BR 1996 Connecting with patients: The personal experience of professional helping. The Occupational Therapy Journal of Research 16: 245–260

Baum CM 1980 Occupational therapists put care in the health system. American Journal of Occupational Therapy 34: 505–516

Beck J 1995 Cognitive therapy: Basics and beyond. New York, Guilford Press

Bing RK 1981 Eleanor Clark Slagle lecturership 1981 Occupational therapy revisited: A paraphrastic journey. American Journal of Occupational Therapy 35: 499–518

Blair SEE, Daniels MA 2006 An Introduction to the Psychodynamic Frame of Reference. In: EAS Duncan (ed) 2006 Foundations for Practice in Occupational Therapy. Elsevier, Edinburgh

Bockoven JS 1971 Occupational therapy – a historical perspective: Legacy of moral treatment – 1800s to 1910. American Journal of Occupational Therapy 25: 223–225

Clark F 1993 Occupation embedded in a real life: Interweaving occupational science and occupational therapy, 1993 Eleanor Clarke Slagle lecture. American Journal of Occupational Therapy 47: 1067–1078

Cole B, McLean V 2003 Therapeutic relationships re-defined. Occupational Therapy in Mental Health, 19(2): 33–56

Crepeau EB 1991 Achieving intersubjective understanding: Examples from an occupational therapy treatment session. American Journal of Occupational Therapy 45: 1016–1025

Devereaux EB 1984 Occupational therapy's challenge: The caring relationship. American Journal of Occupational Therapy 38(12): 791–798

Duncan EAS 2006 (ed) Foundations for Practice in Occupational Therapy. 4th Ed. Churchill Livingstone, Edinburgh

Fleming MH 1991 The therapist with the three-track mind. American Journal of Occupational Therapy 45(11): 1007–1014

Forsyth K, Sommerfield G, Taylor RR, submitted. A survey of use of self among therapists in the United Kingdom

Gilfoyle EM 1980 Caring: A philosophy for practice. American Journal of Occupational Therapy 34(8): 517–521

Jonsson H, Josephsson S, Kielhofner G 2001 Narratives and experience in an occupational transition: a longitudinal study of the retirement process. American Journal of Occupational Therapy, 55(4): 424–432

Kielhofner G 1997 Conceptual foundations of occupational therapy, 2nd edn. FA Davis, Philadelphia, PA

Kielhofner G 2007 The Model of Human Occupation, Theory and Application, 4th edn. Lippincott, Williams and Wilkins, Maryland

Kielhofner G 2004 Conceptual Foundations of Occupational Therapy, 3rd edn. FA Davis, Philadelphia, PA

King LJ 1980 Creative caring. American Journal of Occupational Therapy 34(3): 522–528

Lyons KD, Crepeau EB 2001 The clinical reasoning of an occupational therapy assistant. American Journal of Occupational Therapy 55(5): 577–581

Mattingly C 1991 The narrative nature of clinical reasoning. American Journal of Occupational Therapy 45(11): 998–1005

Mattingly C 1994 The narrative nature of clinical reasoning. In: C Mattingly, MH Fleming (eds) Clinical Reasoning: Forms of inquiry in a therapeutic practice, pp. 239–269. Davis, Philadelphia, PA

Mattingly C, Fleming MH 1994 Clinical Reasoning: Forms of inquiry in a therapeutic practice, pp. 178–196. Davis, Philadelphia, PA

Mattingly C, Gillette N 1991 Anthropology, occupational therapy, and action research. The American Journal of Occupational Therapy 45(11): 972–978

Mosey AC 1970 Three Frames of Reference for Mental Health. Slack, Thorofare, NJ

Peloquin SM 1989a Moral treatment: Contexts considered. American Journal of Occupational Therapy 43(8): 537–544

Peloquin SM 1989b Sustaining the art of practice in occupational therapy. American Journal of Occupational Therapy 43(4): 219–226

Peloquin SM 1990 The patient–therapist relationship in occupational therapy: Understanding visions and images. American Journal of Occupational Therapy 44(1): 13–21

Peloquin SM 1993 The depersonalization of patients: A profile gleaned from narratives. American Journal of Occupational Therapy 47(9): 830–837

Peloquin SM 1995 The fullness of empathy: Reflections and illustrations. American Journal of Occupational Therapy 49(1): 24–31

Peloquin SM 2002 Reclaiming the vision of reaching for heart as well as hands. American Journal of Occupational Therapy 56(5): 517–526

Peloquin SM 2003 The therapeutic relationship: Manifestations and challenges in occupational therapy. In: EB Crepeau, ES Cohn, BA Boyt Schell (eds) Willard & Spackman's Occupational Therapy, Tenth Edition, pp. 157–170. Lippincott, Williams & Wilkins, Philadelphia, PA

Rogers JC 1983 Clinical reasoning: The ethics, science, and art. 1983 Eleanor Clarke Slagle lecture. American Journal of Occupational Therapy 37(9): 601–616

Schell BA 2003 Clinical reasoning: The basis of practice. In: EB Crepeau, ES Cohn, BA Boyt Schell (eds) Willard & Spackman's Occupational Therapy, Tenth Edition, pp. 131–152. Lippincott, Williams & Wilkins, Philadelphia, PA

Schell BA, Cervero RM 1993 Clinical reasoning in occupational therapy: An integrative review. American Journal of Occupational Therapy 47(7): 605–610

Schwartz KB 2003 The history of occupational therapy. In: EB Crepeau, ES Cohn, BA Boyt Schell (eds) Willard & Spackman's Occupational Therapy, Tenth Edition, pp. 5–13. Lippincott, Williams & Wilkins, Philadelphia, PA

Schwartzberg SL 2002 Interactive reasoning in the process of occupational therapy. Pearson Education, Upper Saddle River, NJ

Shannon PD 1977 The derailment of occupational therapy. American Journal of Occupational Therapy 31: 229–234.

Sommerfield G, Forsyth K, Taylor RR 2007 Therapeutic Use of Self within Paediatric Practice. Manuscript submitted for publication

Taylor RR 2008 The Intentional Relationship: Occupational Therapy and Use of Self. FA Davis, Philadelphia

Taylor RR, Lee S, Kielhofner G et al in press A Nationwide Survey of Therapeutic Use of Self in Occupational Therapy. American Journal of Occupational Therapy

Townsend E 2003 Reflections on power and justice in enabling occupation. Revve Canadienne D'Ergotherapie 70: 74–87

Yerxa EJ 1967 Authentic occupational therapy [Eleanor Clarke Stagle Lecture]. American Journal of Occupational Therapy 21: 1–9

Yerxa EJ 1980 Occupational therapy's role in creating a future climate of caring. American Journal of Occupational Therapy 34(8): 529–679

Problem-solving

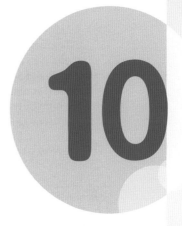

Edward A.S. Duncan

Highlight box

- The pragmatic focus of occupational therapy lends itself to taking a problem-solving theoretical approach in practice.
- The problem solving approach is essentially a form of clinical reasoning.
- Using problem-solving theory enables practitioners to form an objective approach to understanding a client's problems.
- The problem-solving approach is essential, but insufficient in its own right. The information it gains must be considered together with the client's perspective when forming shared decisions in practice.
- The problem-solving process is a flexible clinical intervention that can be used with a wide variety of clients.
- This chapter outlines the problem-solving process and highlights various issues to consider at each stage.
- The problem-solving process helps clients to resolve challenging difficulties and teaches a method of self care for dealing with other challenges in the future.

Introduction

The Chambers dictionary (1994) defines a problem as, 'a matter difficult to settle or solve' and problem-solving behaviour as 'the use of various strategies to overcome difficulties in attaining a goal' (p. 1366). A problem is generally something that is blocking something from being achieved. It can also be something that occurs when a person does not know how to resolve a situation. In other words, 'a problem arises when someone wants to do something but either does not know how or is in someway blocked from implementing a known solution. Thus, the problem is the gap that separates individuals from where they are now and where they want to be' (Robertson 1996: 178). The practical nature of occupational therapy lends itself to naturally take a problem-solving approach to intervention. Consider the following scenarios:

- A lady has suffered a stroke and is currently in a rehabilitation ward. She is having difficulty getting dressed in the morning and wishes to be able to do so independently so she has control over this when she returns home.
- A husband is having difficulty caring for his wife who has dementia. She frequently gets up at night to go to the toilet. Often her husband finds her wandering around the house disorientated and upset as she cannot find the bathroom.
- A 45-year-old taxi driver has been off work for 3 years with low back pain and depression; he would like to return to work but lacks confidence and doesn't know where to start as he is unable to return to his old job.

Each of these scenarios present people who are likely to come into contact with occupational therapy and have problems of various forms that they need to resolve.

This chapter is divided into two main sections that present the key ways in which practitioners use problem solving in practice. The first section presents problem solving as a general theoretical approach to practice (Roberts 1996, Robertson 1996, Dutton 2000, Hagedorn 2001). The second section draws on theory from the cognitive behavioural frame of reference (see Duncan 2006) to present how problem solving can also be used as a specific therapeutic intervention.

Problem solving as a theoretical approach in practice

As a theoretical framework for occupational therapy practice, problem solving can be understood as a form of clinical reasoning (Roberts 1996, Paterson and Summerfield-Mann 2006). Dutton (2000) presented problem solving as the practical manifestation of practitioners' cognitive abilities to break down clients' difficulties and problems in to small steps. Robertson (1996) examined problem solving in practice and presented it as a form of cognitive information processing. This approach views problem solving as a rational and logical process that describes how practitioners understand a problem and work to solve it (Robertson 1996). Whilst occupational therapists often focus on resolving problems, Robertson (1996) emphasised that it is worth initially spending considerable time to conceptualise how the problem is understood as these ideas will shape the future interventions a practitioner will use to resolve the problem.

Hagedorn (2001) argued that the whole occupational therapy process can be viewed in terms of problem solving and suggested that it entailed the following stages:

- Information collection
- Problem identification
- Identification of the desired outcome
- Solution development
- Evaluation and selection
- Development of an action plan
- Implementation and evaluation of results.

Opacich (1991) had, however, already outlined a similar series of stages to describe the occupational therapy process. And although Opacich (1991) considered these in terms of a clinical reasoning process, Paterson and Summerfield-Mann (2006) suggested they can also be viewed in terms of a problem-solving process. Opacich's (1991) stages are:

- Framing the problem – selecting the theoretical model or frame of reference, considering which assessments to use, etc.
- Delineating the problem – organising assessments to collect information and analysing the findings from assessments that are carried out
- Forming a hypothesis – understanding the findings of the results in light of the selected theoretical perspective and developing a written summary of this
- Developing intervention plans – forming goals for intervention and considering the environment in which the intervention will take place
- Implementing intervention – continual assessment to support, alter or dismiss the hypothesis that has already been generated.

Opacich's (1991) and Hagedorn's (2001) approaches to the occupational therapy problem-solving process have clear similarities. Both approaches are essentially forms of hypothetico-deductive reasoning; which is centred on how a professional builds a hypothesis and forms a sequential series of actions. Unsworth (1999) stated that hypothetico-deductive reasoning is an inadequate clinical reasoning strategy to employ on its own as, by its nature, it excludes the interactions that occur between practitioner and clients in practice. However, it can also be argued that the hypothetico-deductive reasoning of the occupational therapy problem-solving process, whilst inadequate in isolation, is essential for practitioners to form an objective perspective of a client's problem. This understanding can then be shared with the client and, informed by clients' personal experiences; perceptions; preferences; as well as the views and opinions of meaningful others in the client's life, can help form a shared decision about the direction of occupational therapy intervention (see Figure 10.1). Chapter 4 describes the challenges of undertaking shared decision making in practice.

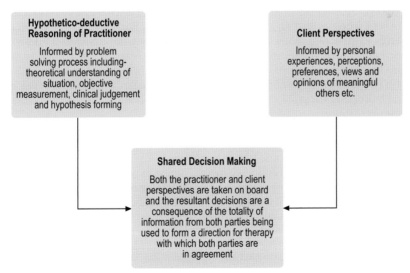

Figure 10.1 Integrating hypothetico-deductive reasoning and client perspectives in a shared decision making model of practice

Using problem solving as a therapeutic intervention

Problem solving in clinical practice is based on the theoretical foundations of cognitive behavioural therapy. Occupational therapists may find that they use this process intuitively, yet it has a strong theoretical basis (D'Zurilla and Nezu 1999, 2000). Whilst the problem-solving process originally developed within mental health settings, its applications are broad and should not be considered as an intervention for mental health settings alone (see Vignette 10.1). As a therapeutic skill and method of intervention, problem solving has several strengths. It is relatively brief, is applicable to a wide range of issues in differing clinical situations, and aims to empower clients to resolve their own personal issues and challenges without seeking professional assistance in the future.

Problem solving has been identified as being useful for two types of individual. The first are people who generally cope well, but perhaps due to an illness or the nature of the problem they are facing are not currently coping with a specific situation. The second are individuals who generally find it difficult to deal with life, or may be said to have generally insufficient coping resources (e.g. strong self-esteem, occupationally involved lives, solution-focused mentality, supportive social network, etc.) (Hawton and Kirk 1989). Whilst the problem-solving process can be used with both groups of individuals, it is likely take longer to instil and be successful with the latter population.

There are various situations in which practitioners may use the problem-solving process outlined in this chapter. A specific situation may arise during a session and the occupational therapist may decide that assisting the client to develop a problem-solving strategy would be useful (for example during the break of a social skills group a teenage girl who has anorexia tells her practitioner of her anxiety about going to a friend's 'sleep over' where there will be lots of food). Alternatively, the problems may already be apparent and the practitioner could introduce the concept of the problem-solving process to a client and agree with him/her that it would be useful to focus on problem solving as part of their agreed goals (for example, discussing discharge and return to work with a client who has had an above-knee amputation). Finally, practitioners may find themselves in crisis situations with clients who they may not know well and who are distressed and would benefit from a problem-solving process to assist them to develop solutions for their immediate issues (for example, working in crisis teams, or on the duty desk of a community mental health team). Therefore, regardless of the practice setting that one is working in, problem solving is a skill that should be in every occupational therapist's repertoire.

Of course, despite its broad potential for application, problem solving is not the panacea to all situations and is not always an appropriate intervention. There are situations in which problem solving should not be considered. A person who has marked learning difficulties or a severe and enduring mental illness may well be cognitively unable to complete the stages of the problem-solving process (Hawton and Kirk 1989). Similarly an individual who has suffered from a stroke or external head injury may (depending on the nature of the event) be unable to complete the stages of the problem-solving process (see Figure 10.2). And whilst problem solving can be very useful for people experiencing a crisis, in extreme situations (such as in the case of suicidal intent) it is more important to deal with the presenting difficulties, hopelessness and personal disorganisation (thereby ensuring the person's safety) before attempting to introduce a problem-solving intervention.

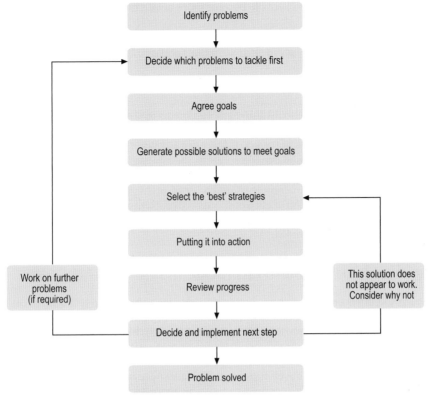

Figure 10.2 The problem-solving process

The problem-solving process

Identifying problems

The identification of client's problems is perhaps the most crucial step of problem solving and time should be taken to make sure that all the problems are identified and clearly specified. This is a collaborative process between the practitioner and client (Hawton and Kirk 1989). Identifying problems may seem straightforward, after all clients are unlikely to be seeing an occupational therapist if they did not have any. Often, however, problem identification is not as straightforward as it may first appear. There can be several reasons for this. Clients can present with problems that are unclearly specified (for example 'difficulty coping at home', or 'unhappy on the ward'). In these situations, it is important that the practitioner helps the client to be more specific about the precise nature of the problem. The aim of this process is to help the client be able to specify exactly what the problem is (for example, 'I am unable to cook dinner for my family and keep the house tidy enough', or 'I am finding sharing a living space with strangers very difficult as they want to watch different TV programmes and ask me personal questions I would rather not answer'). Alternatively, clients may present with a range of clinical conditions (such as depression or anxiety, etc.), but be unable to see how these relate to their personal circumstances, or how addressing certain life situations may help their clinical condition.

Several strategies can assist clients to become more aware of their underlying problems (Hawton and Kirk 1989):

- Ask the client to keep a diary of their symptoms and see if these relate to any specific area of life functioning.
- Gently probe the client for further information about how they feel (e.g. 'what makes you most upset?').
- Take the first step and try to list the client's problems as you see them, from what they have said. Then discuss this list with the client and change, add or amend as they suggest. Remember to ask at the end if there are any other problems that have not been mentioned that should be.

When the above has been completed and a list of problems has been developed, it is vital that a detailed description of each of the agreed problems is developed. Only then will the practitioner and client be able to set meaningful goals together. Table 10.1 presents an example of a client's problem list.

Decide which problems to tackle first

Problem solving is an empowering therapeutic process and ultimately it is up to the client to decide which issue to address first. This should be achieved with support from the practitioner. A client may present a lengthy problem list and it is therefore important that clients prioritise their problems. It is also important that the client commences with a problem that is relatively straightforward to address. An early success in problem solving can increase a client's self belief and, because success with smaller problems can encourage clients that the bigger ones can also be addressed, maintains motivation for the approach. An example of this can be seen in Jack's problem list (Table 10.1). Whilst Jack is almost certain to view his continued detention in a secure hospital as his main problem, this is a significant and challenging life issue that is likely to take some time to address and will necessarily involve 'smaller' problems to be dealt with first. Helping Jack to achieve his discharge would be better addressed, initially, by supporting him to tackle a more manageable issue (e.g. his boredom) in the present moment. Successfully dealing with that issue may encourage Jack to use a similar problem-solving strategy with other problems and will ultimately support him in his goal of being discharged from hospital.

Table 10.1 Jack's problem list

1. Detention in a hospital of high security
2. Frustration at being unable to control his own environment and need for privacy – secondary to problem 1
3. Difficulty concentrating due to schizophrenia and medication side-effects
4. Boredom as unable to carry out activities that he was used to prior to admission and diagnosis of schizophrenia – secondary to problems 1 and 3
5. Loss of contacts with friends and family
6. Has been unable to discuss personal issues with ward key-worker

Agree goals

Having established the priority problems that are going to be addressed, both client and practitioner should then turn their concentration to developing detailed goals to address the identified priority problem. Goal setting in general is discussed in detail elsewhere in this book (see Chapter 8). For the purposes of specific goal setting within the problem-solving process, three key aspects should be kept in mind:

- Goals should be positive
- Goals should be well defined
- Goals should be realistic.

Goals should always be framed in positive terms (for instance what a client will achieve, rather than what they will not do). Setting out goals in this way encourages clients to see that they are moving towards a solution and not avoiding a problem. Goals should be well defined, so that clients know when they have achieved them; well-defined goals are both observable and measurable. Finally, goals need to be realistic, so that they can be achieved. Consider your own experience when you have set personal life goals such as dieting, exercising, etc. Have you ever set unrealistic personal goals? How did you feel when you failed to meet them? Consider what this would be like for some of the clients you work with. To re-emphasise, setting unrealistic goals has the danger of becoming a negative experience for clients and is likely to discourage them from developing their problem-solving skills further.

Generate possible solutions to meet goals

In this stage, the client, with support from their practitioner, lists ways in which their goals could be met. Clients should spend some time on this aspect of the problem-solving process to consider how best to meet their goal. It may be that the most immediate solution is not the best; apart from anything else, it may already have been considered by the client and quite possibly tried before. Strategies for developing lists of possible solutions include brainstorming where the client is asked to write down (or dictate if they have difficulties in writing) all the potential tasks that could result in the target goal being achieved. Clients should be encouraged to list all potential solutions – however implausible. This can lead to a fairly light-hearted component of the session, where a client lets their imagination fly! A side-effect of this process is that the generation of extreme solutions can lead clients to consider possibilities they would otherwise have dismissed (Hawton and Kirk 1989). Once this process has been achieved, clients should list the strengths and weaknesses of each listed solution. Don't dismiss any idea outright.

At times it may appear that there are two or more equally viable solutions. In such cases it can be useful to generate a list of pros and cons for each solution (Table 10.2). This involves assisting a client to generate and list the advantages and disadvantages of each solution. A further step (which may not always be necessary, but further clarifies the importance of items on the list) involves asking the client to weight each listed item. This is achieved by giving Likert-scale-style ratings to each item listed. The complete pros and cons list therefore gives further information about the potential of a solution by listing both the number of advantages/disadvantages that would result as well as their weight in terms of importance to the client.

Table 10.2 Jack's pros and cons list, with Likert scale weightings

Goal: Address boredom: Become more involved in activities in current environment
Potential Solution: Participate three times a week on activities offered to client by occupational therapist

Advantages	Disadvantages
Will distract me from my current situation (4)	I don't like the activities that are being offered (8)
Will sometimes involve getting out of the ward (7)	I don't feel like doing anything (2)
Will keep my multidisciplinary team happy (2)	I feel scared about meeting different people (3)
Will get to meet different people (3)	

Likert scale weighting: 1 = not at all important, 10 = extremely important.

Selecting the 'best' strategy

Having developed a list of potential solutions, and where necessary considered their strengths and weaknesses, you then have to decide which strategy is most likely to help solve the problem/achieve the goal. It is important to remember, however, that this is a best-guess scenario. That is, it is the best guess of the person involved (and ideally of all involved) that the strategy selected is the most likely to work. But it remains a process of trial and error; so keep all the potential solutions to hand – the client may yet need to come back and try another!

It is important, however, to choose a strategy that is likely to work. Practitioners should help clients to carefully weigh up the options, balancing the potential of a strategy to succeed with consideration of the personal resources that it requires, and whether a specific strategy is achievable in practice; it may appear the best solution, but if it is not achievable then the client will not be able to carry it out (Figure 10.3). However sometimes the 'best' strategy can be very apparent; concrete facts or issues can constrain the options available and the selection of a strategy is therefore limited, or other options may carry too much risk to be realistic in practice.

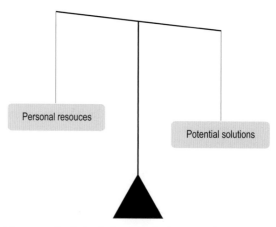

Figure 10.3 Weighing up potential solutions against personal resources

Putting it into action

Once clients have chosen their strategy, it is time to put it into action. Often this stage is viewed simplistically and skimmed over in problem-solving literature. However, this is the central moment of the problem-solving process; implementing action to solve problems is challenging. The chances are if this were simple clients would already have solved the problem. The fact that a client seeks help to resolve a problem means that, at some level it is difficult. Closer consideration of this stage of the problem-solving process is therefore required.

It is important to understand the factors that can influence clients who are about to put their problem-solving plan into action, and consider ways of supporting them to ensure their greatest chance of success. To do so, practitioners can draw on both the Theory of Planned Behaviour (Ajzen and Manstead 2007), and Task Analysis Theory (Hagedorn 2000).

The Theory of Planned Behaviour

The Theory of Planned Behaviour (Ajzen and Manstead 2007) is a well-established psychological theory that links attitudes with action (behaviour). It can help to inform some of the aspects that make it more likely that a client will be able to undertake their selected problem-solving strategy:

- The client should put the selected strategy into action as soon as possible. This is because a person's intention is more closely related to their behaviour when the time interval between them deciding to do something and doing it is low (Ajzen and Manstead 2007). In other words, it is relatively easy for a client to say they will do something, but much harder to actually do it. And it gets harder as time passes.
- A client is more likely to undertake a chosen action if they believe that others who are of importance in their lives (e.g. family) support their action. The Theory of Planned Behaviour describes this as the 'subjective norm' (Ajzen and Manstead 2007). The subjective norm is the client's perception of the beliefs of relevant others that he/she should or should not undertake the chosen strategy. If a client believes he/she has the social support of his family or friends to solve his/her problems and that they are in support of the chosen strategy, they are more likely to put their plan into action.
- A final factor that increases a client's probability of putting the chosen strategy into practice is their 'perceived behavioural control' of the situation. Perceived behavioural control is a construct that describes a person's perception of the ease or challenge that a particular task brings. The easier they feel it is to achieve, the more likely they will undertake the strategy (Ajzen and Manstead 2007). Strategies should therefore appear realistic and achievable in practice.

Putting a problem-solving strategy into action is most likely to be successful therefore when it is done quickly, has the social support of meaningful others in the client's life, and the client believes that what they are about to do is achievable.

Task analysis

Whilst the selected strategy may be the solution to the problem it is usually stated in the form of an overall action (e.g. 'Go to the gym'). To put the strategy into action requires the task to be broken down into manageable parts: a process known as task analysis. Doing so not only clarifies what has to be carried out, but also makes the task appear more achievable thereby increasing the amount of perceived behavioural control a client has and consequently increasing the chances that it will succeed! Hagedorn (2000) differentiated task analysis from activity analysis (see Chapter 7) as task analysis focuses on larger-scale activities (for example 'get fit') whilst activity analysis addresses more focused activities (for example 'having a bath').

Hagedorn (2000) presented a six-question system of task analysis that is useful to consider when putting the problem-solving process into action:

- What is to be done?
- Who is involved?
- How is it performed?
- Where will it take place?
- When will it be done?
- Why are you doing it (A useful reminder!)?

Reviewing progress and implementing the next step

Having put the selected strategy into action, both client and practitioner should evaluate how successful it has been. This can normally be easily measured by asking if the client has solved their problem. If the answer to this question is yes, then the process may naturally come to an end; though it can be worth spending some time with the client looking at how to maintain what has been achieved. Alternatively it may be appropriate to select another problem and commence the process again.

If the problem has not been resolved then the client and practititoner should stop and consider why it did not work and what they can learn from the experience: was the strategy wrong, or was it not implemented as planned? Is more time required, or more intensity of whatever was being done? It may be that the answer to these questions is that it was indeed the wrong strategy, but it is worth stopping and taking some time to consider why it did not work. If necessary another strategy can then be selected (taking into account what has been learnt from the last strategy) and the process worked through again. In this way the implementing of strategies to solve problems can be looked on and communicated by the practitioner to the client as a learning process.

Vignette 10.1

Leon is a 43-year-old man. He is married to Eleanor and has one son, Theo (aged 15). Leon was diagnosed with a relapsing/remitting form of multiple sclerosis at the age of 31. Initially he had managed to continue to work in his office, however he changed his hours to part-time last year as he was becoming increasingly tired. Ten months ago Leon suffered a further relapse in his condition and has since been off work completely.

Leon's GP has referred him to see an occupational therapist. The occupational therapist visited Leon at home.

Identifying problems

In discussion, Leon states that he is having a variety of problems and lists them, in no particular order, as follows:

1. **General weakness:** Leon is now spending almost all of his time in his wheelchair. He is experiencing problems in transferring from his bed to his chair and is also having difficulty getting on and off the toilet.

2. **Fatigue:** Leon reports feeling very tired and spending increasing amounts of time in his bed. At times Leon starts a task, but is unable to finish as he lacks stamina. This leaves him feeling frustrated and 'down'.

Vignette 10.1 continued

3. **Social isolation:** Leon used to enjoy his work. It gave him a sense of purpose, reward and meaningful social contact. Since he has been off work he rarely leaves his house and has missed contact with others.

4. **Financial problems:** Leon is concerned about his future as his 'sick pay' will finish in two months and he is unsure how he will cope financially.

Decide which goals to tackle first

In discussion with Leon, it is agreed to refer to social work to assist with his financial concerns and to focus initially on his fatigue.

Agree goals

Leon wishes to maximize his time awake to look after his self care, and be less tired. Looking after the house is less important to Leon. The following goal is agreed:

1. Leon will have a shower each day before lunch for a week.

Generate possible solutions to meet goals

Leon considers the following potential solutions to meet his goals:

1. Set his alarm clock for 11 am each day to remind him to have a bath.
2. Go to bed each evening no later than 10.30 pm to maximize his energy levels the following day.
3. Promise himself a reward if he manages to achieve his goal for the whole week.

Selecting the best strategy

Leon considers that all possible solutions have worth, and in fact are not mutually exclusive. However, he decides to focus on going to bed no later than 10.30, as he has been reading some information about energy conservation that his general practitioner had given him.

Putting it into action

Leon's occupational therapist encourages him to put his strategy into action as soon as possible. Eleanor thinks Leon's plan is a great idea and says she will encourage him to stick to it. Leon himself acknowledges that going to bed sounds easy, but that he is a creature of habit and enjoys watching American police dramas late at night on digital TV. To manage his strategy he will have to change some habits.

Leon's occupational therapist works with him to develop a wind-down routine for each evening. The aim of this is to help Leon develop new routines and manage his way around the perceived loss of TV. The occupational therapist suggests that Leon could record the programmes he is missing, but Leon dismisses this idea as he says there are so many repeats these days it would not be worthwhile. Instead, Leon decides to switch off the TV at 10 pm each evening and spend the last half an hour getting ready for bed.

Reviewing the progress

The practitioner leaves Leon to implement his plan of going to bed earlier and arranges to return in one week's time. When she returns, Leon reports that he had had a shower six days out of seven and that he had managed to get to bed before 10.30 pm four nights out of seven. On discussion Leon agreed that it was not necessary to think of an alternative strategy at this stage: he could see the benefits that going to bed earlier made on his energy conservation the following day and felt confident that he would be able to at least maintain his performance of the previous week, and potentially improve. Together Leon and his practitioner decided to move on and consider the other issues.

Summary

Problem solving is central to occupational therapy practice. It is used both as a theoretical framework to describe the general process of occupational therapy and as a specific technique, based on the cognitive-behavioural frame of reference, that is applicable for use with a wide range of clients.

The problem-solving basis of occupational therapy has been described and presented as a hypothetico-deductive approach (Opacich 1991, Hagedorn 2001) which has been criticised as insufficient for occupational therapy practice (Unsworth 1999). The danger of such criticism is that hypothetico-deductive reasoning may come to be no longer valued within occupational therapy. Instead, this chapter has presented the problem-solving hypothetico-deductive approach as one arm of the decision-making process (see Figure 10.1) and a central component to the process of shared decision making in practice (see Chapter 4).

The problem-solving process was presented as a useful therapeutic skill and intervention. The aim of working through the problem-solving process is twofold: firstly to help clients resolve problems that have proven too challenging to cope with without support. Secondly, to help clients learn the process of problem solving so that they are able to implement it without specific structured support in the future. Whilst routinely associated with working in mental health settings, the problem-solving process is in fact useful in a variety of settings with clients with a range of conditions. Whilst the problem-solving process appears intuitively obvious various factors can be taken into consideration to improve the manner in which this intervention is delivered.

References

Ajzen I, Manstead ASR 2007 Changing health-related behaviors: An approach based on the theory of planned behavior. In: K van den Bos, M Hewstone, J de Wit et al (eds) The Scope of Social Psychology: Theory and Applications, pp. 43–63. Psychology Press. New York

Chambers 1994 The Chambers Dictionary. Chambers Harrap Publishers, Edinburgh, UK

Duncan EAS 2006 The Cognitive Behavioural Frame of Reference. In: EAS Duncan (ed.) Foundations for Practice in Occupational Therapy 4th edn., pp. 217–232. Elsevier/Churchill Livingstone, Edinburgh, UK

Dutton R 2000 Clinical reasoning in physical disabilities, 2nd edn. Williams and Wilkins, Baltimore, MD

D'Zurilla TJ, Nezu AM 1999 Problem-solving therapy: A social competence approach to clinical intervention, 2nd edn. Springer, New York.

D'Zurilla TJ, Nezu AM 2000 Problem-solving therapies. In: KS Dobson (ed.) Handbook of cognitive-behavioral therapies, 2nd edn. Guilford, New York

Hagedorn R 2001 Foundations for Practice in Occupational Therapy, 3rd edn. Churchill Livingstone, Edinburgh, UK

Hagedorn R 2000 Tools for Practice in Occupational Therapy. Churchill Livingstone, Edinburgh, UK

Hawton K, Kirk J 1989 Problem-solving. In: K Hawton, PM Salkovskis, JW Kirk et al (eds) Cognitive behaviour therapy for psychiatric problems: a practical guide, pp. 406–426. Oxford Medical, Oxford, UK

Opacich KJ 1991 Assessment and informed decision making. In: C Christiansen, C Baum (eds) Occupational Therapy: Overcoming Human Performance Deficits, pp. 355–374. Slack, Thorofare

Paterson M, Summerfield-Mann L 2006 Clinical reasoning. In: EAS Duncan (ed.) Foundations for Practice in Occupational Therapy, 4th edn., pp. 315–335. Elsevier/Churchill Livingstone, Edinburgh, UK

Roberts AS 1996 Clinical reasoning in occupational therapy: Idiosyncrasies in content and process. The British Journal of Occupational Therapy 59(8): 372–376

Robertson LJ 1996 Clinical reasoning. Part 1: The nature of problem solving, a literature review. The British Journal of Occupational Therapy 59(4): 178–182

Unsworth C 1999 Cognitive and Perceptual Dysfunction: A Clinical Reasoning Approach to Evaluation and Intervention. FA Davis, Philadelphia, PA

Educational skills for practice

Tammy Hoffmann

Highlight box

- Education is a core component of all areas of occupational therapy practice and should be treated like any other intervention, with appropriate consideration given to its planning and evaluation.
- As well as imparting knowledge, education can also aim to alter clients' behaviour, attitude, beliefs, confidence, skills and decision-making ability.
- Appropriate education empowers clients and enables them to take responsibility for and participate in their health care.
- Educational theories, models and principles can serve as useful guides for therapists when they are planning educational interventions.
- When planning an educational intervention there are many decisions that therapists need to make and deliberation should be given to issues related to the content, format, timing and evaluation of the intervention, as well as clients' health literacy and any impairments that may impact the understanding of information.

Overview

The provision of educational interventions to clients is a major component of occupational therapy practice, regardless of the type of clients or setting. Educational interventions should be given the same level of regard as other occupational therapy interventions and planned, delivered and evaluated with an appropriate level of consideration and skill. Historically this has not always been the case, but awareness of the importance of effective client education has improved over recent years. This chapter overviews some of the issues that therapists need to be aware of and decisions that they need to make when providing educational interventions. This chapter introduces and overviews some of the major relevant educational theories that therapists should be aware of and guided by when providing client education. Some of the practical skills that therapists need and decisions that they need to make when planning an educational intervention are also discussed. Topics covered include: how to identify educational needs and establish educational objectives, considerations when making decisions about the format and timing of the education, how to assess clients' literacy levels and ensure that written health education materials are appropriately designed, and how to evaluate the outcomes of educational interventions.

The importance of client education and its historical context

Client education is a core component of occupational therapy practice and is an intervention that therapists provide frequently in their day-to-day work with clients. In a survey of Australian occupational therapists who work in physical dysfunction settings, education was identified by participants as one of the most frequently used interventions (McEneany et al 2002). Although there is limited research available that has explored the extent to which education is used in other areas of practice, there is no doubt that client education is an indelible component of all areas of clinical occupational therapy practice.

Client education should be considered as an intervention in its own right and when planning it, therapists should give it the same level of thoughtful consideration as they do other interventions. That is, relevant theoretical principles should be used to guide its design and provision, a collaborative client-centred partnership should be involved, consideration should be given as to the optimum timing and method of delivery of the educational intervention, and decisions about how the effectiveness of the educational intervention will be evaluated should be made prior to providing the intervention.

Unfortunately, client education is often not given the same level of consideration that is given to other occupational therapy interventions. McKenna and Tooth (2006a) have suggested some possible reasons for this. Therapists may not perceive education to be a specific treatment medium and consider it secondary to 'real' interventions that directly relate to the care and treatment of clients. Therapists may lack an understanding of educational theories and principles and the crucial role that education can have in empowering clients. Finally, therapists may consider education to be a basic and straightforward skill that does not require specialised planning or consideration. However, the success of many occupational therapy interventions depends on the client receiving effective education and if occupational therapists are to use education effectively in their daily practice, they need to understand the theories of client education and be knowledgeable about the practical considerations associated with providing education.

Historically, the practice of client education has not received much attention in occupational therapy. Until recently, occupational therapy textbooks have not explicitly addressed the issue of client education or provided readers with all of the knowledge and skills they need to provide effective educational interventions. Although texts have generally acknowledged that client education is an important component of occupational therapy practice and it has been mentioned as a component of occupational therapy intervention in many areas of practice, it has typically not been considered as an intervention in its own right that therapists need to have particular knowledge about and skills in. Similarly, the skills needed to provide effective client education have historically not been explicitly taught to occupational therapy students. Fortunately, this situation is changing. In recent years, there has been a growing number of journal articles published by occupational therapists that address the issue of client education, the topic of client education has been included as a separate chapter in occupational therapy textbooks and some university occupational therapy programmes now contain courses that are aimed at providing students with the knowledge and skills that they need to be effective client educators.

There are theories and models that can provide therapists with a broad framework for approaching and planning educational interventions. This chapter will overview some of the theories and models that are useful to consider when planning educational interventions and suggest some of the ways in which their principles can be practically applied. This chapter will also outline some of the practical issues that therapists need to make decisions about in order to provide effective educational interventions to their clients.

What is meant by client education?

Client education is often assumed to be merely about providing clients with information; however it is far more than that. Client education has been defined as '...a planned learning experience using a combination of methods such as teaching, counselling, and behaviour modification techniques which influence [clients'] knowledge and health behaviour' (Bartlett 1985: 323). The definition continues and highlights that client education is '... an interactive process which assists [clients] to participate actively in their health care' (Bartlett 1985: 323). This definition emphasises that it is changes in both knowledge and behaviour which are targeted by educational interventions. However, increased knowledge does not necessarily and automatically lead to behaviour change and there are some additional variables that often need to be targeted in an educational intervention. For example, therapists may also need to provide education that is aimed at: increasing a client's confidence in their ability to undertake the targeted behaviour/s, altering a client's attitudes or beliefs, facilitating a client's acquisition of skills, or enabling a person to make health-related decisions (van der Borne 1998, Tones 2002).

There are many ways in which education can occur. It can be incidental or planned, formal or informal. Often it is a one-to-one interaction between a therapist and a client. At other times it may take the form of a formal group education programme that a therapist conducts for a number of clients who have similar educational needs. There are also various formats that can be used to provide education, such as verbal, written, audio, video, computer-based or a combination of these. Considerations for the use of these formats are discussed later in the chapter.

Client education is often accompanied by family or carer education, in which therapists also provide education to clients' family or friends. Some of their informational needs may be the same as those of the clients, but they often also have their own specific needs that the therapist needs to address. As with clients, the educational needs of family or friends may extend beyond just knowledge needs and include needs such as learning new skills and developing confidence in performing particular tasks.

Vignette 11.1

Mr M is a 71-year-old gentleman who underwent a total hip replacement 2 days ago. He first met his occupational therapist at the preadmission clinic that he attended 6 weeks before his surgery. At that time, the therapist conducted an initial interview to gather information about his functional ability, home environment and social situation. During that session, the therapist explained the hip movement precautions that Mr M would need to adhere to in the weeks after surgery, the importance of doing so, and showed him some of the assistive devices that he would probably need to use after his surgery. When the occupational therapist sees Mr M for the first time after his surgery, he is anxious about his ability to return to doing self-care activities independently and can not remember any of the movement precautions.

Identifying educational needs

During initial consultation with clients, occupational therapists need to establish their clients' educational needs. One of the most effective methods of doing this is by asking the client (Lorig 2001). In Vignette 11.1, Mr M identifies that he would like to be reminded of the movement precautions and wants to know how he will be able to return to performing self-care activities independently. For clinical situations where there is a large number of topics that clients may wish to receive information about (for example, in stroke rehabilitation), therapists may find the use of a checklist of topics useful as this ensures that no topics are overlooked. There are a number of possible sources that therapists can use when compiling a checklist. These include: the therapist's and his/her colleagues' experience with similar clients, a survey or focus group of clients, and published research studies which have explored the educational needs of the client group.

Therapists may also wish to use more formal methods of evaluating clients' educational needs, such as questionnaires, scales or tests. One advantage of using a formal assessment is that it can be used as a baseline measurement and the assessment readministered after the educational intervention has been provided, as a way of evaluating the educational intervention. As highlighted at the beginning of this chapter, the aim of client education is to achieve more than just increasing a client's knowledge. Consequently, therapists will typically need to assess more than just the informational needs of the client. Formal assessments can be useful ways of doing this. For example, a therapist may use a combination of a knowledge test, self-efficacy scale and health behaviour checklist with a client in order to comprehensively identify the client's educational needs.

Although planning for an educational intervention commences with identification of a client's educational needs, therapists need to be aware that these needs are not static. Clients' needs will change over time, according to many variables such as the nature and stage of their medical condition and their readiness to change. Unless the therapist is only providing a one-off consultation to a client, a client's educational needs should be continually re-evaluated while the therapist is working with the client.

Setting educational objectives

Following identification of a client's educational needs, therapists should set objectives for the educational intervention. Objectives typically contain three elements: the *behaviour or action* that is to be achieved, the *condition* under which the behaviour/action will be achieved, and the extent *(criterion)* to which the behaviour/action should occur to consider the objective achieved (McKenna and Tooth 2006b). For Vignette 11.1, one of the objectives that the therapist sets for an educational intervention with Mr M may be as follows: 'After one 10-minute session that demonstrates hip movement precautions and also verbally explains them (condition), Mr M will be able to demonstrate the hip movement precautions (behaviour) correctly and without prompting from the therapist (criterion)'. The therapist could also set objectives for the other identified educational needs such as being able to independently use long-handled assistive devices. Setting guidelines enables therapists to impartially evaluate if the objective has been met at the conclusion of an educational intervention.

Deciding when to provide the information

Providing appropriate education to clients at the appropriate time is critical and can greatly impact the effectiveness of the educational intervention. The extent of information that is provided at any point in time will vary according to many factors. Clients may only want to receive brief information that is relevant to their immediate concerns when they are seriously ill, recently admitted to hospital, or recently diagnosed with a health condition. Later, they may want to receive more detailed information. Anxiety can prevent clients from absorbing and processing information (Theis and Johnson 1995). Therapists should consider clients' coping level and style each time that they provide information and be guided by clients' readiness to digest information. The optimum time to provide information will vary according to each client, their circumstances and needs, and the type of information being provided. The comprehension and recall of information can be facilitated if the information is provided in more than one format (such as verbal and written), repeated over time, and opportunities for reinforcement and clarification are provided (Theis and Johnson 1995).

Choosing the format of the educational intervention

Through discussion with the client, the therapist needs to determine the client's preferences regarding the format of the education and make decisions accordingly. Where possible, therapists should aim to use a combination of formats as this can often be more effective than using a single format (Theis and Johnson 1995). In addition to considering the client's preferences, other factors that therapists should consider when deciding on format include: the educational resources available to the therapist; the type of content being provided; and the client's cognitive abilities, educational level, impairments, preferred learning style (for example, visual or auditory), cultural background and primary language. Any impairment/s that clients may have (such as hearing, visual, cognitive or speech and language) can particularly influence therapists' choice of format as these impairments impact on how clients are able to process information. There are a range of strategies that therapists can use to facilitate communication with clients who have one or more of these impairments and further reading related to strategies specific to each impairment is recommended (refer to Further Reading section at the end of this chapter for details).

Although verbal education is the most frequently used format, Vignette 11.1 highlights one of the potential difficulties associated with verbal education which is that people frequently forget what they are told (Kitching 1990). It has been estimated that most people remember less than a quarter of what they have been told (Boundouki et al 2004). Consequently, verbal education should ideally be accompanied by written information that supplements or reinforces the main points that were made verbally (Hill 1997). The reinforcement that is provided by written materials can have a positive impact on the effectiveness of the educational intervention (Theis and Johnson 1995).

Written materials have a number of advantages such as: message consistency, reusability, portability, flexibility of delivery, permanence of information and they are economical to produce and update. In a client focus group that explored education, Tang and Newcomb (1998) found that clients sought answers to their questions at the time they formulate their questions. This usually occurred after the client had seen the health professional, not during the encounter. To some extent, written materials may be able to assist clients in answering the questions that occur when they are not interacting with a health professional. A further benefit of written materials is that clients can choose the level and amount of information that best suits them as their level of coping changes (Weinman 1990). Prior to deciding to use written materials with a client, the therapist needs to consider the factors listed earlier, such as the client's cognitive abilities, primary language, vision and reading ability. If a therapist chooses to proceed and use written materials with a client, it is essential that appropriate attention is given to the readability and design of the written materials.

Assessing clients' literacy levels

Prior to making a decision to provide a client with written information, therapists may wish to assess his/her literacy level. This can also provide therapists with information about the type and style of written information they should use with the client and enables therapists to alter their educational intervention according to the client's literacy level

(Weiss et al 1995). Therapists should be aware that people with poor literacy often use a range of strategies to hide literacy problems (Weiss et al 1995) and are often reluctant to ask questions so as not to appear ignorant (Wilson and McLemore 1997). Although asking about a client's education level may provide the therapist with some information about the person's reading ability, reading skill has not consistently been found to be dependent on educational attainment (Weiss et al 1995). Therefore, therapists should consider also assessing a client's reading ability formally (Weiss et al 1995, Wilson and McLemore 1997), using one of the published tests that have been designed for this purpose. Commonly used tests include: the Rapid Estimate of Adult Literacy in Medicine (REALM) (Murphy et al 1993), the Test of Functional Health Literacy in Adults (TOFHLA) (Parker et al 1995), and the Medical Achievement Reading Test (MART) (Hanson-Divers 1997). All of these tests evaluate a client's ability to understand medical terminology and are quick and straightforward to administer and score.

Readability of written materials

The reading level, or readability, of a written material refers to how easy it is to read. Written materials should be written simply, at the lowest level that conveys the information accurately (Hoffmann and Worrall 2004). Unfortunately, it is quite common for health education materials to be written at a reading level that is higher than the reading ability of the majority of the clients who received the materials (Sarma et al 1995, Beaver and Luker 1997, Griffin et al 2006, Hoffmann and McKenna 2006a).

If the reading level of the intended recipients of the material is known (see previous section for how to assess this), the reading level of the material should be two to four grades lower than the average reading level of recipients (Boyd 1987). If the reading level is unknown, a 5th–6th grade reading level (typically equivalent to 10–11 years of age in the Australian education system) is recommended (Doak et al 1996, Weiss et al 1998).

There are a number of readability formulas that allow the calculation of an estimate of the reading grade level of the material. Readability formulas are multiple regression equations and usually involve a calculation of one or more of: average word length in syllables, average sentence length in words, proportion of common words used, proportion of words with three or more syllables, and proportion of words which are monosyllabic (Ley and Florio 1996). Two well-known readability formulas are the SMOG (McLaughlin 1969) and the Flesch Reading Ease formula (Flesch 1948). The latter is available through some word processing programs such as Microsoft Word.

The SMOG is fast and simple to use, widely used in health research, and has been recommended as one of the best readability formulas for assessing health education materials (Meade and Smith, 1991). The SMOG readability formula calculates readability using the number of long words, defined as words of three or more syllables, in 30 sentences (McLaughlin 1969). In the SMOG, 30 sentences are selected from the material that is to be assessed – 10 consecutive sentences from near the beginning, 10 consecutive from the middle and 10 from the end of the written material. For this purpose, a sentence is any string of words punctuated by a period, an exclamation mark or a question mark. From the 30 sentences, words of three or more syllables are counted, including repetitions. From the word count, grade levels are then obtained by using the SMOG conversion table (most easily obtained from the Internet) or by determining the nearest perfect square root of the total number of words of three or more syllables and then adding a constant of 3 to the square root. For example:

Total number of words containing three or more syllables	67
Nearest perfect square	64
Square root	8
Add 3	11

In this example, the grade level of the material is 11 (typically equivalent to approximately 16–17 years of age in the Australian education system).

Design of written materials

Readability is only one element that contributes to the appropriateness of written health education materials. When designing new written materials or evaluating existing materials, there are a number of features in addition to readability that should be considered. Appropriate written health education materials contain content and design features that are designed to maximize the effectiveness of the written material. Ley (1988) summarised this issue simply by noting that for written information to be effective, it needs to be noticed, read, understood, believed and remembered.

When considering the content and design features that should be used in written health education materials, the following categorisation system can be a way of grouping the features: content, language, organisation, layout and typography, illustrations, and learning and motivation (Doak et al 1996). After reviewing literature concerning the design of written health education materials, Hoffmann and Worrall (2004) compiled a list of recommended content and design features that should be followed when designing written materials. The features are shown in Box 11.1. There are checklists available that therapists can use to evaluate the suitability of written materials that they have developed

Box 11.1

Recommendations for designing effective written health education materials

- Involve all key stakeholders, including clients, in the development and testing of the written material

Content
- Clearly state the purpose of the material
- Focus on providing information that is behaviour-focused (e.g. It is important that you do the exercises every day)
- Ensure that the content is accurate, up-to-date, evidence-based, and sources appropriately referenced
- Include the authors' names on the material and the publication date

Language
- Avoid judgemental or patronising language
- Aim for a 5th to 6th grade reading level (typically equivalent to approximately 10–11 years of age in the Australian education system)
- Use short sentences, expressing only one idea per sentence
- Use short words, preferably one to two syllables, where possible
- Use common words wherever possible. Avoid the use of jargon or abbreviations. Include a glossary if jargon or unfamiliar words are necessary
- Write in the active voice and in a conversational style
- Write in the second person (e.g. 'you' rather than 'the client')
- Structure sentences so that the context or old information is presented before new information. (e.g. 'To lower your risk of stroke {context}, you will need to make changes to what you eat' {new information})

163

(Continued)

Box 11.1—Cont'd

Organisation

- Sequence the information so that the information that patients most want to know is at the beginning
- Use subheadings
- Present the information using bulleted lists where possible
- Group related information into lists, list no more than 5 points in each list, and label each list descriptively
- Keep paragraphs short and express only one idea per paragraph
- Summarise the main points, either at the end of sections or end of the material

Layout and typography

- Use a minimum 12 point font size
- Avoid the use of italics and all capitals
- Only use bold type to emphasise key words or phrases
- Ensure good contrast between the font colour (e.g. black) and the background (e.g. white)

Illustrations

- Only use illustrations if they will enhance the reader's understanding
- Use simple-line drawings that are likely to be familiar to the reader
- Use an explanatory caption with each illustration

Learning and motivation

- Incorporate features that actively engage the reader (e.g. blank space to write questions down, short quiz, list 3 things that you should do)

(From Hoffmann T, Worrall L 2004 Designing effective written health education materials: considerations for health professionals. Disability and Rehabilitation 26:1166–1173, with permission from Taylor and Francis Journals. Available at: http://www.informaworld.com)

or those that have come from other sources and they are considering using them. Two of these checklists are the Suitability of Assessment of Materials (SAM) (Doak et al 1996) and a checklist of content and design characteristics that was developed by Paul et al (1997).

Adult learning theory

Vignette 11.1 involving Mr M is a useful case study to illustrate one of the theories, namely the Adult Learning Theory, that occupational therapists should be aware of and where possible, use to guide their provision of educational interventions to adults. Even paediatric occupational therapists need to provide education to adults; typically those who are significant in the child's life, such as their parents and teachers. The central premise of the Adult Learning Theory is that the learning process of adults differs to children and for successful adult learning, adherence to certain principles is necessary. The key principles are described below, along with some of the implications for practice:

- Adults *need to know why they need to learn something before beginning to learn it* (Knowles et al 1998). Planning of an educational intervention should commence with an assessment of the needs of the individual/s that are to receive the education. Education should meet the expressed needs of clients and their families.

Ironically though, clients often are not aware of their need for information, and if they do not know that they are lacking information, they may not perceive a need for it (Buckland 1994). Consequently, to facilitate a client's engagement in the learning process, therapists may need to initially educate a client about the reasons for needing to learn and the benefits of it, prior to conducting a needs assessment.

- Adults need to be *actively involved in learning*, rather than passive recipients of information (Knowles 1980), with the goal of empowering learners and encouraging them to become self-directed and responsible for their learning (Wyatt 1999). This can be assisted by encouraging clients to provide input into the design and delivery of educational experiences as much as possible and grading the goals and activities that are set so that confidence and success develop (Neufeld 2006).
- Adults have a *problem-centred orientation to learning* (Knowles 1980). It is important that the practical application of the concepts being learned is emphasised. This can be achieved by providing how-to information and opportunities for the practice of newly learnt skills.
- Adults enter the learning process with *prior experience* and it is important that clients' life experiences are acknowledged and utilised throughout the learning process (Knowles et al 1998). Therapists should identify clients' prior health experiences and other life experiences and establish their existing knowledge, skills and attitudes and plan educational interventions accordingly.
- Adults' *readiness to learn* will impact on the outcomes of their learning (Knowles 1980). Consequently, educational interventions should meet clients' expressed needs, be sequenced according to their readiness to learn, and appropriately target the clients' current confidence levels.
- Adults are most *motivated to learn when they see the content as relevant* (Knowles et al 1998). Providing education that meets clients' expressed needs, explaining how the education they receive will help to achieve their goals, what practical steps they can take to implement the information that they are receiving, and providing feedback on their progress can all assist in enhancing clients' motivation to learn.

Transtheoretical model

Occupational therapists often provide clients with education where the emphasis is on providing education that will enable clients to make longer-term behavioural or lifestyle changes. In addition to making decisions about the practical considerations of providing an educational intervention (such as educational needs, format and timing), there are other decisions that the therapist needs to make when the education aims to encourage

Vignette 11.2

Mr S is a 53-year-old gentleman who recently experienced a myocardial infarction. He has been discharged from hospital and is now attending an outpatient cardiac rehabilitation programme for the next 8 weeks. Mr S has been a cigarette smoker for the last 20 years, is about 15 kg overweight, does not participate in regular exercise, and has recently begun experiencing breathlessness on exertion. Part of the role of the occupational therapist on the cardiac rehabilitation team is to provide Mr S with information and strategies that will enable him to alter his lifestyle behaviours in order to improve his health and quality of life. Through careful questioning, the occupational therapist identifies that Mr S is currently in the preparation stage of change (as described below in the Transtheoretical Model).

the client to make lifestyle changes. The occupational therapist needs to establish how ready the client is to change as this will subsequently alter the educational intervention. The transtheoretical model can be a useful guide for therapists when planning an educational intervention, particularly when the ultimate aim of the education is behaviour change.

The transtheoretical model considers the transition points in behaviour change and the underlying factors that facilitate change from one stage to another (Prohaska and Lorig 2001). According to the transtheoretical model, change is a process that consists of six discrete stages and individuals move through these stages, although not necessarily in a linear fashion, as they adopt a behaviour (Prochaska et al 1992). Another element of this model is the process of change component, which states that there are specific activities that individuals use to progress through the stages (Prochaska et al 1992). The six stages, along with some strategies (Prochaska et al 1992, Neufeld 2006) that can be used to assist clients to move through the stages, are listed below.

- *Precontemplation* – the individual has no intention to change behaviour within the next 6 months. Strategies are aimed at increasing awareness and include activities such as providing information about the risk and the need for change.
- *Contemplation* – the individual has an awareness of a problem that needs action and intends to take action within the next 6 months. In this stage, the aim is to increase the individual's confidence and motivation to change by reemphasising the benefits of change, discussing possible action plans along with potential barriers and solutions to coping with them, and where appropriate, incorporating the support of family and friends.
- *Preparation* – the individual intends to change behaviour within the next month and in the past year has taken significant action towards the desired behaviour. The focus of this stage is initiating action and this can be facilitated by deciding on an action plan, breaking it into small steps and using goal setting to incrementally achieve each step, and implementing strategies to increase the individual's self-efficacy.
- *Action* – the individual has made observable behaviour change, to a specified criterion that is sufficient to reduce risks to health, within the past 6 months. The goal at this stage is to help the individual commit to the change. Possible strategies include providing encouragement and support, discussing and problem-solving any difficulties that have arisen, enlisting the support of family and friends, and planning to prevent relapse.
- *Maintenance* – the individual has changed behaviour for more than 6 months and is striving to prevent relapse. Strategies are aimed at helping the new behaviour become a lifestyle habit and include activities such as joining self-help groups (if applicable), exploring coping strategies, and implementing steps to prevent relapse.
- *Termination* – the individual has total self-efficacy regarding the behaviour and regardless of the situation, does not revert to previous undesirable behaviour. Self-efficacy in this model refers to an individual's confidence to cope in high-risk situations and not revert to engaging in undesirable behaviours (Prochaska et al 2002).

In the case of Mr S, he is currently aware that he needs to make changes to his lifestyle in order to improve his health and wellbeing and to reduce his risk of subsequent cardiac events. Mr S indicated to the therapist that he is interested in starting to make changes straightaway but that he is not sure how he should go about doing this and what he should do first. Part of the therapist's role with Mr S would be to collaboratively decide on which behaviour he would like to target first (e.g. stopping smoking, losing weight or exercising regularly), discuss the incremental steps that are involved in achieving the target behaviour, and convert each of those steps into specific and measurable goals.

Partnerships with clients

The case study with Mr S highlights the fact that educational interventions should be a collaborative partnership between the therapist and client and that educational interventions should be designed so that client participation is facilitated. The principle of collaborative practice and active participation by clients in their health care is also at the heart of client-centred care (Law and Mills 1998), which is a guiding philosophy of modern occupational therapy practice.

Historically, clients have had a passive role where they have been provided with only the information that the health professional thinks they need to know (Coulter 1997). However, over recent years there has been growing recognition of the need for clients to be active partners in their own learning. There are now various models of client–health professional relations that promote the active involvement of clients in their care, such as the active participation model (Roter 1987), client-centred care model (Coulter 2002), the chronic care model (Bodenheimer et al 2002) and when the focus is on making decisions, the shared decision-making model (Coulter 2002).

Involving clients as active partners in managing their health is an important contributor to the empowerment of clients (Coulter et al 1998). Results of research studies suggest that by increasing clients' sense of control and participation in medical care, they may be more motivated to manage their illness and perform the desired healthy behaviours, which may in turn lead to better outcomes (Greenfield et al 1988, Wyatt 1999). To become empowered and active participants in their care, clients need to be provided with information that they can use to manage their health. Without appropriate information, they cannot make informed decisions (Coulter 2002). However, establishing a client–therapist partnership requires more than just the provision of education that is tailored to the client's needs. It also involves a collaborative, two-way relationship between the therapist and client, where the client's beliefs, prior experiences, knowledge and preferences for receiving education contribute to the relationship, in addition to the therapist's expertise (McKenna and Tooth 2006a). It is important to note that while the above section has focused on the importance of actively involving clients in their own care, not all clients may desire this level of involvement and some may prefer a more passive role. This is a legitimate choice that should be respected (Coulter 2002). However the opportunity to be actively involved should be available for all who want to take it (Tones and Tilford 1994).

Health Belief Model

In addition to the Transtheoretical Model, there is another model that occupational therapists may find useful when planning educational interventions, particularly those where the aim is behaviour change. According to the Health Belief Model (Becker 1974, Glanz et al 2002), individuals are more likely to change their behaviour if they believe that:

- they are susceptible to the condition *(perceived susceptibility)*
- the condition is serious and if untreated will impinge on their lives *(perceived severity)*
- there are benefits of taking health action *(perceived benefits)*
- any negative aspects of the health action or barriers to undertaking it are outweighed by the benefits of the action *(perceived barriers)*.

Therapists can provide information that specifically targets each of the four main components of this model. In the case of Mr S, he has already experienced a myocardial infarction and was very unwell in hospital for a number of days as a result. He has therefore already experienced events which have provided him with evidence of his susceptibility and the seriousness of the condition. As a result of the education that he received while in hospital, he is also aware of the benefits of making lifestyle changes. However, he is uncertain as to whether the benefits will outweigh the barriers and costs of making the changes. As part of her role, Mr S's therapist could provide him with an action plan that contains specific how-to information, discuss potential barriers to implementation of the action plan, and in conjunction with Mr S, brainstorm solutions to overcome or cope with these barriers. If Mr S then decides that the benefits of taking action outweigh the tangible and psychological costs of taking action, it is likely that he may undertake the desired behaviour changes.

Self-efficacy

When clients have the necessary knowledge to undertake behaviour change, yet they do not change their behaviour, as is the case with Mrs C, it may be that their self-efficacy is low. Self-efficacy refers to an individual's judgement of his or her ability to perform an action to reach a desired goal (Bandura 1986). Because one of the goals of health education is behaviour change, self-efficacy has an important role to play in health education. Therapists should be cognisant of the important role of self-efficacy and where possible, should evaluate clients' self-efficacy (see section below on evaluating outcomes).

According to self-efficacy theory, a person is more likely to perform a particular behaviour if engaging in that behaviour is expected to result in desired outcomes (Bandura 1986). Even if individuals recognise the value in changing their behaviour, they also need to develop the confidence to carry out the behaviour prior to attempting the behaviour (Bandura 1986). Self-efficacy has been found to be a major determinant in the initiation and maintenance of behavioural change (Strecher et al 1986, Bandura 1997). Self-efficacy influences the amount of effort that an individual will put into a task and the length of time that he or she will persevere with the task in the face of obstacles (Bandura 1977). According to self-efficacy theory, self-efficacy can influence the acquisition of new behaviours, inhibition of existing behaviours and disinhibition of behaviours (Bandura 1977). It has been demonstrated that self-efficacy can be enhanced through education and that higher self-efficacy is related to successful attempts at behaviour change and improved health status (Lorig et al 1989, Clark et al 1992).

Therapists should realise that self-efficacy refers to specific behaviours in particular situations (Bandura 1977). It is not a global trait or personality characteristic and unlike personality characteristics which are difficult to alter, self-efficacy is malleable and able to be altered (Lorig and Holman 1993). When a therapist is attempting to alter self-efficacy, using the strategies described below, it is important that the therapist is specific about the change sought, as self-efficacy is specific to each behaviour (Glanz et al 2002). There are a number of strategies that therapists can use to enhance a client's self-efficacy (Strecher et al 1986, Prohaska and Lorig 2001), such as:

Vignette 11.3

Mrs C is a 49-year-old woman who was recently diagnosed with rheumatoid arthritis. Due to increasing pain in the joints of her upper limbs, she has been experiencing difficulty in performing basic and instrumental activities of daily living. She has been referred to an occupational therapist at her local community health centre. Her therapist identifies that Mrs C has a reasonable amount of knowledge about rheumatoid arthritis and how it affects joints, but she has not yet made any changes to the way in which she performs activities or commenced an exercise programme. Discussion with her therapist reveals that she is lacking confidence in her ability to incorporate these changes into her life.

- *Performance accomplishment or skill mastery* – this strategy involves using incremental goal-setting, breaking the desired behaviour into smaller steps, and ensuring the client achieves success in performing the easier steps before attempting the more difficult steps. The therapist working with Mrs C may use this strategy when teaching her joint protection techniques to enable her to perform activities of daily living with minimal discomfort.
- *Modelling* – this strategy involves clients observing other people who appear similar, such as their peers, performing the desired behaviour. If written information is used as part of the educational intervention, it is important that the modelling strategy is also applied to the written material and that it contains illustrations of people similar to the client in terms of characteristics such as age, body shape and ethnicity.
- *Verbal persuasion* – in this strategy, therapists talk with clients and emphasise the importance of performing the behaviour.
- *Reinterpreting signs and symptoms* – in this strategy, therapists clarify information with clients, correct any myths or misconceptions that they have, and aim to lessen clients' fear and anxiety about physiological signs and symptoms by explaining how to reinterpret them.

Additional formats for providing education

The case of Mrs C is a good example of how therapists may find formats other than verbal and written information valuable when providing educational interventions. For example, the use of demonstration, in addition to written and verbal information, when educating Mrs C about exercises, would be invaluable. The use of video cassettes or digital video discs (DVDs) that contain educational material can be useful, particularly when the education involves demonstrations, such as of movements, techniques, exercises or activities. For example, a DVD that demonstrates how to carry-out joint-protection and energy-conservation techniques while performing self-care and household activities may be useful to provide to Mrs C as it will reinforce information that has already been provided face-to-face by the therapist. By providing her with a DVD, Mrs C can review the information as many times as needed and at any time that she needs to. DVDs can also be useful when the topic being covered requires graphics to more effectively explain the content. Video presentation of information caters to clients with auditory learning styles, as well as those with visual learning styles and can assist clients who have low functional health literacy or English as a second language to understand the content being conveyed. Audio, video and written materials all have the added advantage that clients can share them with their family members, so that even if family were not present when the therapist was providing the information, they can still receive the information.

Another educational format that can be useful for supplementing and/or reinforcing information that is provided by therapists is computer-based materials. There are a number of ways in which computer programs can be used as an educational intervention, such as providing clients with interactive information (see for example, Stromberg et al 2002), helping clients to make health-related decisions (see for example, Hochlehnert et al 2006), or providing clients with tailored printed information that is customised according to their informational and visual needs (see for example, Hoffmann et al 2004). Although it depends on the features of the software being used, there can be advantages to using computer programs to provide information such as: they can enable clients to interact with the information, view it at their own pace, and view only information that is relevant to them, they often contain graphics that clients can interact with and this can assist with understanding the information, learning tools such as knowledge quizzes can be incorporated into them, and some computer programs enable clients to print out the information that they have viewed on screen, which therefore provides them with a resource that they can refer back to at any time. Computer programs should be designed so that they are user-friendly and able to be operated by individuals who do not

169

have computer experience. A recent systematic review of computer-based programs for people with coronary heart disease found that the programs were effective in increasing patients' knowledge and that they were generally well accepted by patients (Beranova and Sykes 2007).

In addition to computer-based programs, the Internet is also influencing the provision of education to clients. Health information is one of the most frequently searched topics on the Internet (McMullan 2006). Clients who wish to be active consumers of health information will have a need to seek out their own information either before and/or after they have seen their therapist (McMullan 2006). Therapists may find that clients will come to them with information that they have found on the Internet and wish to discuss. Therapists need to be aware that 'Internet-informed' clients will affect the traditional therapist–client relationship, and therapists should acknowledge clients' search for information, answer questions they have about information that they have found, and assist by directing them to reliable and accurate Internet sites (McMullan 2006).

Evaluating the outcome of educational interventions

Although therapists are accustomed to measuring outcomes and evaluating the effectiveness of interventions that they provide, they often do not apply the same process to educational interventions. Therapists should evaluate the outcome of any educational intervention that they provide, as they would after providing any other intervention, to determine whether the education had the intended effect and whether the stated objectives have been met. This information enables therapists to decide whether further education or reinforcement of the content is needed and whether the objectives, content and/or delivery methods of subsequent educational interventions should be altered to improve effectiveness (Hoffmann and McKenna 2006b).

The evaluation can be done either informally or formally, depending on factors such as the objectives of the educational intervention, the purpose of the evaluation, and the time and resources available. Methods of informal evaluation include seeking feedback from clients, ascertaining if they have understood the information that the therapist has provided to them, if their informational needs have been met, and if they have any unanswered questions.

In the case of Mrs C, an example of an informal evaluation would be asking Mrs C to correctly demonstrate the joint protection techniques that she was taught to use when doing household activities.

Formal evaluation typically requires administration of formal outcome measures and therapists must decide which outcome/s they will measure, which outcome measure/s they will choose, and when and how the outcome measure will be administered. Decisions about which outcome/s to measure should be guided by the objectives of the educational intervention. As one of the objectives in Vignette 11.3 was to improve Mrs C's self-efficacy for incorporating joint protection techniques into her daily routine, a self-efficacy instrument would be an appropriate outcome measure.

Decisions about which outcome measures/s to use will depend on whether there is an existing outcome measure that will adequately measure what the therapist needs to. There are many published health education measures (such as measures of knowledge for various conditions, satisfaction, self-efficacy, health behaviour, emotional health and quality of life) and many of these are freely available. The Redman (2003) resource that is listed in the Further Reading section at the end of this chapter overviews many of the published health education measurement tools. However, for many of the educational interventions that are provided by occupational therapists, an existing outcome measure will not exist. In this case, therapists will need to adapt an existing outcome measure or create their own. There are some general guidelines to follow when adapting or creating outcome measures and these are described in the Hoffmann and McKenna (2006b) reference that is listed in the Further Reading section at the end of this chapter.

After deciding which outcome measure/s to use, therapists also need to decide when the measure/s will be administered. Decisions about timing will be guided by the original objectives that were set for the educational intervention. For example, for educational interventions that had the objective of improving knowledge it is appropriate to evaluate them shortly after, such as on the same day the education has been provided, whereas it may be more appropriate to evaluate an educational intervention that aimed to change behaviour at a later time, such as a number of weeks after the intervention, so that clients have the chance to implement what they learnt. An advantage of formal evaluation is that therapists can readminister the same formal assessment that was used earlier when they were establishing clients' educational needs, and then compare changes in client's performance on the assessment (a pre-test post-test approach) that likely occurred as a result of participating in the educational intervention. Because the same outcome measure may be used at both the beginning and end of an educational intervention, when initially planning an educational intervention, therapists should also plan how they are going to evaluate the intervention.

Before proceeding with the evaluation, therapists also need to decide how it will be administered. There are many available methods and choice will depend on factors such as the information sought, the clients' needs and abilities, and the time and resources available (Hoffmann and McKenna 2006b). Use of a combination of methods is often most appropriate. Some of the most common methods of measuring outcomes include observation, interview, client self-report, open-ended questioning, questionnaires, scales, tests and diaries (Hoffmann and McKenna 2006b).

Summary

Client education is an important component of occupational therapy practice and for it to be effective, therapists need to have knowledge and skills in this area. Education aims not only to improve knowledge, but can also aim to alter clients' skills, behaviours, confidence and attitude. Therapists should design educational interventions according to relevant theoretical principles and give thoughtful consideration to practical issues such as the objective/s, format, timing and evaluation of the educational intervention. Where possible, there should be collaboration between the therapist and client and the provision of education should be guided by decisions that are made by this partnership so that clients are empowered to actively participate in their own health care.

171

Further reading

Fleming J, Onsworth T 2006 Educational partnerships with clients who have cognitive impairment. In: McKenna K, Tooth L (eds) Client Education: A Partnership Approach for Health Professionals, pp. 246–269. University of New South Wales Press, Sydney

Hickson L 2006 Educational partnerships with clients who have hearing impairment. In: McKenna K, Tooth L (eds) Client Education: A Partnership Approach for Health Professionals, pp. 226–245. University of New South Wales Press, Sydney

Hoffmann T, McKenna K 2006b Evaluation of client education. In: McKenna K, Tooth L (eds) Client Education: A Partnership Approach for

Health Professionals, pp. 159–182. University of New South Wales Press, Sydney

McKenna K, Liddle J 2006 Educating older clients. In: McKenna K, Tooth L (eds) Client Education: A Partnership Approach for Health Professionals, pp. 183–205. University of New South Wales Press, Sydney

Redman B 2003 Measurement Tools in Patient Education. Springer, New York

Worrall L, Howe T, Rose T 2006 Educating clients with speech and language impairments. In: McKenna K, Tooth L (eds) Client Education: A Partnership Approach for Health Professionals, pp. 206–225. University of New South Wales Press, Sydney

References

Bandura A 1977 Self-efficacy: Toward a unifying theory of behavioural change. Psychological Review 84: 191–215

Bandura A 1986 Social foundations of thought and action: a social cognitive theory. Prentice Hall, Englewood Cliffs, NJ

Bandura A 1997 Self-efficacy: The Exercise of Control. WH Freeman, New York

Bartlett E 1985 At last, a definition. Patient Education and Counselling 7: 323–324

Beaver K, Luker K 1997 Readability of patient information booklets for women with breast cancer. Patient Education and Counselling 31: 95–102

Becker M 1974 The Health Belief Model and personal health behaviour. Health Education Monographs 2: 324–508

Beranova E, Sykes C 2007 A systematic review of computer-based softwares for educating patients with coronary heart disease. Patient Education and Counselling 66: 21–28

Bodenheimer T, Lorig K, Holman H et al 2002 Patient self-management of chronic disease in primary care. Journal of the American Medical Association 288: 2469–2475

Boundouki G, Humphris G, Field A 2004 Knowledge of oral cancer, distress and screening intentions: longer term effects of a patient information leaflet. Patient Education and Counselling 53: 71–77

Boyd M 1987 A guide to writing effective patient education materials. Nursing Management 18:56–57

Buckland S 1994 Unmet needs for health information: a literature review. Health Libraries Review 11: 82–95

Clark N, Janz N, Dodge J et al 1992 Self-regulation of health behaviour: the 'take PRIDE' program. Health Education Quarterly 19: 341–354

Coulter A 1997 Partnerships with patients: the pros and cons of shared clinical decision making. Journal of Health Services Research and Policy 2: 112–121

Coulter A 2002 The autonomous patient: ending paternalism in medical care. The Nuffield Trust, London

Coulter A, Entwistle V, Gilbert D 1998 Informing patients: an assessment of the quality of patient information materials. King's Fund, London

Doak C, Doak L, Root J 1996 Teaching patients with low literacy skills, 2nd edn. JB Lippincott, Philadelphia, PA

Flesch R 1948 A new readability yardstick. Journal of Applied Psychology 32: 221–233

Glanz K, Rimer B, Lewis F 2002 Health behaviour and health education: theory, research, and practice, 3rd edn. Jossey-Bass, San Francisco, CA

Greenfield S, Kaplan S, Ware J et al 1988 Patients' participation in medical care: effects on blood sugar and control and quality of life in diabetes. Journal of General Internal Medicine 3: 448–457

Griffin J, McKenna K, Tooth L 2006 Discrepancy between older clients' ability to read and comprehend and the reading level of written educational materials used by occupational therapists. American Journal of Occupational Therapy 60: 70–80

Hanson-Divers E 1997 Developing a medical achievement reading test to evaluate patient literacy skills: a preliminary study. Journal of Health Care for the Poor and Underserved 8: 56–59

Hill J 1997 A practical guide to patient education and information giving. Baillieres Clinical Rheumatology 11: 109–127

Hochlehnert A, Richter A, Bludau H et al 2006 A computer-based information tool for chronic pain patients: computerised information to support the process of shared decision-making. Patient Education & Counselling 61: 92–98

Hoffmann T, McKenna K 2006a Analysis of stroke patients' and carers' reading ability and the content and design of written materials: recommendations for improving written stroke information. Patient Education and Counselling 60: 286–293

Hoffmann T, McKenna K 2006b Evaluation of client education. In: McKenna K, Tooth L (eds) Client Education: A Partnership Approach for Health Professionals, pp. 159–182. University of New South Wales Press, Sydney

Hoffmann T, Worrall L 2004 Designing effective written health education materials: considerations for health professionals. Disability and Rehabilitation 26: 1166–1173

Hoffmann T, Russell T, McKenna K 2004 Producing computer-generated tailored written information for stroke patients and their carers: system development and preliminary evaluation. International Journal of Medical Informatics 73: 751–758

Kitching J 1990 Patient information leaflets: the state of the art. Journal of the Royal Society of Medicine 83: 298–300

Knowles M 1980 The Modern Practice of Adult Education. Cambridge, New York

Knowles M, Holton E, Swanson R 1998 The Adult Learner, 5th edn. Gulf Publishing Company, Houston, TX

Law M, Mills J 1998 Client-centred occupational therapy. In: Law M (ed) Client-centred Occupational Therapy, pp. 1–18. SLACK, Thorofare, NJ

Ley P 1988 The use of written information. In: Ley P (ed) Communicating with Patients, pp. 125–140. Chapman & Hall, London

Ley P, Florio T 1996 The use of readability formulas in health care. Psychology, Health and Medicine 1: 7–28

Lorig K 2001 Patient Education: A Practical Approach, 3rd edn. SAGE Publications, CA

Lorig K, Holman H 1993 Arthritis self-management studies: a twelve-year review. Health Education Quarterly 20: 17–28

Lorig K, Chastain R, Ung E et al 1989 Development and evaluation of a scale to measure perceived self-efficacy in people with arthritis. Arthritis and Rheumatism 32: 37–44

McEneany J, McKenna K, Summerville P 2002 Australian occupational therapists working in adult physical dysfunction settings: what treatment media do they use? Australian Occupational Therapy Journal 49: 115–127

McLaughlin H 1969 SMOG grading: a new readability formula. Journal of Reading 12: 639–646

McKenna K, Tooth L 2006a Client education: an overview. In: McKenna K, Tooth L (eds) Client Education: A Partnership Approach for Health Professionals, pp. 1–12. University of New South Wales Press, Sydney

McKenna K, Tooth L 2006b Planning educational interventions. In: McKenna K, Tooth L (eds) Client Education: A Partnership Approach for Health Professionals, pp. 112–127. University of New South Wales Press, Sydney

McMullan M 2006 Patients using the Internet to obtain health information: how this affects the patient–health professional relationship. Patient Education and Counselling 63: 24–28

Meade C, Smith C 1991 Readability formulas: cautions and criteria. Patient Education and Counselling 17: 153–158.

Murphy P, Davis T, Long S et al 1993 REALM: a quick reading test for patients. Journal of Reading 37: 124–130

Neufeld P 2006 The adult learner in client-practitioner partnerships. In: McKenna K, Tooth L (eds) Client Education: A Partnership Approach for Health Professionals, pp. 57–87. University of New South Wales Press, Sydney

Parker R, Baker D, Williams M et al 1995 The Test of Functional Health Literacy in Adults: a new instrument for measuring patients' literacy skills. Journal of General and Internal Medicine 10: 537–541

Paul C, Redman S, Sanson-Fisher R 1997 The development of a checklist of content and design characteristics for printed health education materials. Health Promotion Journal of Australia 7: 153–159

Prochaska J, Di Clemente C, Norcross J 1992 In search of how people change: applications to addictive behaviours. American Psychologist 47: 1102–1114

Prochaska J, Redding C, Evers K 2002 The transtheoretical model and stages of change. In: Glanz K, Rimer B, Lewis F (eds) Health Behaviour and Health Education: Theory, Research, and Practice, pp. 99–120. Jossey-Bass, San Francisco, CA

Prohaska T, Lorig, K 2001 What do we know about what works? The role of theory in patient education. In: Lorig K (ed) Patient Education: A Practical Approach, pp. 21–55. SAGE publications, CA

Redman B 2003 Measurement Tools in Patient Education. Springer, New York

Roter D 1987 An exploration of health education's responsibility for a partnership model of client–provider relations. Patient Education and Counselling 9: 25–31

Sarma M, Alpers JH, Prideaux DJ et al 1995 The comprehensibility of Australian educational literature for patients with asthma. The Medical Journal of Australia 162: 360–363

Strecher V, McEvoy B, Becker M 1986 The role of self-efficacy in achieving health behaviour change. Health Education Quarterly 13: 73–91

Stromberg A, Ahlen H, Fridlund B 2002 Interactive education on CD-ROM: a new tool in the education of heart failure patients. Patient Education and Counselling 46: 75–81

Tang P, Newcomb C 1998 Informing patients: a guide for providing patient health information. Journal of the American Medical Informatics Association 5: 563–570

Theis S, Johnson J 1995 Strategies for teaching patients: a meta-analysis. Clinical Nurse Specialist 9: 100–105

Tones K 2002 Reveille for radicals! The paramount purpose of health education? Health Education Research 17: 1–5

Tones K, Tilford S 1994 Health Education: Effectiveness, Efficiency and Equity, 2nd edn. Chapman & Hall, London

van den Borne H 1998 The patient from receiver of information to informed decision-maker. Patient Education and Counselling 34: 89–102

Weinman J 1990 Providing written information for patients: psychological considerations. Journal of the Royal Society of Medicine 83: 303–305

Weiss B, Reed R, Kligman E 1995 Literacy skills and communication methods of low income older persons. Patient Education and Counselling 25: 109–119

Weiss B, Coyne C, Michielutte R et al 1998 Communicating with patients who have limited literacy skills: report of the National Work Group on Literacy and Health. Journal of Family Practice 46: 168–175

Wilson F, McLemore R 1997 Patient literacy levels: a consideration when designing patient education programs. Rehabilitation Nursing, 22: 311–317

Wyatt T 1999 Instructional technology and patient education: assimilating theory into practice. The International Electronic Journal of Health Education 2: 85–93

Group skills for practice in occupational therapy

12

Sharan L. Schwartzberg

Highlight box

- Essential leader functions are correlated to successful group outcomes.
- Group structure and process influence group outcomes.
- Effective leadership considers the individual, subgroups and the group as a whole.
- Problems in a group are not the fault of the member but rather a misconstruction in the leadership, membership and group process.
- Groups follow a developmental pattern. Leader skills and activity group processes employed are best geared to the group's phase of development.

Overview

Groups have been used in occupational therapy since the beginning of practice. There are a variety of skills needed to fulfil the essential functions of the leader role. These skills take into account the individual member's needs, concerns of the group as a whole, the environment and problematic forces within the group. By employing skills in a strategic manner the leader can be effective in helping both the individuals and the group function at its highest level. The leader must consider the group's phase of development in the types of process and activity suggested as well as role in the group. In early stages of a group the members will rely more on the leader for defining the purpose of the group and its process. As the group matures the leader may be able to be less active if the members are able to assume the leadership roles to support each other and complete the task.

Historical context

Occupational therapists have used groups in their practice from the outset. The types of groups have been influenced by changes in health-care delivery, needs of individuals

Table 12.1 Eras of group work in occupational therapy (Howe and Schwartzberg 2001)

Project era: 1922–1936

Socialisation era: 1937–1953

Group dynamics – Process era: 1954–1961

Ego building – Psychodynamic era: 1962–1969

Adaptation era: 1970–1990

Wellness era: 1990–2000+

and populations, and shifts in theoretical models for practice. Howe and Schwartzberg (2001) identified six eras of group treatment in occupational therapy (Table 12.1).

The skills needed for practice have shifted from focus on the activity and therapeutic relationship to incorporating research evidence as a basis for practice. The technical skills for intervention presented in this chapter require reasoning about needs of the client, the group as a whole and environment. These skills need to be adapted to the type of setting where occupational therapists employ groups. Intervention programmes using groups include: schools, hospitals, outpatient clinics, community agencies and natural environments such as families, organisations, work teams and living facilities.

Leadership functions and skills

Critical leadership functions

Yalom and Leszcz (2005) identified four empirically researched significant leadership functions. These include:

1. '*Emotional activation* (challenging, confronting, modelling by personal risk-taking and high self-disclosure)
2. *Caring* (offering support, affection, praise, protection, warmth, acceptance, genuineness, concern)
3. *Meaning attribution* (explaining, clarifying, interpreting, providing a cognitive framework for change: translating feelings and experiences into ideas)
4. *Executive function* (setting limits, rules, norms, goals; managing time; pacing, stopping, interceding, suggesting procedures)' (p. 536).

These basic leadership functions were derived from observing leader behaviours (not what they say they do) and were found to have a significant relationship to outcome. 'The most successful leaders, then – and this has great relevance for therapy – were those whose style was moderate in amount of stimulation and in expression of executive function and high in caring and meaning attribution' (Yalom and Leszcz 2005: 537).

How to compose a group and establish a group contract

Before starting a group the leader should survey the population and individual member needs. The survey should include an assessment of functioning in cognitive, social-emotional and physical motor areas. Population-based needs are more general and

Table 12.2 Schwartzberg 'Need and Ask' group criteria checklist

- Need: Belonging with others to validate concerns and learn ways to compensate
- Ask: Are there individuals with like diagnosis, disability or impairment who would feel validated by being with others in a similar situation to gain support and learn new coping mechanisms?
- Need: Disability leaves individual socially isolated
- Ask: Are there individuals who are alone because they lack the ability to seek out others because of problems in functioning in daily activities?
- Need: Functional ability impairs performance in social roles such as worker, student, retiree, homemaker and volunteer
- Ask: Are there individuals who can no longer function in a social role because of a functional impairment?

require assessing community resources and the impact of disease, disability or prevention on individuals with common problems such as post-traumatic head injury, chronic illnesses effecting function, mental illness, learning problems and so on. The Schwartzberg 'Need and Ask' Group Criteria Checklist can help determine the need for a group (Table 12.2).

Once you determine a need for the group you should decide three basic things:

1. How many members will you have in the group?
2. Will it be closed to new members once started or will it be open for new members?
3. How many sessions will the group meet?

In beginning a group the leader frequently presents a group contract to members. This may be discussed in an individual session with the client or in the group itself. Group contracts include things such as (a) expectations for participation and potentially payment, (b) consequences for lateness and absences, and (c) expectations about confidentiality, putting thoughts into words and not actions, and outside contact between members. A group contract helps to promote safety and caring through clear boundaries and predictable expectations. Contracts can be written or verbal agreements. They are often tested and need to be openly discussed and followed through within reason. The overall aim of the contract is to provide an emotional container so the work of the group can be accomplished.

How to select members and activities for a group

In deciding on what type of group to conduct leaders should assess the level of member ability and determine group goals. The selection of modality would depend upon members needs. Modalities range from educational groups, activities of daily living, arts and crafts, horticulture, expressive and constructive activities, and leisure interest and vocational activities. No matter the modality the activity is adapted to member need and functioning. Other factors that require consideration are the leader's role and the group's phase of development.

Leaders may need to be highly directive in selecting an activity or can facilitate a group to make decisions about the activity programme. Where members need a lot of emotional support the leader may need to take on roles of encourager and mediator while validating the value of the individual to the group's process. It is usually advantageous to work with a co-leader to share in the task and emotional aspects of facilitating a group especially when members are highly limited in functioning.

How to structure the overall group and individual sessions

Howe and Schwartzberg (2001) have designed several protocols to help with assessing needs, planning and evaluating groups. These protocols include: group history, assessments of members, a general group plan protocol and session evaluation protocol (Schwartzberg et al 2008).

Creating the group

Vinogradov and Yalom (1989) identify essential tasks in creating a group. These tasks include (a) building group culture and climate (pp. 43–55), (b) patient selection and composition (pp. 43–47), and (c) pre-group preparation (pp. 47–50). These leader activities need to be modified depending upon the setting and programme structure.

Building group culture and climate

The leader creates the atmosphere by setting expectations. It is the leader's responsibility to foster an environment that is therapeutic. In occupational therapy this often involves matching the task to member ability and function. The leader must ensure that the space is adequate for the activity and accessible to accommodate a range of abilities. Establishing clear norms for procedures are a part of building the group culture. These norms may include things such as who has responsibility for setting up the activity and clean-up. An example of the impact of group culture on process and realignment of the dynamics is given in Vignette 12.1.

Patient selection and group composition

In selecting group participants the major challenge is matching individuals so that they all can function well together to perform the task. Alternatively the group may have heterogeneous membership to augment learning from others who are different. The leader may decide to compose the group with individuals who are similar to heighten feelings of belonging and to make an easier match between the demands of the task and member functioning. See Table 12.3 for group inclusion criteria in occupational therapy.

Vignette 12.1

Building a group culture and climate (by Jenni Guest)

When new facilitators took on an art group for patients with mental illness, they observed that members were always late. Members never stayed for the continuous duration of the group, often popping in and out throughout the session and weekly attendance was sporadic. The new facilitators were concerned about these trends, as it was creating an unsettled climate within the group. When raised for discussion with group members the main comments made centred around the behaviour of the previous facilitators, stating that 'the previous leader was never on time, often cancelled sessions with no warning and was always leaving the group for a cigarette break or for a phone call'. This highlighted the impact that the facilitators' behaviour and attitudes had on how group members used and treated the group. The new facilitators realised that they had to reestablish the group culture. They chose to do so through formally ending the original group, having a short break and then starting a new art group and all of this was discussed and agreed with group members. The facilitators asked the group members to name the new group, in the aim of encouraging a climate of ownership and commitment, and ensured that the group always started on time, with no facilitator breaks for cigarettes or phone calls.

Table 12.3 Occupational therapy group inclusion criteria

- Able to tolerate participating in activity with others
- Able to concentrate on task in the presence of others
- Willingness to arrive on time and stay in the group for the session
- Functional ability in cognitive, psycho-social, motor and language skills to engage in task

Vignette 12.2

Pre-group preparation (by Jenni Guest)

When auditing a music group being facilitated by two other occupational therapists, I remember watching the look on a new group member's face when the first activity was introduced. The activity involved listening to a piece of music and then on the second listen using movement and dance to demonstrate how the music made you feel. This particular member looked totally shocked and horrified at the idea of dancing or using movement within a group of people who she did not know. At the end of the session when talking to this client it became clear that her understanding of a music group had been very different than what she had encountered. She had thought the group focused on music appreciation and it turned out to be more of an exploratory use of music to express emotions. Sadly this confusion led to her choosing to not access any group services through the centre.

Pre-group preparation

The aim of preparing the member in advance of the first session is to help members understand the purpose and tasks of the group. This may involve explaining the reasons why the group will be helpful, clarifying expectations for participation, and allaying fears of group participation. To avoid member drop out it is good practice to carefully explain the nature of the group activities and the value to the individual. Vignette 12.2 illustrates the impact of lack of preparation on a group member.

If at all possible it is a good idea to meet with a new group member prior to group participation. See Table 12.4 for topics to include in occupational therapy pre-group preparation meeting.

How to engage individual members and the group as a whole

There are many techniques to use for engaging individuals in a group. A few that you may find useful are: bridging activities, communicating with the individual in relation to the group theme, and showing and telling how the activity matches with the group purpose.

Bridging

The technique used to bring people in closer connection and to develop a powerful group identity is called 'bridging' (Ormont 1990). In occupational therapy clients often lack the social skills and emotional or cognitive capacity to easily form emotional and social

Table 12.4 Occupational therapy pre-group preparation meeting topics

- Explain purpose of group and its expected value
- Describe expectations for participation, including things such as: regular attendance, beginning and ending times of meeting, putting thoughts and feelings into words (no verbal or physical abusive behaviour), procedures in event of illness or other unexpected absence, payment (where appropriate), confidentiality, and prohibitions about out of group socialisation, if any
- Describe what to expect in the sessions, necessary preparation before or after the meetings, the relationship of the group to other interventions, the leader and member roles

connections. Using members as 'bridge builders' is most desirable (Ormont 1990) although not always feasible given the level of function of clients. The members may lack the insight or emotional attunement to sense the perspective of others. It is the leader's task to role model and facilitate group members to become bridge builders. Three methods of leader initiated bridging are suggested (Boxes 12.1, 12.2, 12.3): (1) 'by open-ended questioning', (2) 'by directed questioning', and (3) by 'questioning a member about an interaction taking place between two others' (Ormont 1990: 8–9).

As with any technique bridging should be used judiciously. Ormont warns against its use (1) when focusing on an individual will be traumatic or frightening to the person, (2) at the end of a session with a person who is timid, (3) when two members are communicating well and adding a third would be a hurdle, and (4) as a means to protect the therapist who is challenged by a difficult group situation such as feeling attacked.

Box 12.1

Open-ended questioning

Asking one member about how he or she thinks another member feels (Ormont 1990):
'What do you think Tim feels when he leaves the room before we finish the activity?'
Asking one member about another member's pattern of behaviour (Ormont 1990).
'What happens with Tim when he does not get help on his project from Sarah?'

Box 12.2

Directed questioning

Asking a question so that it sounds like an interpretation to invite another member to comment (Ormont 1990).
'I wonder if you are aware that Tim feels very disappointed when he is not asked to talk about his painting?'

Box 12.3

Questioning a member about an interaction taking place between two others

Asking an important question of a third member to help create a bridge between two other members (Ormont 1990).
Leader asks John, 'What feeling is Tim keeping from Sarah at this moment'?

Communicating with the individual in relation to the group theme

Group members may have difficulty understanding how the process is relevant to their situation. The leader can take an active role in explaining how the process or content of a session relates to their intervention goals or situation. When the member is capable the leader may encourage the client to explore the meaning of the themes.

'Showing and telling' how the activity matches with the group purpose

In occupational therapy the group activity, whether it be what Mosey (1970) calls a 'parallel' or 'cooperative' one, has a therapeutic purpose. In a parallel group members work side by side on individual tasks. The leader structures the activity and supports members' social emotional needs. In a cooperative level group the leader is in an advisory role. The group is likely to have more consistent attendance, successful outcomes, and client satisfaction when the activity matches the understood purpose of the group. In Vignette 12.3 the group leader introduces an activity that would seem ordinary, perhaps even silly or confusing, without an explanation of its therapeutic value given the group's purpose.

181

How to structure process from formation stage to ending stages of a group

Groups are known to go through various phases of development (Agazarian and Gantt 2003). Although there are several configurations of group development, there are broadly five stages of development (Tuckman 1965, Tuckman and Jensen 1977):

1. 'Forming' stage – developing trust and goals
2. 'Storming' stage – resisting leader authority
3. 'Norming' stage – finding common goals and expectations
4. 'Performing' stage – working on group goals
5. 'Adjourning' stage – separating, consolidating gains, planning for future.

In leading a group the leader assumes a more active role in the beginning stage. This may involve setting up the activity room and explaining specific procedures. In order to facilitate development of trust the leader needs to maintain the group's boundaries and be

Vignette 12.3

'Showing and telling': How the activity matches with the group purpose (by Jenni Guest)

While facilitating a group known as 'Making Changes' we often used what appeared to be random games and activities as tools to introduce a deeper topic or theme that the group was addressing. When working through a series on self-esteem and confidence I remember using an altered version of 'spin the bottle' to introduce the session. It involved the spinning of the bottle and whoever the bottle landed on the group member had to compliment them or thank them for something that they appreciated or had noticed about that member during their time in the group. The member being complimented then had to acknowledge and thank the person for the comment. Each member found this challenging on some level and there was a high level of laughter.

The purpose of the activity had been three-fold, firstly, to 'break the ice' at the beginning of session introducing the topic for the week with some fun, secondly, to introduce the concept of giving and receiving compliments and identifying good characteristics in those around you. And lastly, to allow members to experience others making compliments about them and introduce a discussion on how members felt receiving them and whether people felt comfortable accepting what people had said. The function of the activity was only utilised when the facilitator discussed the activity with group members exploring what its aim and purpose was, and providing a wider discussion platform concerning self esteem, compliments and confidence.

---

consistent in expectations and availability. As the group is able to assume more leadership the activity may be shared as well as the responsibility for deciding on the activity, materials needed, group process, and preparations for ending the session. In Vignette 12.4 a group leader describes her experience of turning points in variety of groups and their development.

Vignette 12.4

How to structure group process from forming stage to adjourning stage (by Jenni Guest)

Introducing from the start of a group meeting the idea of group closure can be a useful way of managing the stages of a group. However this is only appropriate in certain groups, such as those where members have a limited number of sessions – for example, anxiety management, anger management, and symptom and medication management groups on an inpatient unit. With more vulnerable group populations or groups that have an undefined length the therapist intervenes as individual members terminate participation.

When starting a new gardening group an effective way I found of encouraging the group to develop trust and establish goals was for the first group session to be spent at the garden centre. As a group the members chose the items to use and reviewed the

Vignette 12.4 continued

purpose of what the time in the group would be. As a facilitator my main contribution was providing both the opportunity and finances, and driving the mini-bus. Instantly from the start the group had a sense of purpose, ownership, and began establishing effective communication and trust relationships.

Whether to mark the closure of a group is something that the group needs to decide as a whole, but to acknowledge the closure is something the facilitators have responsibility to ensure happens. One group I was a member in, not facilitator, acknowledged the closure through having a photograph taken of the whole group. It was almost a way to taking part of what you had gained and learned through the group process away with you. When ending a group because of leaving a post I have found this substantially different and harder, and attempted to avoid taking responsibility for it. The group, however, took the initiative and decided themselves to mark the ending, through the sharing of cards and a time of sharing what they had gained from being a part of the group.

Self-disclosure

Group leaders must decide how much to share in the group of their own personal reactions and situation. Storytelling is a common technique used in occupational therapy to convey information, develop a personal connection and establish rapport (Schwartzberg 2002). Therapists exchange stories with clients to promote alliances and collaborative relationships (Mattingly and Fleming 1994). They must make explicit decisions about how much to share based on the best interests of clients. Vignette 12.5 illustrates the process of clinical reasoning used in leader self-disclosure.

Vignette 12.5

Therapist self-disclosure (by Jenni Guest)

When facilitating my first anger management group, the format of the sessions meant that in the last 15 minutes of each session I asked the group to share openly about their own personal experiences of anger, and dependent on the topic discussed that week on the worksheets, to reflect on a specific example relevant to that topic. At these moments in the group sessions, I remember being mystified as to why the group dynamics changed so dramatically. The process moved from a talkative and engaged group to one that was unresponsive and appeared to have completely disengaged.

During session number 4 I followed the same format of the group, however when silence descended again in the last 15 minutes I decided that I needed to address this to the group through reflecting my concerns. At this point one particular member addressed me directly and asked 'Why each week do you ask us to share with you our experience, when you haven't shared anything personal with us in the last 3 weeks'?

He was right. On reflection I could see that his statement was true. I had up until that point followed, almost word for word, the pre-designed worksheets that the previous occupational therapist had left for me. Not once had I used a personal illustration to support the topics we had discussed. As a relatively new occupational therapist at the time I spent the remainder of that week wrestling with the conflict in my mind between the member's statement and the professional theory I thought I was adhering to, always maintain clear therapist and patient boundaries. However, the question that remained clear to me was why should they share with me, someone

Vignette 12.5 continued

who purely sits, listens and asks them to participate in tasks or answer questions but never discloses any information or completes any of the tasks for themselves? How would I act if I were a group member and not the occupational therapist facilitating it?

Within the next anger management group session I decided to start the session differently and opened by reflecting to the group my thought process following the member's question from the previous session. I then continued to introduce, using a personal experience as an example, the topic for discussion during the session that week. Slowly during that and the subsequent remaining five sessions, the group and I gained comfort and confidence in confiding personal experiences within the group. The group began to discuss these situations and identify with each other, relating similar scenarios that they had experienced. The use of appropriate self disclosure by the occupational therapist within the group led the way for other members to share more openly their stories and ultimately allowed the group to evolve into what I viewed as a more effective vehicle to assist its members to learn and explore new techniques to managing their anger.

Process comments

To enhance members' capability to self-monitor the leader can summarise observations and then ask members to explain what they see happening in the group (Vinogradov and Yalom 1989). For example, the leader notes, 'I notice that half the group is doing the project at one end of the table and the other at the far side of the room. I wonder, what do you see happening?' Yalom and Leszcz (2005) explain that through process comments the client goes through a sequence in the change process as follows:

1. 'Here is what your behaviour is like' (p. 180).
2. 'Here is how your behaviour makes others feel' (p. 180).
3. 'Here is how your behaviour influences the opinions others have of you' (p. 180).
4. 'Here is how your behaviour influences your opinion of yourself' (p. 181).

The use of process commentary is very helpful in supporting members to take the initiative in directing their own behaviour rather than relying on the therapist or blaming others. A clear example of the value of process comments is illustrated in Vignette 12.6 where family members learn to observe and process their own behaviour.

Reality testing

Understanding the patterns of one's own behaviour through getting impressions from others is commonly referred to as 'reality testing'. This process can take place through hearing other members' and the leader's observations. Similar to process comments, reality testing focuses on opportunities in the group for consensual validation of the member's own observations with others in the group (Howe and Schwartzberg 2001, Schwartzberg et al 2008).

Reframing

In order to create a safe and positive group environment the leader tries to minimise conflict and increase a sense of support (Vinogradov and Yalom 1989). By reframing, the leader puts things in a way that emphasises the member's positive intentions, efforts

Vignette 12.6

Process comments (by Jenni Guest)

When I first graduated and working with experienced group workers I remember panicking when people discussed process comments, and wondered what I was doing that day when it was covered at university. On reflection it is something we do all the time, just within a different context. When working on a ward for patients with severe and enduring mental illness I remember observing one particular family interaction when they visited their son, the picture and rhythm of interaction was almost identical on every visit. When one family member started to talk, another would interrupt until finally one member would get frustrated and leave the situation.

During the end of his stay on the ward the patient's family requested some family work to be completed prior to him moving into the community from hospital. This was offered and the group comprised of providing information, promoting effective communication within the family unit and supporting discussion and problem solving of concerns the family and patient had about him moving from hospital. When first starting the sessions it was clear that the interaction between members in the family unit was going to be the same within the group as what had been observed on the ward. Therefore to try to develop a culture and climate of listening within the sessions the facilitators used process comments to reflect back to the family what behaviour and patterns of interaction were being observed. For example, a process comment was, 'I've been observing that every time someone starts to talk they are interrupted, and was wondering how that makes you all feel'?

For the first four sessions with the family the majority of facilitator time was spent reflecting back that the group boundaries to listen to one another were not being adhered to and reflecting the effective communication that happened when they were listening. By the fifth session the family themselves were reflecting back process comments about how they were interacting and praising individual members of the family. In the family work evaluation one of the points of feedback given concerned their interaction, and how until someone had reflected back to them as a group their pattern of communication they had not realised what they were doing. But stating that both within and outside of the family work sessions they feel more able to talk and communicate as a family.

and contributions. For example, a member in a loud voice demands another member turn over supplies needed to complete an activity. The therapist may say, 'Mary, you seem in a big rush and putting pressure on John to finish quickly. I know you really want to bring home your project and show your family what you have accomplished in occupational therapy. In this group we have enough supplies for everyone. Come with me and I will show you the cabinet where you can get your own supplies next time you need something'. By reframing the situation the leader again reinforces the member's own capacity to do and thereby enhancing the member's self-esteem and defusing what could become an explosive interaction in the group. A poignant story is told in Vignette 12.7 where a group and a member's behaviour when given context or reframed changes meaning.

Giving feedback

The process of feedback is stating your reaction to another person (Howe and Schwartzberg 2001). For example, the group leader says, 'as much as I would like to help you with your project, Fred and I are both occupied. I notice that when someone else in the group needs my help you immediately ask for my assistance. Although

Vignette 12.7

Reframing (by Jenni Guest)

Within a gardening group on an elderly neuro-rehabilitation unit I remember being faced with one gentleman who repetitively made statements within the group that focused on other members of the group deliberately behaving in a way to isolate or annoy him. Such complaints included not passing him items that he wanted, not talking to him within the group, or choosing to sit next to other people in the group. The member's belief around these situations and scenarios was firmly focused on the others' behaviour being deliberately negative towards him. Specifically he believed people did not want him in the group and that this was evidenced as group members never passed him items that he asked for when completing activities.

As group facilitator, I took the lead on working with the member within the group to look at the situation and try to reframe his belief and thinking around this situation. The phrase 'I appreciate how you feel, but do you think there is another way of looking at that' being one of the most useful phrases at that time. This simple statement both acknowledged his feelings and position, whilst also encouraging a time of thinking around the situation and providing an opportunity to reframe the situation in a more realistic and true manner.

In truth, some of the origins of the member's frustrations were quite grounded. He often did not get passed what items he asked for in the group. When thinking it through we were able to identify the real reason and therefore reframe his belief that ignoring him was a personalised and deliberate act. The true answer was quite simple; he had badly slurred speech and was only able to talk quite quietly, whilst others in the group were hard of hearing. This was discussed within the group, and a new way of sharing items amongst group members was agreed that included thinking about how each member could communicate in a manner to accommodate all members' individual needs.

I feel under pressure to help you immediately it may take a few moments until I can. Taking turns can take some practice'. Feedback is best timed when members are calm, not defensive, and as close to the event as possible. If the feedback is not well received, the member appears anxious, angry or is defensive; it is best to stop and try to reframe the situation.

Structured exercises versus open process

The leader needs to think about when it is to the group's advantage to use structured exercises and when it is preferable to listen and attend to themes as well as needs emerging in the session. In settings where there is a quick turnaround for group participation standardised group activity protocols have advantages. The risk is in missing important process themes necessary to successful outcomes for individuals and the group as a whole. For example, the loss of a group member or staff member may be emotionally difficult for a group. To proceed ahead with a standard activity would aid in the denial and separation with the individuals.

Leaders are best off seeking a balance between structure, product and process. The main question to gauge these choices is: What is in the best interest of the clients and group as a whole? By structuring the group task to the members' level of capability therapeutic outcomes are more likely. The leader should take into consideration the members' level of functioning in domains of cognitive, social, motor and communication. Environmental factors such as the size of the room, type of furniture, noise level, distractions and physical climate should also be monitored and adjusted to the needs of group members. For example, a predictable arrangement of furniture and materials enhances a sense of safety. The hazards of overly structuring a group are illustrated in Vignette 12.8 along with an example of group-centred use of structure and open-ended process.

How to intervene with problematic forces in a group

It is the leader's responsibility to maintain as cohesive a group as possible. This means addressing diminished group functioning when subgroups form, individuals become a scapegoat for group issues, and there is competitiveness, lateness, absenteeism, boundary violations, or anger in the group. It is the leader's obligation to maintain the safety of each member by, for example, sticking to the contract and stated expectation of the group such as when to begin and when to end. By helping members to see commonalities as much as possible projections are diminished. Vignette 12.9 illustrates the value of establishing a contract with members around expectations.

The leader's success in intervening is highly dependent on self-awareness and knowing aspects of the member's behaviour that trigger idiosyncratic responses in the leader. The member's behaviour may also call upon a common reaction from others. By understanding these factors the leader can better modulate the response to the group and members.

Problematic group forces

Problematic behaviours often arise in a group. Rather than see these as destructive elements, or what Nitsun (1996) calls 'anti-group' phenomena, as he suggests, the leader can mobilise the group to enhance its creative potential. See Box 12.4 for examples of problematic forces in a group and self-reflective questions for the leader.

Summary

In this chapter the nature of group work in occupational therapy was explained. The leader's role in composing, leading and evaluating a group were summarised. Protocols for planning and evaluating a group were identified; techniques for engaging the individual and group as a whole were summarised. Common issues that are problematic in a group were identified. Finally, the value of leader self-awareness was stressed.

Vignette 12.8

Structured exercises versus open process (by Jenni Guest)

When asked to provide feedback following a group session one set of patients described the experience as 'the blind leading the blind'. In this case the facilitators were standing in for other members of staff and followed the session plans left word for word throughout the group session. However the rigidity that this brought to the group, on reflection, did not allow for the group to take ownership of the material and mould how they were going to work through the session material that week. In this example the balance was wrong between structure and openness. Even when using structured exercises, as facilitators, there is a need to react and interact with the group continuously moulding the materials available to meet the needs of the group that session.

In one anger management session, this meant that only the first activity that had been formally planned was completed that session. The group discussion that came out of that activity was so productive and relevant for the group at that time it would have been wrong to force them to move onto the next item on the plans list.

Vignette 12.9

Establishing a contract (by Jenni Guest)

Recently, during a course on group work, I was involved in setting up a short-term group for children within a pre-school. During the pre-planning discussion with management it had been emphasised to us that the philosophy of the centre was to positively reinforce good behaviour but to not reprimand or discipline children for inappropriate behaviour. On arrival at the pre-school and meeting the children my co-worker and I were excited by the prospect of spending time there and optimistic about what we could offer them during our time there. However, it became clear through the first two sessions that this was going to pose a difficulty for us. During the sessions we found ourselves as leaders purely crisis managing the behaviour of our group of five children aged between three and five, as opposed to running the activities we had planned. The children's behaviour was not the only difficulty; consistently throughout the group the children wanted to leave and then return, interrupting any flow of activity that we had managed to establish.

At this point my co-worker and I decided we needed to take a proactive stance at establishing a set of ground rules with the children that when in the group would be followed. On reflection I think we had not done this on group commencement because the children were so young and we had assumed that as leaders we could just enforce group rules on the children. How wrong were we? During the next group session we set out a large piece of paper on the floor, and started the session with all the children sitting around it. Then taking turns around the circle we all got to put down items on the paper about how we through the group should run the group and how our behaviour should be within the group. In honesty, the children who had been the most challenging were providing some of the most powerful statements, such as 'we should keep our hands to ourselves' and 'we should turn our listening ears on when someone else is talking'. It was agreed, or contracted, amongst the group members that if you decided to attend the group that you could only leave and return to the group if you were going to the toilet, otherwise if you chose to leave you had to wait until the next week to come into the group again. It was amazing to watch how the children appeared to enjoy setting themselves rules for the sessions, and during subsequent sessions we started each session revisiting our list and checking if there were any statements that needed to be changed or added. The process probably took less than 10 minutes during that third session, but it set the scene for how the children knew they were to behave when in the group and allowed us to make the most of the limited time the group was together. It also meant on the occasions when behaviour became an issue and jeopardised the groups' safety and the purpose of the session, it was possible to discuss the 'ground rules' that the child had agreed to on entering the group and made consequences for this behaviour much simpler to handle.

Acknowledgement

I sincerely thank Jenni Guest, Occupational Therapist, Oxford, UK, for her case vignettes and sharing her reflections on practice. Her vignettes aptly illustrate concepts central to group process and show the value of clinical reasoning. At the time of this writing Jenni was a post-professional master's degree student at Tufts University, Department of Occupational Therapy, Medford, Massachusetts, USA.

Box 12.4

Problematic group forces and leader self-reflection

Problematic force: Anger.
There is an angry outburst in the group. What should the leader do and why?
Problematic force: Avoidance and withdrawal.
A group member hides in the cloakroom 10 minutes into the session. What should the leader do and why?
Problematic force: Attacks on members and leader.
Group members are blaming an individual for mistakes in a group activity. One group member verbally attacks the leader for the problem. What should the leader do and why?
Problematic force: Conflict between members.
Group members cannot come to an agreement about how to proceed with an activity. What should the leader do and why?
Problematic force: Lack of group cohesiveness.
The members of the group are divided into subgroups and unwilling to cooperate with each other. What should the leader do and why?

References

Agazarian Y, Gantt S 2003 Phases of group development: Systems-Centered hypotheses and their implications for research and practice. Group dynamics: Theory, Research, and Practice 7(3): 238–252

Gans JS, Alonso A 1998 Difficult patients: Their construction in group therapy. International Journal of Group Psychotherapy 48(3): 311–326

Howe MC, Schwartzberg SL 2001 A functional approach to group work in occupational therapy, 3rd edn. Lippincott, Williams & Wilkins, Philadelphia, PA

Mattingly C, Fleming MH 1994 Interactive reasoning. Collaborating with the person. In: C Mattingly, MH Fleming(eds) Clinical Reasoning Forms of Inquiry in a Therapeutic Practice, pp. 178–196. FA Davis, Philadelphia, PA

Mosey AC 1970 The concept and use of developmental groups. American Journal of Occupational Therapy 24(4): 272–275

Nitsun M 1996 The Anti-group: Destructive Forces in the Group and their Creative Potential. Routledge, New York

Ormont L 1990 The craft of bridging. International Journal of Group Psychotherapy 40(1): 3–17

Schwartzberg SL 2002 Interactive reasoning in the practice of occupational therapy. Prentice-Hall, Saddle River, New Jersey

Schwartzberg SL, Howe MC, Barnes MA 2008 Groups: Applying the functional group model. FA Davis, Philadelphia, PA

Tuckman BW 1965 Developmental sequence in small groups. Psychological Bulletin 63: 384–399

Tuckman BW, Jensen MA 1977 Stages of small-group development revisited. Group and Organization Studies 2(4): 419–427

Vinogradov S, Yalom ID 1989 Concise Guide to Group Psychotherapy. American Psychiatric Press, Washington, DC

Yalom ID, Leszcz M 2005 The Theory and Practice of Group Psychotherapy, 5th edn. Basic Books, New York

Record and report writing

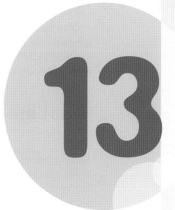

Lisa McCaw and
Jane Grant

Highlight box

- Accurate care records and good-quality report writing are essential skills for practice.
- Care records include any material concerning a client. They provide an accurate record of the client's condition over time detailing the assessment, planning and care delivery and its evaluation. They must demonstrate everything that has been done for or with a client and show practitioners' clinical reasoning.
- Care records can be kept in various formats. Recent developments include client-held records, integrated care pathways and electronic care records.
- Regardless of clinical setting, the occupational therapy process (from initial referral to discharge) must be comprehensively and accurately reported.
- Ensuring good standards of record keeping is an important aspect of service quality. Clinical audit helps services to monitor the quality of record keeping.
- Current legal issues pertinent to recording and report writing include documenting risk assessment and child protection reports. Practitioners may also be asked to provide evidence in court.

Introduction

Recording and report writing may not initially appear to be the most engaging aspect of clinical practice; however, it is a vital component within all settings. It is the professional duty of all occupational therapists to maintain accurate and up-to-date records, but little evidence or attention has been paid to this subject within the literature.

This chapter outlines the purpose and process of maintaining records and creating reports. Current themes in recording and format of care records are discussed. Aspects of recording and reporting the occupational therapy process are explored and examples provided. Finally, quality assurance and legal issues in recording and report writing are highlighted.

The focus of this chapter is on UK guidelines and standards, however, the principles are valid for good report writing internationally. Readers from other nations are recommended to follow this chapter up by consulting the specific guidance from their own professional body, national guidelines, standards and legislation.

What are records

The College of Occupational Therapists states that 'care records include any material that holds information regarding an individual, collected as part of their care provision. Such material can be written, electronic, auditory or visual, and include computer or digital data, images, auditory or visual recordings, letters, notes, e-mails and duplicate copies' (College of Occupational Therapists 2006a: 1).

In addition, there are some less obvious types of information that should be incorporated into care records. The occurrence, content and outcomes of any decisions made after discussions within supervision, or during official or unofficial discussions concerning the client, should be recorded in care records. If the practitioner is following specific national or local guidelines, procedures, care pathways or other standard process, this should also be demonstrated and recorded in the care record. It is also important to document fully all activity, including frequent and repetitive activities, otherwise they cannot be proven to have occurred. A client's response to all outcomes should be recorded. Similarly, if a planned intervention does not occur, perhaps due to client non-attendance, this should be recorded with an explanation if possible. 'This demonstrates that the therapist's planning and care was disrupted for unavoidable reasons and that it was not withheld, or not provided, due to lack of organizational skills or lack of competence' (College of Occupational Therapists 2006a: 5).

Purpose of records

The Department of Health states that, as high-quality information underpins the delivery of high-quality evidence-based health care, all information needs to be accurate, up to date and accessible in order:

- 'To support patient care and continuity of care
- To support day to day business which underpins delivery of care
- To support evidence-based clinical practice
- To support sound administrative and managerial decision making, as part of the knowledge case for NHS services
- To meet legal requirements, including requests from patients under subject access legislation
- To assist clinical and other audit
- To support improvements in clinical effectiveness, and support archival functions by taking into account the historical importance of material and the needs of future research'

(Department Of Health, 2006)

Care records should provide an accurate record of a client's condition over time, detailing the assessment, planning and delivery of the care provided and its evaluation. In turn this will:

- Provide an objective basis to determine the appropriateness of, need for and effectiveness of intervention
- Demonstrate the practitioner's professional reasoning and the rationale behind any care provided
- Highlight problems and changes in the client's condition at an early stage
- Facilitate better communication and dissemination of information between members of health and social care teams
- Protect the welfare of service users by promoting high standards of care.

(College of Occupational Therapists, 2006a:2)

Content and quality of records

The Professional Standards for Occupational Therapy Practice require that practitioners in all settings, keep records of 'all occupational therapy activity and intervention made with, or on behalf of, the service user' (College of Occupational Therapists 2003: 35).

Records must demonstrate everything that has been done for or with a client, including the clinical reasoning behind the care planning and provision. Occupational therapists need to demonstrate the outcomes of the care they have provided for the benefit of the client and others in the care team who have access to the records (College of Occupational Therapists 2006a).

To ensure good-quality care records, the Department of Health (2005) states that all organisations need to ensure that their staff are fully trained in record creation and maintenance, including having an understanding of what they are recording and why; how to validate information with the client or against other records to ensure that the correct data are recorded and how to correct errors. It is also important that staff understand what the records are used for and why accuracy is so important (Department of Health 2005).

The College of Occupational Therapists (2000) provides clear guidance for occupational therapists and occupational therapy services in relation to the content of care records. They state that all staff must:

- 'Clearly identify the client by name, address and date of birth on all records kept
- Document details of all key people involved in the client's care, both professionals and family/carers
- Document all referral details, including date and source of referral and reason for referral when given
- Document any social, medical or rehabilitative history
- Document, date and time all assessments made, methods used and resulting outcomes
- Document and date the views and wishes of the client about goals or treatment plans, and any timeframes suggested
- Document the consent and nature of consent given to intervention
- Document, date and time all interventions planned and carried out in connection with the client, and the resulting outcomes
- Document and date all reviews, and alterations to goals, treatment plans or timeframes
- Document all interventions or decisions made by members of the multidisciplinary team when it impacts upon the occupational therapy care given, including decisions taken in clinical supervision
- Incorporate in the records all correspondence, telephone conversations and reports related to the client's care

- Document and date interventions or contact with family and carers and any outcomes
- Document all information and advice provided to the client and their family/carers
- Document all discharge, closure or transfer details
- Document the destination of onward referrals or care transfers and any information that needs to be considered in handover (with the knowledge and consent of the service user)'

(College of Occupational Therapists (2000) cited in the Professional Standards for Occupational Therapy Practice (2003: 35)).

The importance of accurate and full record keeping is further highlighted by the Health Professions Council Conduct and Competency Committee who regard record keeping as a competency and can take action 'against practitioners where the care records demonstrate a lack of competence, either in the record keeping itself, or in their practice'. This includes an 'unacceptable standard of record keeping, false or failed entries, or there being no evidence of activities such as assessment, treatment planning or the provision of information' (College of Occupational Therapists 2006a: 4).

Legal and professional requirements

It is primarily the employer's responsibility to ensure that care records created or used by their employees meet legal, national and local requirements, and that all staff have access to professional guidance and support appropriate to their roles, responsibilities and needs (College of Occupational Therapists 2006a).

The Health Professions Council Standards of Proficiency for Occupational Therapists (2003) states that registrant occupational therapists must be able to maintain records appropriately and:

- 'Be able to keep accurate, legible records and recognize the need to handle these records and all other clinical information in accordance with applicable legislation, protocols and guidelines
- Understand the need to use only accepted terminology (which includes abbreviations) in making clinical records.'

(Health Professions Council 2003a: 12).

It is important to remember that clinical notes have two purposes. Firstly to provide a clinical record of interventions with clients, and secondly (and only infrequently) they may be used as evidence in court proceedings. The College of Occupational Therapists (2003b) provides useful further guidance on the contents of good clinical notes from the perspective of their potential to be used as legal evidence.

In addition to guidelines from professional bodies, occupational therapists should follow local procedures and protocols when completing care records, meeting all the regulatory body requirements set for the workplace and for themselves as professionals (College of Occupational Therapists 2006a).

Signing and countersigning

It is a professional requirement for occupational therapists to 'provide a clear signature, designation and date with all entries, additions or amendments' (College of Occupational

Therapists 2000 cited in The College of Occupational Therapists 2003: 36). If using an electronic record-keeping system, it is important to ensure that electronic records clearly identify the member of staff making the record, in the absence of a signature to meet the same standards as written records.

Previously qualified staff were also required to countersign entries into records which were completed by students or support staff in order to ensure and demonstrate their accuracy (College of Occupational Therapists 2003). This however inferred that the practitioner had witnessed the treatment encounter and could ensure that the record accurately reflected the event that took place. By countersigning, this also identified the practitioner as the individual responsible for the events recorded. The College of Occupational Therapists recognised that it is not always possible to ensure that record entries are accurate, if the activities themselves have not been witnessed. It is therefore recommended that practitioners 'meet local or regulatory body requirements for countersigning student or support staff entries in the records' (Health Professions Council 2003b).

Use of acronyms and abbreviations

In their guidance on record keeping, the College of Occupational Therapists (2006a) highlight that abbreviations and acronyms are useful when trying to record in a concise way, especially if it can be assumed that the other members of the multi-disciplinary team will understand the terms used. However it should be remembered that a client has the right to access their records upon request and should be able to read and understand what is written in them. In addition, the use of certain terms and acronyms may change over time, and are likely to differ across different service providers. It is suggested that occupational therapy services should consider having an agreed number of acronyms or abbreviations in use and should ensure that these are defined fully within each set of care records (College of Occupational Therapists 2006a).

Timing and dating entries

It is necessary to record the date and time of the care provided to each client. This allows the therapist to document and demonstrate that the care was appropriate and proceeded as planned (or not). In addition, it allows the frequency of care to be monitored. It is important to remember that this may serve as a vital piece of evidence should care records be examined at a later date.

Timely record keeping

The longer the time lapse between an event occurring and it being recorded, the greater the chance of inaccuracies or omissions in the records. Records should be chronological and contemporaneous, made at the same time as the event being recorded, or immediately afterwards (College of Occupational Therapists 2003b).

Confidentiality and consent

In general client information must not be shared without consent from the individual themselves. However, there are exceptions to this rule. Disclosure is permitted if it is in the interest of the public to know the information and where a legal duty exists (College of Occupational Therapists 2006a). Practitioners should always manage client information in a way that respects their confidentiality, consent, right to access and best interests (College of Occupational Therapists 2006a). In 1997, a review of client-identifiable information within the National Health Service (NHS) in England, was chaired by Dame

Fiona Caldicott. This review explored how patient information was being used and high-lighted the potential of risk to confidentiality. A number of recommendations were made regarding information passing between organisations for reasons other than direct care, research or as a legal requirement. The aim was to ensure that client information is only ever shared for valid reasons and that the minimum necessary information was shared (Department of Health 2006). Following the review, the Caldicott committee developed six principles that should be followed when sharing client information.

- Principle 1 – the purpose of using the information must be justified
- Principle 2 – share only when it is absolutely necessary
- Principle 3 – use the minimum amount of information required
- Principle 4 – access should be strictly on a need to know basis
- Principle 5 – everyone must understand their responsibilities
- Principle 6 – those seeking to share information should understand and comply with the law (Department of Health 2006).

Senior officers within health and social care services are now chosen to be Caldicott Guardians. They are responsible for ensuring that organisations achieve the highest standards possible for handling client-identifiable information (Department of Health 2006).

Documenting consent

Once consent, for assessment or intervention, is obtained from a client, it should be recorded and regularly confirmed. The nature of consent given (for example verbally, in writing, through a guardian or advocate, or by other means) should be recorded. All written consent forms should be kept in the client's records. Consent should also be gained before a student observes or provides an intervention, and again the consent and nature of the consent should also be documented. A client's refusal to consent to occupational therapy should also be documented, along with their reasons, if given (College of Occupational Therapists 2003). There are times when documenting consent may be difficult, for example when working with children or adults who may experience impaired capacity to make informed decisions. In such situations individuals should refer to national good practice guidelines or local standards.

Correcting errors

It is important that any errors noted are corrected immediately and initialled by the practitioner. Information should not be added or altered at a later date, and if any additions are essential, these should be noted as a separate or supplementary note or entry, dated and signed. Correction fluid should never be used to correct errors; instead they should be scored out with a single line so that the original text is still legible.

Format of care records

Care records may be kept in a variety of different ways, some of which are outlined below. Current developments in record keeping include the integration of care records across services, the move from paper-based records to electronic systems, and patient-held notes. Regardless of such innovations, the same standards of record keeping should be applied across all types of records.

One example of a specific record-keeping system used in some services is problem-orientated medical records. This system was first proposed in 1968 by Lawrence Weed in an attempt to improve the structure of the medical record by encouraging a more logical and clearer way of communicating information about an individual to another clinical professional (NHS Information Authority 1999). 'SOAP' notes, Subjective-Objective-Assessment-Plan, are the preferred format for note writing within this structure. This type of record keeping is frequently found in physical health settings, and is based upon a problem-solving approach which aims to gather information, appraise it, plan an action and evaluate an outcome. This system can be useful as it enables the reader to gain a quick understanding of a client's functioning. However Blijlevens and Murphy (2003) critiqued SOAP notes and stated that they are too mechanistic and as they are based predominantly on a medical model do not necessarily fit with a holistic, client-centred philosophy of occupational therapy. In their review of the SOAP note-writing structure within their service, they found that the clients, 'appeared to be regarded as made up of damaged body parts that needed to be restored to enable that person to perform fundamental activities in their home, and the notes did not reflect "who the client was in terms of their meaningful occupations and in what context these normally occurred"' (Blijlevens and Murphy 2003: 4). As an alternative, they propose a structure based upon a more client-centred approach.

A large proportion of record-keeping systems are now multi-professional. There is now an increasing development of uni-professional and multi-professional integrated care pathways (ICPs) and the expansion of ICPs from health into social and community settings. ICPs are designed to provide an evidence-based plan of care for a client that incorporates appropriate national and local guidelines. They form a single, multi-professional record of care in an attempt to ensure best practice, co-ordination and consistency. They contribute to clinical governance procedures by providing an 'expected pathway' against which outcomes and interventions can be measured. This information and information on any variations from the expected pathway can provide opportunities to improve practice and improve the quality and outcomes of a client's care (College of Occupational Therapists 2005). Duncan and Moody (2003) provide a useful overview of care pathways in general, and outline the development of an occupational therapy integrated care pathway in a mental health setting. An illustration of an occupational therapy integrated care pathway is given below (Figure 13.1).

Electronic care records

There is an international trend towards the introduction of electronic care records. Within the health service in the UK, development and use of electronic health records is a key part of the plan to develop an improved information system within the NHS. The proposed 'NHS Care Records System' will connect GPs with acute, community and mental health trusts in a single system, and will aim to replace existing paper-based systems by 2010. A national database will contain a summary of all records, making important service user information available at all times.

Garner and Rugg (2005) state that the use of electronic care records is likely to become 'the major national programme strand to have an impact on occupational therapy' in the near future, with an aim 'to integrate records across multiple agencies including health and social care' (p. 132).

In 1998, the College of Occupational Therapists and the Chartered Society of Physiotherapy commissioned 'The Garner Project' to explore the use of information and communication technologies within the allied health professions. The project specifically focused on the implementation of electronic care records within the two professions. The most recent phase of this ongoing project has assisted in identifying key themes for the occupational therapy profession to consider and respond to in light of the move towards electronic systems. These include organising client records, focusing on client's views, involving staff, developing new ways of working, acknowledging problems of access and learning from others' experience of using electronic records. Garner and Rugg (2005)

Name:						DOA	Transfer	Destination
DOB inc CHI No:			Unit No:					
Consultant:								
OT Service:								
Occupational Therapist:								

	Yes	No	N/A	Date	Initials	Variance	Actions to be carried out/Comments
REFERRAL.							
Risk assessment received.							1) Assess appropriateness 2) If not received contact referrer
Appropriate							1) Not appropriate–complete referral refusal form 2) Inform referring agency within 5 days 3) Inform Senior/Head OT–letter to GP
Waiting list							1) Complete waiting list proforma 2) Inform referred within 10 days 3) Review waiting list weekly 4) Re-contact referrer within 3 months if case not allocated
Initial assessment							1) To be carried out: -
							Routine: Acute - 7 working days Community/Day Hospital - 20 working days *Urgent* Acute - 3 working days Community/Day Hospital - 5 working days Long stay - 20 working days
CONSENT							
Was consent to assessment/ treatment given?							
Verbally							
Written							
Advocate/Guardian							
Other							
Was individual advised regarding withdrawal of consent							1) Advise consent can be withdrawn at any time and this will not affect OT treatment
Consent to share information							1) Explain role in MDT and need to share information 2) Complete and gain signature for consent of information
Consent for student to observe/take part in patient treatment							1) Complete student observation/treatment form and gain signature

Figure 13.1 Integrated care pathway. From NHS 2008.

ASSESSMENT TREATMENT						
Community						1) Complete standardised assessment form
Kitchen						2) Forward copy to relevant individuals in accordance with consent to share information
PADL (self-care, etc.)						3) Any action carried out on carer's behalf should be noted
DADL (laundry, etc.)						4) Refer to Social Work for Carer's Assessment
Home visit						5) Record unmet needs
Functional needs assessment						
MOHOst						
Claudia Allen						
MEAMS						

	Yes	No	N/A	Date	Initials	Variance	Actions to be carried out/Comments
ASSESSMENT TREATMENT							
OSA							
HADS							
Other							
Identify unmet needs							
Single shared assessment							
Completed							
Requested							
Forwarded to call centre							
Carers assessment							
Carer informed							

Figure 13.1—Cont'd

Referral to Social Work								
GOAL SETTING/ TREATMENT PLANNING								
Discuss goal setting/treatment plan with patient/client								1) Ensure interventions are in accordance with evidence based practice 2) Where applicable issues copies of treatment plan in accordance with sharing of information
Carer								
MDT								
Advocate/Guardian								
EVALUATION								
Review treatment plan in accordance with timescales								*Maximum period:* In-patients (Acute) 4 weekly Day Hospital and Community 4 monthly Continuing Care and Rehab 6 monthly 1) Amend plan as required 2) Discuss with patient/client/MDT as per consent to share information 3) Consider need for discharge, closure or transfer of case
DISCHARGE, CLOSURE OR TRANSFER								
Write discharge date on progress notes								1) Identify unmet needs 2) Requirement for assistive devices/support 3) Recommend follow-up or re-assessment 4) Forward completed discharge summary to referrer/referring agency and others in line with consent to share information 5) If required complete Single Shared Assessment
Complete discharge summary								

Reproduced with permission of NHS Fife Occupational Therapy Mental Health Service

Figure 13.1—Cont'd

suggest a number of actions that occupational therapy services can begin to take now, in order to prepare for the move towards electronic record-keeping systems in the future.

Patient-held records

In today's health-care climate there is considerable emphasis upon providing cost-effective services. Patient-held records are thought to be a cost-efficient way of improving the care and outcome for those experiencing severe mental illness (Henderson and Laugharne 1999). Such records have become normal practice in some clinical settings, particularly obstetrics, paediatrics and chronic disease or disability management (Henderson and Laugharne 2005). Patient-held records may be particularly useful if an individual is receiving care from a variety of professionals. In addition, it is thought that they may allow the individual to be a more active participant in their care; for example being able to have the information that shows what has worked or been unhelpful in the past. This information may be useful in mental health settings when discussing issues such as relapse. It has been suggested that patient-held records also reduce any possible 'coercive' elements of treatment (Henderson and Laugharne 2005). However, possible difficulties exist. These include confidentiality issues, reliability of the client to carry the information and keep records safe and duplication of the information (Warner et al 2000). Practitioners are advised to follow local policy regarding whether or not duplicate records should be retained by the professional. If policies restrict the keeping of such records, it is the responsibility of that organisation or authority to accept any possible consequences (College of Occupational Therapists 2006a). According to Warner et al (2000), patient-held shared care records had no significant effect upon mental state or satisfaction of mental health service users. The uptake of the scheme was low by both staff and clients and it appeared that those experiencing a psychotic illness were less likely to use the records. In relation to the use of patient-held records in palliative care, a study by Cornbleet et al (2002) also found no significant evidence to support the introduction of such a scheme. There appeared to be no improvement in information giving or sharing, or to the degree to which the family were involved in decision making. However, most individuals who had a record found it to be of some benefit. Clearly this is an area that requires further investigation.

Recording and reporting the occupational therapy process

Referral

It is the practitioner's responsibility to record or retain the referral details in the appropriate occupational therapy records (College of Occupational Therapists 2003). This should include the source and date of referral. There is also a requirement to inform the referring agency should the referral be declined. Justification should be provided. A documented system for prioritising referrals should be evident. At the same time, optimum use of resources should be sought. If the referral is considered inappropriate, it may be recommended that the client's details are passed on to an alternative service. Should this occur, informed consent must be documented (College of Occupational Therapists 2003). Figure 13.2 illustrates an example of an occupational therapy referral form.

Assessment

All assessments including both standardised and non-standardised interview and observational assessments should be recorded. A description of the client factors, circumstantial aspects and features of the activity that allow or impinge upon performance should be acknowledged. The therapist's confidence in the assessment results should also be included (American Occupational Therapy Association 2003). Should variables exist that would affect the results (for example a client's tiredness), such factors should also be documented.

Within practice, many different types of assessments are used (see Chapter 6). If a standardised assessment is used the aims and procedures must be clearly stated. Any variation during the assessment that would affect the standardised process, must be recorded. The type of assessment used will depend upon the clinical area and needs of the client. Examples may include, but are not limited to, a comprehensive initial assessment, home visit assessments, workplace/vocational assessments, dressing assessments and kitchen assessments.

Stancliff (1998) suggests that private (or insurance-based) services provide further issues for consideration; demonstrating the value and effectiveness of an intervention through accurate documentation is particularly important for clients, services and con-

**Mental Health
Occupational Therapy Service – Referral form**

Patient/Client details	Care groups (physical, mental health, learning disability, addictions)
Date of referral	Consultant
Name	
DOB M ☐ F ☐	Base
Address/Ward	Keyworker (CPN/Medic/Health Visitor/District Nurse/Social Work/OT)
Postcode	Contact No
Tel (Day)	GP Details
Referrer details	Name
Name of referrer	Address
Designation	Tel No
Address	Emergency Contact
Tel No	Contact No

Presenting problems (including mental/physical health)

Any other difficulties

Medical alerts (e.g. diabetes, angina, epilepsy, addiction history)

Medication

Additional information e.g. MH Act status

Client aware of referral to Occupational Therapy   Yes/No

Home circumstances (lives alone, family, carer, etc)

Reason for referral (to be completed by referrer)

Personal Activities of Daily Living (ADL) Assessment ☐
Vocational/Lifestyle Assessment ☐
Domestic ADL Assessment ☐
Feeding Assessment ☐
Home Assessment ☐
Other (specify) ☐

Structured use of time ☐
Specific activity programme (please specify) ☐
Community integration ☐
Social skills/communication ☐
Coping strategies ☐
Groups (if known specify) ☐

Risk factors

NIL ☐
History violence/aggression ☐
Self harm ☐
Suicide ☐
Forensic history ☐
Absconding risk ☐
Self neglect ☐
Other (specify) ☐

Data collection (for official use only)

Date of referral:
Date received:
Outcome: Accepted/rejected/diverted/client refused OT involvement
Date 1st contact:
Date of initial assessment:
Client remains on caseload: Yes/No
Date discharged:

Figure 13.2 Referral form from NHS. Greater Glasgow and Clyde Mental Health Partnership 2008.

tractors. McGuire (1997) proposes that occupational therapy reports must firstly focus upon function and highlight clearly the occupational performance area being addressed. Furthermore, practitioners should precisely record the relationship between any medical diagnosis/problem and function. However, it may be that a diagnosis is not always known. And by viewing the individual in a medical and compartmentalised way, practitioners may depersonalise the individual and exclude their knowledge, meanings and experiences (Blijlevens and Murphy 2003).

Recording progress

McGuire (1997) states that reports should clearly indicate progress made. Documentation should focus upon function. When using narratives in progress notes, practitioners should emphasise the functional focus by organising the content in relation to the overall performance area being addressed within the treatment plan (McGuire 1997). The practitioner should then clearly document the relationship between medical problem and occupational functioning. Progress in performance components (cognitive, sensorimotor, psychological) must be related directly to the client's functional goals established within the performance areas (ADL, work/productivity, leisure) (McGuire 1997). As safety issues are particularly important these issues should be clearly documented (McGuire 1997). Furthermore, therapeutic expectations regarding improvement in the client's safety or functional ability should also be documented. Reasons for slow or lack of progress must also be included. Finally, the skilled component of occupational therapy must be recorded, showing the clinical reasoning, and therapeutic strategies or principles used (McGuire 1997). Whilst these issues are important in all record keeping, they are particularly relevant when practitioners are concerned with demonstrating effectiveness to third-party payers.

Documenting clinical reasoning

Practitioners should document the clinical reasoning behind their care planning and service provision (College of Occupational Therapists 2006a); a task, it has been argued, that they are not always good at (Stancliff 1998).

Neidstadt (1996) suggests that mostly pragmatic and procedural reasoning styles are used within medical, physical health-orientated environments. However, narrative reasoning engages the individual in a life history story-telling process that ultimately places the practitioner in a better position to understand their client's subjective experiences, values and goals for the future. By gathering and reporting this information, practitioners ultimately build a picture of the person through what they do. As a result, meaningful client-centred goals can be established (Neidstadt 1996).

Reflecting theory within documentation is a powerful method of communicating professional reasoning and rationale. Not only does it allow us to communicate to other professionals, or significant others, the aims, interventions and outcomes of therapy it also allows us to enhance professionalism and credibility amongst colleagues (Forsyth and Kielhofner 2002). However, it can be difficult to effectively communicate profession-specific models and perspectives within client reports. Forsyth and Kielhofner (2002) acknowledges that a disadvantage of professional terminology is that the language is not common to all professionals, clients or families/carers. However, they also suggest that practitioners do not use terminology due to lack of confidence rather than any contention from colleagues.

By documenting a clear relationship between the assessment outcomes, goals and proposed treatment plan, practitioners educate others regarding the varied scope of occupational therapy intervention (Kyle and Wright 1996). Efficient reporting should be organised and comprehensible. It should provide descriptive characteristics of the client and the context in which the assessment or intervention occurred. Documentation is particularly useful for sharing small, gradual and hard-to-detect changes. Evidence should be recorded either quantitatively or qualitatively (Tickle-Degnen 2000).

All assessment results should be recorded and comprise all decisions made including not to continue intervention either by the client or relevant other. It is important to remember that assessment results are shared jointly with the client and practitioner and that, within the bounds of legality, it is the client's choice to share the information with relevant others or to withhold consent (Creek 2003).

Goal setting and treatment plans

Following an initial screening and subsequent assessment, collaborative goals are established (see Chapter 8 for further information) and should be recorded. Any needs or aims that cannot be addressed must also be recorded and reasons for this given (Creek 2003).

Despite this, a study carried out by Anderson et al (1991), expressed concern at the noticeable lack of goals within occupational therapy documentation. Without clear, measurable goals it is not possible to evaluate their achievement. Perhaps more worryingly, it is also suggested that there was little evidence to suggest that clients were involved in the treatment planning process (Anderson et al 1991); hopefully this situation has improved significantly in the intervening years. Occupational therapists are required to record each client's assessed needs and subsequent goals and intervention plan (College of Occupational Therapists 2003). It is possible that existing resources may impact upon a practitioner's ability to carry out the ideal, fully comprehensive treatment plan. In such cases, the practitioner should identify and record the objectives that must be achieved in order to provide a service that is considered to offer a minimum level of satisfaction and safety to clients and significant others (Creek 2003).

It is not only crucial that goals be clearly documented and client-centred but also measurable and, therefore, provide a means for evaluating therapy. Forsyth and Kielhofner (2002) state that measurable goals must contain the action to be carried out to demonstrate achievement of the goal. They should also specify the environment in which the goal relates to. Furthermore, the level of independence/degree of support needed should be recorded, and a clear timeframe should be specified.

Reassessment/alteration to treatment plans

In addition to documenting a clear treatment plan, all subsequent occupational therapy interventions and contacts must be documented. As assessment and evaluation of interventions are an ongoing process any changes to them should also be recorded.

Discharge planning

Clearly, discharging an individual from therapy will depend upon the clinical area and timescale. Creek (2003) states that practitioners usually write a short informative report when an individual is discharged. More detailed reports are produced when required. However, the depth of these reports will vary from location to location.

Any plans for a client's discharge, case closure or transfer of care should be recorded within their treatment plans (College of Occupational Therapists 2003).

When considering discharge or transfer from the service, the practitioner should assess progress made towards agreed goals, and record the level of support or assistance needed in any areas of functioning. They should also make recommendations for future support or interventions if appropriate and propose any follow up or further assessment needed (College of Occupational Therapists 2003).

Ensuring standards of record keeping

Ensuring good standards of record keeping is an important aspect of service quality. Audits enable organisations to evaluate and monitor the services they provide, and allows the identification of potential areas of risk, inefficiency or ineffectiveness providing opportunities to take any necessary action to improve the quality of services provided The involvement of clients in the audit process is now actively encouraged, in order to gain their views as recipients of care. The College of Occupational Therapists (2004) has published a useful briefing paper to assist services in involving clients in such activities.

Gibson et al (2004) developed a retrospective audit tool of 61 standards from the College of Occupational Therapists core standard on record keeping. They used this tool to conduct an audit of 320 client records across many clinical specialisms within a service. The audit identified many areas of good practice, and areas which did not meet the standards were used to form the basis of a number of service action plans, highlighting how the audit process should be used as a learning opportunity. Participation in audit is now a clinical governance requirement, and many audit tools are now available to assist services in this process (College of Occupational Therapists, 2005b).

Legal issues in documenting and report writing

Practitioners should also consider their involvement in documentation that is not occupational therapy specific. These may include involvement in risk assessment and risk management, child protection reporting, and legal reports for court.

Risk assessment

In mental health settings, changes within legislation and highly publicised tragedies have led to increasing emphasis on accurate risk assessment and risk management (Newell 2001). Several clinical risk assessment tools have been developed and practitioners should select the most suitable tool for their clinical area and working environment, and for which they have received appropriate training.

Practitioners must assess the possibility of any health and safety risks and clearly document the outcomes of any risk assessment carried out. Contingency plans should be developed for risks that cannot be eradicated and any decisions made by the practitioner based upon their assessment should be documented (College of Occupational Therapists 2003). For example, practitioners should ensure that appropriate risk management policies and incident reporting procedures have been developed. However, Mandelstam (2005) describes a reduction of practitioner confidence in such decision making due to worries of legal action. This can lead to inaccurate perceptions of risk and overly defensive practices.

Child protection

Practitioners may have to be aware of possible involvement in scenarios whereby child protection issues are raised. The 'Hidden Harm' agenda (Scottish Executive 2006) reinforces the importance of effective communication and information sharing between agencies when working with individuals who may misuse drugs or alcohol. Confidentiality policies can present barriers to sharing relevant information. However, identifying a situation where a child may be at risk overrules any agency rules or obligations. All agencies should have clearly documented child protection procedures.

Court reports

Increasingly, practitioners are involved in claims and legal issues. In relation to clinical work, practitioners may become involved in court cases in the following ways:

- As a witness of fact whereby a report or statement is requested regarding what was seen, heard or known
- As a defendant whereby the practitioner or employer is accused of alleged negligent practice
- As a claimant whereby the practitioner is attempting to sue another individual.
- As expert witnesses when they are asked to provide independent opinion on a case.

(College of Occupational Therapists 2003b)

As a witness of fact therapists may be asked to produce a statement or a report. Statements include personal details and professional background. It should also provide a coherent, chronological record of events. Technical jargon should be fully explained.
Reports should be:

- 'Logical
- Objective
- Factual
- Truthful
- Easy to read and understand'

(College of Occupational Therapists 2003b: 21)

Records and notes may be required. The content of the report will differ depending upon the specific case. The referenced guidelines produced by the College of Occupational Therapists (2003) provide a useful example of how to structure a court report. According to Mandelstam (2005: 47), 'the law aside, good professional practice anyway demands a reasonable standard of evidence, reasoning and documentation; if professionals record their decision making it is likely to be of a higher quality'.

Investigations carried out by the Health Professions Council into professional competence frequently centre around the inadequacy of record keeping. The importance of documenting the thoughts and evidence that have led a practitioner to make the decision cannot therefore be overemphasised. In general, the legal system is likely to focus more upon the decision-making process rather than the actual outcome or merits of decisions (Mandelstam 2005). It is of crucial importance that occupational therapists demonstrate their clinical reasoning process and document clearly, how the decision was reached.

Summary

This chapter has provided an overview of the key aspects of recording and report writing. Emerging issues (such as electronic records) have also been acknowledged. Although guidelines produced by professional bodies are available, variations in national and local procedures exist and should be referred to. This chapter provides essential information and guidance to effectively and accurately record clinical information and create reports. It should be treated as an initial introduction to the topic, equipping the reader to develop further skills and continue their reading, reflection and action regarding recording and report writing.

References

American Association of Occupational Therapy Association 2003 Guidelines for documentation of occupational therapy. Cited In: KM Sames 2005 Documenting occupational therapy practice. Pearson, Prentice Hall

Anderson B, Llewellyn G, Bell J 1991 Records: one measure of occupational therapy practice in the field of developmental disabilities. The Australian Journal of Occupational Therapy 38(2): 77–81

Blijlevens H, Murphy J 2003 Washing away SOAP notes: refreshing clinical documentation. New Zealand Journal of Occupational Therapy 50(2): 3–8

College of Occupational Therapists 2000 Occupational therapy record keeping (standards for practice). College of Occupational Therapists, London

College of Occupational Therapists 2003 Professional Standards for occupational therapy practice. College of Occupational Therapists, London

College of Occupational Therapists 2003b The occupational therapist and the court. A step by step guide for occupational therapists and their staff. College of Occupational Therapists, London

College of Occupational Therapists 2004 COT/ BAOT Briefing: 28 service user involvement. College of Occupational Therapists, London

College of Occupational Therapists 2005 COT/ BAOT Briefing: 1 Integrated Care Pathways. College of Occupational Therapists, London

College of Occupational Therapists 2005b COT/BAOT Briefing: 40 Quality Briefing: Audit. College of Occupational Therapists, London

College of Occupational Therapists 2006a Record Keeping. College of Occupational Therapists guidance 2. College of Occupational Therapists, London

College of Occupational Therapists 2006b Record keeping – issues of responsibility COT/BAOT briefing 43. College of Occupational Therapists, London

Cornbleet MA, Campbell P, Murray S et al 2002 Patient-held records in cancer and palliative care: a randomized, prospective trial Palliative Medicine 16(3): 205–212

Creek J 2003 Occupational therapy defined as a complex intervention. College of Occupational Therapists, London

Department of Health 2006 The Caldicott Guardian Manual. London, Department of Health, UK Council of Caldicott Guardians

Department of Health 2006 The Records Management: NHS Code of Practice. www. dh.gov.uk/en/Managingyourorganisation/ Informationpolicy/Recordsmanagement/index. htm Accessed on 07/04/2008.

Duncan EAS, Moody KJ 2003 Integrated care pathways in mental health settings: An occupational therapy perspective. British Journal of Occupational Therapy 66(10): 473–478

Forsyth K, Kielhofner G 2002 Putting theory into practice. In: Kielhofner G 2002 Model of Human Occupation Theory and Application, 3rd edn. Lippincott, Williams and Wilkins, Baltimore

Garner R, Rugg S 2005 Electronic care records: an update on the Garner project. The British Journal of Occupational Therapy 68(3): 131–134

Gibson F, Sykes M, Young S 2004 Record keeping in occupational therapy: Are we meeting the standards set by the College of Occupational Therapists? The British Journal of Occupational Therapy 67(12): 547–550

Health Professions Council 2003a Standards of Proficiency. Occupational Therapists Health Professions Council, London

Health Professions Council 2003b Standards of conduct, performance and ethics. Your duties as a registrant. Health Professions Council, London

Henderson C, Laugharne R (1999) Patient held clinical information for people with psychotic illnesses. The Cochrane Database of Systematic Reviews 4: 1–20

207

Kyle T, Wright S 1996 Reflecting the Model of Human Occupation in occupational therapy documentation. The Canadian Journal of Occupational Therapy 63(3): 192–196

Mandelstam M 2005 Occupational therapy: law and good practice. College of Occupational Therapists, London

McGuire MJ 1997 Excellence and efficiency in documentation. Targeting your audience bridges the gap between services delivered and provider reimbursement. OT Practice 36–41

Neidstadt M 1996 Teaching strategies for the development of clinical reasoning American Journal of Occupational Therapy 50(8): 676–684

Newell S 2001 Clinical risk assessment for an occupational therapy inpatient group programme. The British Journal of Occupational Therapy 64(4): 200–202

NHS Fife 2008 Mental Health Occupational Therapy Service Integrated Care Pathway. NHS Fife

NHS Greater Glasgow and Clyde Mental Health Partnership 2008. Mental Health Occupational Therapy Referral Form. NHS Greater Glasgow and Clyde

NHS Information Authority 1999 Briefing Paper: Problem Orientated Medical Record (POMR) and SOAP

Scottish Executive 2006 Hidden harm. Next steps. Supporting children – working with parents. Scottish Executive, Edinburgh, UK

Stancliff BL 1998 Documentation insurance companies understand. OT Practice July/August: 55–56

Tickle-Degnen L 2000 Monitoring and documenting evidence during assessment and intervention. The American Journal of Occupational Therapy 54(4): 434–436

Warner JP, King M, Blizard R et al 2000 Patient-held shared care records for individuals with mental illness: randomized controlled evaluation. The British Journal of Psychiatry 177: 319–324

Evidence-based and research skills for practice

SECTION

3

Finding and appraising the evidence

14

M. Clare Taylor

Highlight box

- The development of evidence-based occupational therapy.
- The nature of 'evidence' within evidence-based occupational therapy.
- Ensuring the search is clearly structured and has a specific focus.
- Asking the right appraisal questions.
- Identifying ways of sharing and disseminating appraisal.

Overview

The aim of this chapter is to explore ways of both locating and evaluating the evidence that underpins practice. Developing the skills of evidence-based occupational therapy (EBOT) is vital in today's political climate. Without a sound appreciation of the evidence, or lack of evidence, to support occupational therapy interventions and actions then practitioners will be unable to justify the rationale for these interventions and actions.

The chapter will begin by reminding the reader of the background and context of evidence-based practice (EBP) and how EBP has developed into EBOT. The main focus of the chapter will be on exploring both the nature and sources of 'evidence' with practical examples of searches. Having located some evidence, the next step is to appraise the rigour and value of that evidence; this process will then be discussed. However, finding and appraising evidence is often difficult for the busy practitioner, the chapter will, therefore, discuss ways of including appraisal into everyday practice.

Historical context

The need to find and appraise evidence is central to the concept of EBP. The term 'evidence-based practice' is probably very familiar to most readers. However, it is worth spending a little time reviewing the definitions and history of EBP and EBOT in order to provide a context for the remainder of the chapter.

EBP has its roots in the evidence-based medicine (EBM) movement, which began at McMaster University in Canada in the 1980s (Taylor 2007), linked to the use of a problem-based approach to the teaching of medicine. By the mid-1990s EBM had been defined as:

> *the conscientious, explicit and judicious use of current best evidence in making decisions about the care of individual patients (Sackett et al 1996: 71)*

By the late 1990s EBP had begun to seep into the consciousness of the occupational therapy profession, especially in the UK and Canada, with special issues of both the *British Journal of Occupational Therapy* (College of Occupational Therapists 1997, 2001) and the *Canadian Journal of Occupational Therapy* (Canadian Association of Occupational Therapists 1998) as well as books (e.g. Law 2002, Taylor 2007) and articles (e.g. Brown and Rodgers 1999, Bennett and Bennett 2000) on the implementation of EBP in occupational therapy. It is also worth noting that the 1997 Casson Memorial Lecture in the UK (Eakin 1997), the 2000 Eleanor Clarke Slagle Lecture in the US (Holm 2000) and the 2001 Sylvia Docker Lecture in Australia (Cusick 2001) all explored EBP and EBOT and encouraged practitioners to find and use evidence to support their everyday practice.

This interest in EBOT also led to the development of a number of definitions of EBOT, the best known of which defines it as:

> *Client-centred enablement of occupation, based on client information and a critical review of relevant research, expert consensus and past experience* (Canadian Association of Occupational Therapists et al 1999: 267).

However, the essence of EBOT is probably best expressed by Cusick (2001: 103),

> *When we practice with evidence, it means we should ask ourselves the following question: 'am I doing the right thing in the right way with the right person at the right time in the right place for the right result – and am I the right person to be doing it?'*

The challenge for the evidence-based occupational therapist is to find and appraise the relevant evidence. However, the challenge does not end once the evidence has been located. The evidence may indicate that a particular intervention has been shown to be effective. The evidence may also show that there is little or no evidence to support the effectiveness of a chosen intervention and the evidence-based occupational therapy then needs the courage to change practices, that may be long established, and to ensure that occupational therapy is seen as an effective and relevant profession (see Chapter 15). Thus EBOT is a way of thinking critically about every intervention and action and, as such, is just one of the tools of clinical reasoning and reflective practice. However, because of the use of up-to-date best evidence, evidence-based practice is a powerful tool.

Why is appraisal of evidence important?

Whilst the principles of EBOT and a questioning approach to the value of our interventions and activities as practitioners might appear to be a valuable philosophy, and very useful in the abstract, we must also remind ourselves of the reasons that EBOT and the need to appraise evidence are currently seen as vitally important for all practitioners.

EBP has been enshrined into health and social care policy for some time (English examples include *The New NHS: Modern, Dependable* (DoH 1997; National Service Frameworks, DoH, 2000, 2001) and into professional practice at both statutory (Health Professions Council, 2003) and professional levels (College of Occupational Therapists 2003, 2005). However, for many practitioners there has been a resistance to this drive for EBP. Dubouloz et al (1999) found that occupational therapists have been slow to integrate research evidence into their clinical decision-making, although there is some more recent evidence that occupational therapists now believe that EBP is important to practice (Bennett et al 2003).

For many practitioners their own previous experiential evidence has been key to intervention decision-making (Pringle 1999, Upton 1999a, 1999b). EBP does not seek to deny the value of experiential evidence; it seeks to ensure that experiential evidence is not the sole source of evidence for competent decision-making. To be able to make competent decisions about our interventions and action we must be able to incorporate critical reflection on our own experiential knowledge with critical appraisal of the theoretical and research evidence relevant to that intervention or action.

The stages of EBOT

Whilst EBOT can be described as a way of thinking about practice and asking, as Cusick (2001) puts it, the 'right' questions; EBOT is also a problem-solving process, which mirrors both the research process and the occupational therapy process. Sackett et al (1995) articulated the five stages of EBP as:

1. to convert our information needs into answerable questions
2. to track down, with maximum efficiency, the best evidence with which to answer these questions
3. to appraise the evidence critically (i.e. to weigh it up) to assess its validity (closeness to the truth) and usefulness (clinical applicability)
4. to implement the results of this appraisal in our clinical practice
5. to evaluate our performance.

Whilst other chapters focus on the 4th and 5th stage (Chapters 16 and 6 respectively), this chapter will focus on the first three stages of this process:

- asking a question
- finding the evidence
- appraising the evidence.

However, the process of EBOT should not be viewed as a one-off activity: it should run parallel to the process of clinical reasoning and can be applied at each stage of the occupational therapy process to ensure that every action from initial assessment to final evaluation is effective and based on sound reasoning and evidence. Bennett and Bennett (2000) have developed a framework that shows how EBP can be used at every stage of the occupational therapy process. Rappolt (2003) has developed a model of a client-centred EBOT process, which has integrated three strands of evidence (from the client, from research and from professional expertise) into the occupational therapy process in the hope of overcoming the perception that EBP and client-centred practice are mutually exclusive (Taylor 1997).

Asking good questions

The first stage of the EBOT process is to identify and articulate a question that will guide the search for evidence to be appraised. Because of the original medical focus of EBP, questions are often thought of as 'clinical' questions relating to diagnosis, prognosis or treatment (Rosenberg and Donald, 1995) and are phrased in terms of:

What is the evidence for the effectiveness of **x** *(the intervention) for* **y** *(the outcome) in a patient with* **z** *(the problem or diagnosis)?*

This might fit very nicely into medical practice when thinking about whether treatment with aspirin and warfarin will reduce the risk of stroke in an elderly lady with hypertension, but how can it relate to the complexities of occupational therapy practice? Herbert et al (2005: 12) have expanded the application of the clinical question to include:

- the effects of intervention
- the patients' experiences
- the course of the condition, or the life-course of a particular patient group (prognosis)
- the accuracy of diagnostic tests or assessments.

Whilst broadening the idea of the clinical question beyond assessing the potential effectiveness of an intervention, this approach still does not address the totality of occupational therapy practice. However, if we adopt Cusick's (2001) approach of asking the right questions, we can utilise an evidence-based approach to all stages of the occupational therapy process, e.g.:

- Am I the right person?
  - Does this person need to be seen by someone with occupational therapy skills?
  - What are the right skills needed to work with this person?
- Am I doing the right thing?
  - Not only is this the right intervention, but also is this the right assessment tool?
- Am I doing it in the right way and for the right reasons?
  - What is the most effective model or frame of reference?
  - Do I have all of the relevant information that I need to plan this intervention properly?
- Am I doing it with the right clients?
  - Do *all* patients/clients with this problem need to be seen by an occupational therapist, or just those with other particular problems?
- Am I doing it at the right time?
  - Should I see this client in the morning or the afternoon?
  - Should I see them everyday or just once a month?
- Is it being done in the right place?
  - Would I be better working with this patient/client in their own home rather than in hospital?

The anatomy of a well-built question

The task for the evidence-based occupational therapist is to devise a question. This question will arise from practice, possibly by asking oneself one of the 'right' questions outlined above or by articulating or reflecting on a particular incident or client to develop a scenario to help you to develop the final EBP question. Box 14.1 outlines two scenarios, which will be used as illustrations throughout this chapter.

Having identified and articulated a scenario, it is then possible to refine this information further to create and structure a specific evidence-based question. The clearer the structure of the EBP question, the more focused and, hopefully, successful the search for evidence.

As we noted above, an evidence-based question usually consists of a number of elements:

- a problem
- an intervention
- an outcome.

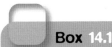

> **Box 14.1**
>
> ## Identifying a scenario
>
> ### Scenario 1
>
> The Stroke Unit where you are working is keen to use 'constraint induced therapy' (CIT) as an intervention. You are unsure of the potential value of this approach, especially in relation to other more established intervention approaches, and decide to explore the literature to find out what evidence exists to demonstrate the effectiveness of CIT.
>
> ### Scenario 2
>
> You have been asked to co-facilitate a fatigue management group for people living with multiple sclerosis (MS). The central philosophy for the group is self-help and empowerment and to use strategies that are informed by experience as well as research evidence. You identify some relevant anecdotal knowledge but want to adopt a more evidence-based approach. You decide to collect evidence from a range of sources to inform your planning of the fatigue management group. You also hope that the evidence will give you ideas about assessing the outcomes and the success of the group.

Richardson et al (1995) refer to these elements as the 'anatomy' of a well-built question, and add a further element: a comparative intervention. The inclusion of a comparative intervention is common practice in the context of EBM where the effectiveness of drug *x* may be compared with that of drug *y*. The inclusion of a comparative intervention may be perceived as having less relevance to many for EBOT, although it may be of value in the context of some EBP questions.

Whilst this approach, commonly referred to as PICO (problem, intervention, comparative intervention, outcome) may seem of limited relevance to EBOT, where there is rarely a comparative intervention and outcomes are not always clearly identified, as Table 14.1 illustrates the elements can easily be applied to occupational therapy especially if the elements are renamed:

- person; rather than problem
- action; rather than intervention
- comparative action; rather than comparative intervention
- application.

This structure can then be applied to any scenario, as Box 14.2 illustrates.

Searching for the evidence

Having articulated the evidence-based question the next task is to search for and locate the evidence to address this question. However, before we can embark on the search it is necessary to understand the concept of 'evidence' and the scope of evidence within EBOT.

What do we mean by 'evidence'?

Sackett et al's (1996) definition of evidence-based practice talks about the need to use 'best evidence' to support the decision-making process. However, the nature of 'best evidence' is perhaps the most contentious and debated area within the concept of evidence-based practice (Sackett and Wennberg 1997, Taylor 2007). The traditional view, drawn from evidence-based medicine, has been to adopt a hierarchy, or levels, of research evidence. Table 14.2 outlines the hierarchy of evidence for evidence-based medicine.

Table 14.1 The elements of a well-built question

Person	Action	Comparative action (if applicable)	Application
Describe your client/patient/ client group and her/his/their problem. This may be a diagnosis, a functional problem or an occupational performance problem. The description should also include all key information e.g. age, sex, occupational status	Describe the main action or activity of interest. This may be an intervention or assessment undertaken by the occupational therapist, but could also be a task/activity/strategy used by the client	Describe the comparative or alternative action/ intervention/ assessment/task. This may also take the form of alternative approaches to the intervention e.g. group or individual sessions; different frequency of intervention	Describe what you hope to achieve, what effect the action may have on your client/patient/ client group or how you hope to apply the action

Box 14.2

Developing an evidence-based question

Scenario 1

person – people experiencing hemiparesis, especially upper limb involvement, following a stroke
action – constraint induced therapy
comparative action – all other current approaches to stroke intervention
application – improved upper limb (UL) function, independence in activities of daily living (ADL), increased meaningful occupational behaviours
evidence based question:
What is the evidence for the effectiveness of constraint induced therapy, in comparison to existing approaches to stroke rehabilitation, in improving UL function/independence in ADL or increasing meaningful occupational behaviours in clients who experience hemiparesis following stroke?

Scenario 2

person – people experiencing fatigue as a consequence of MS
action – living with fatigue; fatigue management
comparative action – not relevant for this question
application – guidelines for facilitating a fatigue management group
evidence based question:
What information can be derived from a range of evidence into the experience of living with MS-related fatigue, in order to facilitate a fatigue management group?

However this approach ignores two major factors. The first is that there is a breadth of potential research approaches, which might be appropriately viewed as 'best evidence'. The second is that many definitions of evidence-based practice include not only research but also the therapist's experiential knowledge and the client's perspective as potential sources of evidence. Table 14.3 identifies the potential range of research approaches that might be seen as evidence.

The question for the evidence-based occupational therapist is, which of this long list might be the 'best evidence' to use to address a particular evidence-based question? As Sackett (1998), Sackett and Wennberg (1997) and Taylor (2007) argue, the nature of the 'best evidence' depends upon the type of evidence-based question being asked and as we have seen the potential varieties of EBOT questions are diverse. Table 14.4 gives an overview of the types of research evidence that might be appropriate for the different types of evidence-based question.

Having established a list of the potential types of research evidence to address a particular question, the evidence-based occupational therapist's next task is to decide whether there is a particular order or hierarchy of the types of evidence, to ensure that the 'best' evidence is found.

Developing a hierarchy of the most appropriate evidence for the effectiveness of interventions is relatively straightforward. The hierarchy, outlined in Table 14.2, was developed to show the value and weighting of evidence for the effectiveness of interventions, with systematic reviews of RCTs seen as the most rigorous and reliable form of evidence. Similar hierarchies have been developed for

- therapy/prevention/aetiology/harm questions
- prognosis questions
- diagnosis questions
- differential diagnosis/symptoms questions
- economic questions (Phillips et al 2001).

Table 14.2 Levels of evidence within EBM

- systematic reviews & meta-analyses of randomised controlled trials
- randomised controlled trials
- non-randomised experimental studies
- non-experimental studies
- descriptive studies
- respected opinion, expert discussion

Table 14.3 Types of research evidence

- Randomised controlled trials (RCTs)
- Systematic reviews of RCTs
- Controlled clinical trials
- Non-randomised experimental studies
- Single case design studies
- Cohort studies
- Cross-sectional studies
- Longitudinal studies
- Correlational studies
- Qualitative research studies
- Systematic reviews of qualitative research
- Surveys
- Delphi studies
- Consensus studies
- Qualitative case studies

Table 14.4 Appropriate research evidence for particular types of evidence-based questions

Effectiveness of interventions

Systematic reviews of RCTs

RCTs

Other experimental designs, e.g. controlled clinical trials

Single subject design studies

Client's experiences and perceptions

Qualitative research studies

Systematic reviews of qualitative research

Descriptive research studies, e.g. surveys

Appropriateness of assessments

Cross-sectional studies

Measurement studies

Prognosis and life-course of a particular condition or group of people

Cohort studies

Longitudinal studies

Qualitative research studies

Correlational studies

The appropriateness of a similar hierarchy for qualitative research is much more questionable, with many authors (e.g. Barbour 2001, Pawson et al 2003) arguing that, whilst it might be possible to critically appraise the rigour and strength of a particular qualitative study is it neither possible nor appropriate to locate different types of qualitative studies within a hierarchy.

The identification of the 'best' evidence is a complex task. The potential range of evidence is broad and should not solely focus on research evidence. Using specific types of research evidence to address particular evidence-based questions may seem the most useful approach. However, it may also act as a constraint to the development of a broad perspective on the 'best evidence' with which to answer evidence-based questions. Certainly an RCT or a systematic review should provide powerful evidence for the effectiveness of a particular intervention, it should not, however, be the only evidence required for clinical reasoning and decision-making. Pawson et al (2003) argue, from a social care perspective, that evidence should include:

* organisational knowledge
* practitioner knowledge
* service-user knowledge
* research knowledge
* policy knowledge

thus acknowledging the breadth and complexity of evidence to be considered, especially within a social care context.

Evidence from research studies can only give a partial answer to any evidence-based question. The research evidence must be balanced with information from the client about their values and perspectives, as well as the therapist's experiential knowledge. The intervention or action decision will also be influenced by contextual factors such as service priorities and resources, as well as local and national policies. Evidence should not be seen in terms of a hierarchy but in terms of pieces of a complex jigsaw, which together provide the 'best evidence' to answer any evidence-based question.

Structuring a search

Having clarified the elements of the evidence-based question, the next stage in the process is to use these elements to provide a clear structure for the task of searching for some evidence, which will then be appraised for its value in the context of the evidence-based question.

Once the evidence-based question has been articulated, there is often a temptation to go straight on to the Internet to find some evidence. However, if you start searching without doing sufficient thinking and planning your search will probably be very frustrating and ultimately unsuccessful. It is much more useful to spend some time thinking about the structure of your search, so that any time spent at the computer or in the library is usefully spent and might also result in the successful location of some relevant and valuable evidence.

Developing a search strategy consists of a number of stages:

- articulating a clear question, which can then be used to identify key words and search term
- identifying the most relevant information sources, which might include specific databases (see below for further discussion of databases) or library collections
- identifying the types of evidence that are most appropriate for the question.

Identifying the key words and search terms is an important task if the search is to be successful. It is always useful to look at the search terms and key words that you have identified and then to think of synonyms or alternative terms, as well as different spellings (many terms have different spelling depending on whether the usage is English or American).

Most databases do not readily understand 'natural language', the colloquial language that we use every day. However, the majority of databases have a thesaurus of accepted terms and key words. Databases use what are known as Boolean operators to help the searcher refine the search question. Operators can be used to focus the search. The most common Boolean operators are:

- AND: used to combine two search terms in order to find articles that contain both of the terms
- OR: allows you to use alternative terms to broaden a search
- NOT: is used to exclude articles with particular unwanted terms, to narrow a search.

It is also sensible to set limits to any search to avoid being swamped by information that is inappropriate, irrelevant or inaccessible. Common limits are the language the article is written in, the age of the article and the type of article.

Table 14.5 provides a summary of the pointers to assist in structuring a search and Box 14.3 illustrates how the questions identified in the previous scenarios can be developed into search strategies.

Where to look

Rather than wandering vaguely around the library randomly selecting interesting-looking books and journals, the evidence-based occupational therapist should focus on the most appropriate resources in the search for relevant evidence. Bibliographic indexes and databases have been developed to help the evidence-based practitioner to locate the most suitable information. However, many databases are only available by subscription,

Table 14.5 Structuring the search

Improving the search terms:

- use synonyms and both English and American terminology; e.g. learning difficulty/ learning disability/mental retardation

- use English and American spellings; e.g. paediatrics/pediatrics

- make sure that you spell words correctly

- use " " for collections of words which collectively have a specific meaning; e.g. "occupational therapy"

- use * or $ (the truncation symbol) to find all terms beginning with … ; e.g. alcohol* will retrieve articles related to alcohol, alcoholic, alcoholics and alcoholism

- use Boolean operators (AND, OR & NOT) to expand or limit the search; e.g. "occupational therapy" OR physiotherapy will retrieve all articles related to occupational therapy and physiotherapy individually, whereas "occupational therapy" AND physiotherapy will retrieve only those articles that relate to combinations of occupational therapy and physiotherapy; and "occupational therapy" NOT physiotherapy will exclude articles that include reference to physiotherapy

Setting limits:

- limiting your search to English language only references means that you avoid identifying a potentially useful reference only to find that you need a translator as the original paper is in German or Japanese

- limiting your search to papers published in the last 5 years will mean that you only access 'current' evidence and not something that was published in 1960, which may have since been refuted, although sometimes historical evidence might be of value

- limiting your search to include only research papers, this means that any opinion pieces or other non-research evidence will be excluded

so it is worth checking with your library to see which databases you might be able to access. The databases most relevant to occupational therapy are identified in Table 14.6. The searches linked to the evidence-based questions outlined above are discussed and illustrated in Table 14.7 and Box 14.4 and the reader might be able to draw some conclusions as to the relative merits of the various databases for their own evidence-based searches.

Databases have different areas of focus. MEDLINE, PubMed (the free access version of MEDLINE) and EMBASE have a very medical focus, whilst CINAHL and AMED focus more on allied health. ASSIA, PsychLit and SocioFile draw heavily on social science literature and ERIC has an educational focus. A number of specific EBP databases now exist. These databases, unlike general databases, employ quality checks, and so will only include citations for work that meets their standards for good evidence. There are also a number of occupational therapy-specific databases, which might be of value. OTSeeker (www.otseeker.com; Bennett et al 2003, McClusky 2006, McKenna 2004, 2005) is a particularly valuable resource as it also incorporates an evidence-based approach and does not require a subscription. Web-based search engines (such as Google, Google Scholar and Ask) are also databases of a sort, although they are less regulated and, therefore, less rigorous than more specific databases. Intute (www.intute.ac.uk) is a relatively new free online service, which aims to give students access to good web-based resources that have been evaluated by a network of subject specialists. Table 14.7 gives an overview of the results of the searches for the two scenarios (constraint induced therapy and MS-related fatigue), in terms of numbers of 'hits' and Box 14.4 provides a commentary on these searches.

Box 14.3

Developing search strategies

Scenario 1

Evidence-based question:

What is the evidence for the effectiveness of constraint induced therapy, in comparison to existing approaches to stroke rehabilitation, in improving UL function/independence in ADL or increasing meaningful occupational behaviours in clients who experience hemiparesis following stroke?

types of evidence:

the question focuses on the effectiveness of an intervention, so the search needs to look for systematic reviews and RCTs

key words:

"constraint induced therapy" OR "constraint induced movement therapy" AND stroke

limits:

English language only

Scenario 2

Evidence-based question:

What information can be derived from a range of evidence into the experience of living with MS-related fatigue, in order to facilitate a fatigue management group?

types of evidence:

the question focuses on people's experiences of dealing with illness as well as the effectiveness of an intervention, therefore a range of evidence including both qualitative research studies and RCTs/systematic reviews will be sought

key words:

"multiple sclerosis AND fatigue OR fatigue management"

limits:

English language only

Table 14.6 Databases relevant to the evidence-based OT

General databases	Specialist evidence-based databases
• AMED	• Cochrane Library
• ASSIA	• DARE
• BIDS	• Campbell Collaboration
• CINAHL	• Best Evidence
• EMBASE	• Clinical Evidence
• ERIC	• Health Technology Assessment database
• MEDLINE	
• PubMed	
• PsychLit	
• SocioFile	

(Continued)

Table 14.6 Databases relevant to the evidence-based OT—Cont'd

OT databases	Web-based resources
• OTSeeker (and its sister physiotherapy database – PEDro) • OTBibSys • OTDBase	• Intute • Google/Google Scholar • Ask

Appraising the evidence

Once suitable research evidence has been identified and located the job of the EBOT is not finished. Research evidence should not be accepted at face value. Whilst many journals use a rigorous process of peer review and critical evaluation prior to the publication of any article, it does not mean that a published piece of research is flawless or that it can be applied to any practice situation.

Having located relevant research evidence, the next stage in the EBOT process is to critically appraise the evidence. Critical appraisal can be defined as

> 'the ability to read original and summarised research, to make judgements on its scientific value and to consider how its results can be applied in practice' (Taylor 2003: 102).

Table 14.7 Search results for the evidence-based question scenarios

	Constraint induced therapy		MS-related fatigue	
	"constraint induced therapy"	AND stroke	"multiple sclerosis" AND fatigue	AND "qualitative research"
AMED	22		50	0
CINAHL	159	98	282	2
MEDLINE	59	42	728	3
PubMed	60	47	748	3
Cochrane Library	33	28	102	n/a
OTSeeker	20	16	10	n/a
Intute	0	0	2	0
Google	24 100	19 600	1 940 000	111 000
Google scholar	750	666	23 800	3170
Ask	2370	1900	604 300	480

Box 14.4

Overview of search examples

Scenario 1

Evidence-based question:

What is the evidence for the effectiveness of constraint induced therapy, in comparison to existing approaches to stroke rehabilitation, in improving UL function/independence in ADL or increasing meaningful occupational behaviours in clients who experience hemiparesis following stroke?

search outcome:

The first choice of databases for this question would be those databases that have a specific focus on systematic reviews and RCTs, such as the Cochrane Library and OTSeeker, with more general databases such as AMED, CINAHL and MEDLINE/PubMed providing access to other types of research evidence and the web-based resources possibly giving access to a range of opinion-based information.

Cochrane Library:

This search only identified RCTs, it did not locate the systematic reviews that were found in the OTSeeker search.

OTSeeker:

This was a highly successful search as all 16 of the citations were potentially relevant to the evidence-based question. One of the strengths of OTSeeker is that all RCTs are critically appraised and rated for their research rigour by a team of researchers, so much of the EBOT's has already been done.

AMED/CINAHL/MEDLINE/PubMed:

Whilst the AMED search resulted in the fewest hits, it was probably the most focused although all of the studies identified in the OTSeeker search were replicated in the AMED search. There was also considerable replication between all of these searches, but also some useful additional material that was not identified in either the Cochrane Library, OTSeeker or AMED searches. However, for both the CINAHL and MEDLINE/PubMed searches the reader would have to spend some time sifting through a number of apparently irrelevant citations, such as a paper on the effects of d-amphetamine injections on the motor training of squirrel monkeys (Barbay 2006). Narrowing the search by including the search terms 'occupational therapy' and 'activities of daily living' resulted in the identification of a smaller number (8) of highly relevant research papers, reminding the reader of the need to have clear and specific key words to avoid being swamped by the search results.

Web-based searches:

These resulted in a large number of hits but little evidence that was of value for the evidence-based question.

Scenario 2

What information can be derived from a range of evidence into the experience of living with MS-related fatigue, in order to facilitate a fatigue management group?

search outcome:

The search for this evidence-based question is rather less straightforward than the previous search. This question has a primary focus on the lived experience of MS-related fatigue but is also interested in the effectiveness of fatigue management as an intervention. The search, therefore, needs to begin with the general databases such as AMED, CINAHL and MEDLINE/PubMed in order to access the qualitative research and

(Continued)

223

Box 14.4—Cont'd

then needs to look at OTSeeker and the Cochrane Library for systematic reviews and RCTs.

AMED/CINAHL/MEDLINE/PubMed:

In terms of the search for qualitative research evidence the MEDLINE/PubMed search was the most effective as all 3 'hits' were highly pertinent to the evidence-based question. Replication of citations was again common across the various databases. The AMED search provided some useful supporting material on the nature of MS-related fatigue and the effectiveness of fatigue management strategies.

OTSeeker:

Not all of the 10 'hits' were relevant to this evidence-based question, but this search did identify relevant papers that the other searches did not find.

Cochrane Library:

This search produced a mixed bag of results. 7 Cochrane reviews were identified, although only 2 were of relevance to the evidence-based question. A further review was identified on DARE (Database of Reviews of Effectiveness) but this proved to be a review of pharmacological interventions. A total of 93 RCTs were identified, however the majority of these were not relevant to the evidence-based question and those that were had already been located in other searches.

Web-based searches:

These searches did reveal some useful material, but only after considerable time and effort had been spent scrutinising the numerous citations.

Critical appraisal provides a structured framework in order to assess the value and trustworthiness of a piece of research within the context of practice. The structure of the critical appraisal process allows the evidence-based occupational therapist to review not just the findings of the research but the whole research process. Critical appraisal should give the reader the opportunity to identify both the strengths and the weaknesses of a particular research paper. The weaknesses of the research should be weighed and evaluated carefully but should be viewed in the context of whether they make you question the conclusions of the researchers. Critical appraisal should be positive rather than negative and viewed with an open mind and the ability to challenge your own, as well as the researcher's, ideas and assumptions.

Adopting a critical appraisal approach to reading the research evidence will encourage the reader not to ignore, or skip over, the 'complicated' sections of a research paper, such as the results section. Skipping over parts of an article may lead to misinterpretation of findings or erroneously accepting (or rejecting) the author's conclusions. Critical appraisal is often more interesting if it is not a solitary activity, so that the findings and ideas can be discussed and ideas and comments can be challenged and reviewed. Journal clubs can be used as a way of sharing critical appraisals of research literature.

The key questions

Critical appraisal is a process of asking a series of structured questions about the rigour and applicability of the research. Any critical appraisal, irrespective of the type of research being appraised, is structured around three essential questions:

- How rigorous/valid/trustworthy is the research?
- What are the findings?
- Can the findings be applied to my particular context and evidence-based question?

All of these questions can be broken down further to explore the research in depth.

The first group of questions addresses the rigour of the research and helps the reader to appraise how good the research is. The second group of questions helps the reader to focus on the research findings and to assess the significance, both statistical and clinical, or strength of the findings. The final group of questions gives the reader the opportunity to explore whether the research and its findings can be used in the context of practice, does the research give any evidence to support or challenge current practice.

Appraising different types of evidence

Whilst the three questions outlined above give an overall structure to any critical appraisal, they have to be adapted to suit different types of research methodology. A common mistake when starting to critically appraise research evidence is to adopt a standard series of questions, in a one-size-fits-all approach to appraisal. This can lead to certain research papers and research methodologies being viewed as less rigorous because the wrong questions have been used to appraise them. Thus, qualitative research papers need to be appraised with a different set of questions from quantitative research papers and systematic reviews should not be appraised with questions relevant to RCTs. Any appraisal calls for some level of understanding and knowledge of the research methodology being appraised.

It is beyond the scope of this chapter to give a thorough and detailed discussion of the questions used to appraise different research types and methodologies. Critical appraisal is usually best facilitated by the use of an appraisal checklist, which will outline the key questions for a particular research type. Numerous examples of checklists and lists of questions are available. Table 14.8 outlines some of the most useful examples.

Including appraisal in everyday practice

Evidence-based occupational therapy is not about *doing* research it is about *using* research evidence to underpin interventions and actions within everyday practice. The challenge is to find space in the busy working week to be able to search for and appraise the relevant research evidence. The chapter will now explore a number of ways that appraisal of evidence can be incorporated into everyday practice.

Journal clubs

Journal clubs have been a regular feature of medical education and practice for many years (Linzer 1987). They usually consisted of someone presenting an overview of a paper that they had read and then attempting to stimulate discussion. However, with the advent of EBM the format of journal clubs began to change (Sackett et al 1997) and evidence-based journal clubs began to be established (Phillips and Glasziou 2004). Evidence-based journal clubs also began to be developed not just amongst medical practitioners but for groups of occupational therapists, nurses and other allied health professionals (Bannigan and Hooper 2002, Sherratt 2005, McQueen et al 2006).

Evidence-based journal clubs provide an opportunity for a group of like-minded colleagues to meet together to discuss and appraise the relevant research evidence linked to a clear evidence-based question, probably using an appraisal checklist as a way of structuring and recording their discussions.

Journal clubs are a useful way of both promoting and recording evidence of continuing professional development. They enable participants to maintain and enhance their critical appraisal skills and their knowledge of the research base for practice. They also provide an opportunity to review and reflect on current practice. The outcome of a journal

Table 14.8 Identifying a useful appraisal checklist

Taylor (2007) gives worked examples of appraisal using separate checklists for:

- RCTs
- Systematic reviews
- Qualitative research
- Surveys
- Web-based information
- Outcome measures

Humphris (2005) gives a brief overview of the questions that might be used to appraise:

- Case-controlled studies
- Cohort studies
- Surveys
- Qualitative research
- Professional consensus papers

Dickson (2005) gives a brief overview of the questions to use when appraising systematic reviews

Craig and Smyth (2002) outline the types of questions to ask when appraising a range of types of evidence, including:

- Studies of intervention effectiveness
- Studies into the value of diagnostic tools and assessments
- Qualitative research
- Systematic reviews
- Guidelines

Greenhalgh (2006) gives a thorough overview of the questions to ask when appraising a variety of medical research approaches, including:

- Drug trials
- Diagnostic & screening tests
- Systematic reviews & meta-analysis
- Guidelines
- Economic analyses
- Qualitative research
- Questionnaire research

Helewa and Walker (2000) give a basic overview of the questions to ask when appraising a variety of research articles:

- Outcome measures & diagnostic tests
- Treatment efficacy & effectiveness studies
- Economic evaluations
- Review articles & meta-analysis

Herbert et al (2005) provide questions for assessing the validity of a number of research types:

- Intervention studies
- Studies about attitudes & experiences
- Evidence about prognosis
- Evidence about diagnosis & assessment
- Systematic reviews
- Clinical guidelines

CASP [www.phru.nhs.uk/Pages/PHD/CASP.htm] have a range of checklists, which can be downloaded from their web site, for:

Table 14.8 Identifying a useful appraisal checklist—Cont'd

- Systematic reviews
- RCTs
- Qualitative research
- Economic evaluation studies
- Cohort studies
- Case control studies
- Diagnostic test studies

McMaster University School of Rehabilitation Science [www.srs-mcmaster.ca/Default. aspx?tabid=546] have general guidelines for reading and appraising research, which can be downloaded from their web site, for:

- Quantitative research
- Qualitative research

Netting the evidence [www.shef.ac.uk/scharr/ir/netting/] has weblinks to a wide range of appraisal resources

club discussion might be to implement changes to current interventions or actions, or just to enhance confidence in the value of those interventions and actions. The journal club can provide a valuable opportunity for groups of colleagues to explore issues, share ideas, consider different perspectives and participate in shaping and developing departmental policy and practice. Specific guidelines for establishing a journal club are beyond the scope of this chapter, but can be found in a number of publications e.g. Taylor (2007), Sherratt (2005) and Phillips and Glasziou (2004).

As the focus of this chapter is on evidence-based occupational therapy, it would seem appropriate to outline the evidence for the value of journal clubs in changing practice and ensuring that all interventions and actions are evidence-based. Sadly, the majority of the evidence is anecdotal or, at best, expert opinion and consensus (McQueen et al 2006). There is evidence to support the value of journal clubs in developing critical appraisal skills (Parkes et al 2001), but there is little research evidence to support the impact of journal clubs on practice development and change. McQueen et al's (2006) small exploratory study indicated that there were some changes in the participants' attitudes and confidence and an increased awareness of the evidence base supporting their interventions and actions. Journal clubs would appear, at face-value, to be useful activities both for developing an evidence-based culture within a department and for ensuring that practice is evidence-based, however it is imperative that the impact and value of journal clubs is researched further.

Evidence-based reflection and case studies

In the discussion on the nature of 'evidence' earlier in the chapter it was noted that experience is often reported as the main source of evidence used by practitioners when making decisions about interventions and actions as part of the clinical reasoning process. However, whilst Enkin and Jadad (1998) put forward a sound and coherent argument for the use of experiential, or, as they term it, 'anecdotal', evidence within EBP, they do not give any practical suggestions as to its use. Rappolt's (2003) model of a client-centred EBOT process mentions both 'client evidence' and 'clinical expertise' but does not discuss how evidence of clinical expertise can be articulated. The evidence-based occupational therapist is, therefore, left wondering how experiential evidence can be brought explicitly into the process of EBOT.

Reflection on action and the use of evidence-based case studies may provide useful tools to help the evidence-based occupational therapist to articulate the experiential evidence used in practice (see Chapter 5). The process of reflection involves describing an event and then looking at the decision-making and reasoning process, which underpin the actions taken within that event. The event concerned can be any interaction with a client. To use these reflections to develop an evidence-based case study the following topics should be addressed:

* description of a case study or incident
* reflection on action and articulate experiential evidence
* explore and appraise the research evidence
* synthesis and dissemination.

Bailey et al (2007) and Smallfield and Lou (2006) are two interesting examples of how evidence-based case studies can be developed and used to incorporate EBOT within everyday practice.

Developing critically appraised papers and critically appraised topics

Many practitioners are developing their critical appraisal skills and becoming involved in the critical appraisal of research papers. It is important to avoid duplication of effort and that appraisal of research evidence is shared and disseminated to the wider practitioner community. Two useful tools for disseminating appraisal are critically appraised papers (CAPs) and critically appraised topics (CATs).

A number of journals are now including CAPs regularly (for example the *Australian Occupational Therapy Journal*, and the *Australian Journal of Physiotherapy*) whilst journals such as *Evidence-based Mental Health* and *Evidence-based Healthcare* contain nothing but CAPs. The importance of these papers is that they include not just a structured summary of a previously published research paper but they also include a commentary, by a practitioner, on the rigour of the research and its usefulness as evidence for practice. CAPs are vital tools in the dissemination of EBOT and wider publication of CAPs should be encouraged within the professional literature.

CATs are short summaries of the research evidence on a topic of interest, usually focused around an evidence-based question. A CAT should be seen as a shorter and less rigorous form of a systematic review; beginning with an outline of the evidence-based question and the search strategy before summarising the best available research evidence on the chosen topic. Usually more than one research study is included in a CAT. CATs are a useful tool for busy practitioners to summarise and share their research appraisals. There are multiple sites on the internet containing CATs. Many have a medical focus, but sites of interest to occupational therapists include:

* OTCATs – www.otcats.com
* McMaster University & University of British Columbia – www.mrsc.ubc.ca/site_page.asp?pageid=98
* Queens University, Canada – critically appraised topics in rehabilitation – www.rehab.queensu.ca/cats/

A major benefit of a CAT is its brevity and simplicity. It is important to note a major limitation of many CATs is the absence of independent peer review, as many CATs published on the Internet are not peer reviewed, it is important to bear this fact in mind if using CATs to guide practice. Readers cannot be confident that a thorough and complete search of the literature has been conducted nor that an accurate interpretation of the methods, results and statistics has been made. However, CATs are useful tools that can be used to guide and inform practice. When appraising the research literature it is worth considering whether the work you are doing can be developed into a CAT.

Summary

This chapter has focused on the first stages of the EBOT process. It began by outlining the nature of EBOT before exploring the nature of 'evidence' in the context of EBOT and discussing ways of searching for research evidence. The chapter then discussed the questions to ask when critically appraising a research paper before concluding by presenting a number of ways of incorporating critical appraisal into everyday practice.

References

Bailey DM, Bornstein J, Ryan S 2007 A case report of evidence-based practice: from academia to clinic. American Journal of Occupational Therapy 61(1): 85–92

Bannigan K, Hooper L 2002 How journal clubs can overcome barriers to research utilisation. British Journal of Therapy & Rehabilitation 9(8): 299–303

Barbay S 2006 A single injection of d-amphetamine facilitates improvement in motor training following a focal cortical infarct in squirrel monkeys. Neurorehabilitation & Neural Repair 20(4): 455–458

Barbour RS 2001 Checklists for improving rigour in qualitative research: a case of the tail wagging the dog? British Medical Journal 322(7294): 1115–1117

Bennett S, Bennett JW 2000 The process of evidence-based practice in occupational therapy: informing clinical decisions. Australian Occupational Therapy Journal 47: 171–180

Bennett S, Hoffman T, McCluskey A et al 2003 Evidenced-based practice forum. Introducing OTSeeker (Occupational Therapy Systematic Evaluation of Evidence): a new database for occupational therapists. American Journal of Occupational Therapy 57: 635–638

Brown GT, Rodgers S 1999 Research utilization models: frameworks for implementing evidence-based occupational therapy practice. Occupational Therapy International 6(1): 1–23

Canadian Association of Occupational Therapists 1998 Special edition on evidence-based practice. Canadian Journal of Occupational Therapy 65(3)

Canadian Association of Occupational Therapists, Association of Canadian Occupational Therapy University Programs, Association of Canadian Occupational Therapy Regulatory Organizations & the Presidents' Advisory Committee 1999 Joint position statement on evidence-based practice. Canadian Journal of Occupational Therapy 66: 267–269

College of Occupational Therapists 1997 Special edition on evidence-based practice. British Journal of Occupational Therapy 60(11)

College of Occupational Therapists 2001 British Journal of Occupational Therapy 64(5)

College of Occupational Therapists 2003 Professional Standards for Occupational Therapy Practice. College of Occupational Therapists, London

College of Occupational Therapists 2005 Code of Ethics and Professional Conduct. College of Occupational Therapists, London

Craig JV, Smyth R L (eds) 2002 The Evidence-based Practice Manual for Nurses. Churchill Livingstone, Edinburgh, UK

Cusick A 2001 2001 Sylvia Docker Lecture: OZ OT EBP 21c: Australian occupational therapy, evidence-based practice and the 21st century. Australian Occupational Therapy Journal 48(3): 102–117

Department of Health 1997 The New NHS: Modern, Dependable. HMSO, London

Department of Health 2000 www.doh.gov.uk/nsf/coronary.htm

Department of Health 2001 www.doh.gov.uk/nsf/mentalhealth.htm

Dickson R 2005 Systematic reviews. In: S Hamer, G Collinson (eds) Achieving Evidence-based Practice, 2nd edn., pp. 43–62, Baillière Tindall, Edinburgh, UK

Dubouloz CJ, Egan M, Vallerand J et al 1999 Occupational therapists' perceptions of evidence-based practice. American Journal of Occupational Therapy 53(5): 445–453

Eakin P 1997 The Casson Memorial Lecture 1997: Shifting the balance – Evidence-based Practice. British Journal of Occupational Therapy 60(7): 290–294

Enkin MW, Jadad AR 1998 Using anecdotal information in evidence-based health care: Heresy or necessity. Annals of Oncology 9: 963–966

Greenhalgh T 2006 How to Read a Paper, 3rd edn. Blackwell Publishing, Oxford, UK

Health Professions Council 2003 Standards of Proficiency, Occupational Therapists. London, Health Professions Council

Helewa A, Walker JM 2000 Critical Evaluation of Research in Physical Rehabilitation. Philadelphia, PA, WB Saunders

Herbert R, Jamtvedt G, Mead J et al 2005 Practical Evidence-based Physiotherapy. Edinburgh, UK, Churchill Livingstone

Holm MB 2000 The 2000 Eleanor Clarke Slagle Lecture – Our mandate for the new millennium: Evidence-based practice. American Journal of Occupational Therapy 54: 575–585

Humphris D 2005 Types of evidence. In: S Hamer, G Collinson (eds) Achieving Evidence-based Practice, 2nd edn. Edinburgh, UK, Baillière Tindall

Law M (ed.) 2002 Evidence-based Rehabilitation. Thorofare, NJ, Slack Incorporated

Linzer M 1987 The journal club and medical education: over one hundred years of unrecorded history. Postgraduate Medical Journal 63: 475–478

McCluskey A 2006 How and why do occupational therapists use the OTseeker evidence database? Australian Occupational Therapy Journal 53(3): 188–195

McKenna K 2004 In practice. OT seeker: facilitating evidence-based practice in occupational therapy. Australian Occupational Therapy Journal 51(2): 102–105

McKenna K 2005 Australian occupational therapists' use of an online evidence-based practice database (OTseeker). Health Information & Libraries Journal 22(3): 205–214

McQueen J, Nivison C, Husband V et al 2006 An investigation into the use of a journal club for evidence-based practice. International Journal of Therapy & Rehabilitation 13(7): 311–316

Parkes J, Hyde C, Deeks J et al 2001 Teaching Critical Appraisal Skills in Health Care Settings. Cochrane Database of Systematic Reviews 2001, Issue 3

Pawson R, Boaz A, Grayson L et al 2003 Knowledge Reviews 3: Types & Quality of Knowledge in Social Care. London, SCIE & The Policy Press

Phillips R S, Glasziou P 2004 What makes evidence-based journal clubs succeed? Evidence Based Medicine 9: 36–37

Phillips B, Ball C, Sackett D et al 2001 Oxford Centre for Evidence-based Medicine Levels of Evidence (May 2001) http://www.cebm. net/index.aspx?o=1025 (accessed 28th October 2001)

Pringle E 1999 EBP: is it for me? Therapy Weekly 25(46): 12

Rappolt S 2003 The role of professional expertise in evidence-based occupational therapy. American Journal of Occupational Therapy 57(5): 589–593

Richardson WS, Wilson MC, Nishikawa J et al 1995 The well-built clinical question: a key to evidence-based decisions (editorial) ACP Journal Club, 123: A12–A13

Rosenberg W, Donald A 1995 Evidence based medicine: an approach to clinical problem-solving. British Medical Journal 310: 1122–1126

Sackett D L 19 March 1998. Shamanism (Was: Pre-test probability). Evidence-based-health [online]. Available from: http://www.mailbase. ac.uk/lists/evidence-based-health/1998– 03/0066.html Accessed 8 June 2000

Sackett DL, Wennberg JE 1997 Choosing the best research design for each question. British Medical Journal 315: 16–36

Sackett DL, Rosenberg WMC, Gray JAM et al 1996 Evidence-based medicine: what it is and what it isn't. British Medical Journal, 312: 71–72

Sackett DL, Richardson WS, Rosenberg W et al 1997 Evidence-based Medicine: How to Practice & Teach EBM. New York, Churchill Livingstone.

Sherratt C 2005 The Journal Club: a method for occupational therapists to bridge the theory-practice gap. British Journal of Occupational Therapy 68(7): 301–306

Smallfield S, Lou JQ 2006 The effectiveness of low vision rehabilitation on quality of life: an evidence-based practice approach to answer clinical questions. Occupational Therapy in Health Care 20(2): 17–30

Taylor MC 1997 What is evidence-based practice?. British Journal of Occupational Therapy 60(11): 470–474

Taylor MC 2003 Evidence-based practice: informing practice and critically evaluating related research. In: G Brown, SA Esdaile, SE Ryan (eds) Becoming an Advanced Practitioner, p. 90–117. Edinburgh, UK, Butterworth-Heinemann

Taylor MC 2007 Evidence-based Practice for Occupational Therapists, 2nd edn. Oxford, UK, Blackwell Publishing

Upton D 1999a Clinical effectiveness and EBP 2: attitudes of health-care professionals. British Journal of Therapy & Rehabilitation 6(1): 26–30

Upton D 1999b Clinical effectiveness and EBP 2: application by health-care professionals. British Journal of Therapy & Rehabilitation 6(2): 86–90

230

Knowledge exchange

Katrina Bannigan

Highlight box

- Knowledge exchange in health and social care focuses on the use of research findings in practice. It involves collaboration, is dependent on interaction, results in mutual learning, and uses a problem-solving process.
- Knowledge exchange is as much a social process (i.e. focused on people) as a technical process (i.e. focused on research) that requires a consideration of context, relevant audiences and the message to be communicated.
- Knowledge brokers are experts who act as mediators to link researchers and decision makers such as policy makers.
- The organizational culture in occupational therapy services (including academic settings) should be shaped to encourage knowledge exchange.
- There is no single approach to knowledge exchange. Interactive rather than passive approaches are more effective in facilitating research use so should form the cornerstone of knowledge exchange activity. All other activity should be tailored to the individual scenario.

Overview

Knowledge exchange (also known as knowledge transfer) involves using research findings to inform clinical practice. The reason knowledge exchange is needed is a substantial amount of time and money is invested by health and social services across the world in generating research knowledge but this knowledge is not always transferred into practice which means the benefits for patients are lost. Knowledge exchange is achieved through collaboration, interaction and using a problem-solving process; all skills occupational therapists use on a daily basis. The key message is that in knowledge exchange interactive rather than passive approaches are needed to achieve change. This process should be facilitated by a knowledge broker.

The principles of change management can be used to support this process (Bryar and Bannigan 2003). The literature on knowledge exchange in occupational therapy is limited but there are examples of it happening.

We live in a knowledge society in which sharing information and collaboration are key survival skills (Knexa 2005). Knowledge transfer is a broad-based approach to sharing information that is reliant on collaboration and so is a growing area of interest. This interest is not confined to the health and social care sector; the literature on knowledge transfer crosses many different disciplines from management to education to nursing (Thompson et al 2006). Universities, for example, are increasingly focusing their attention on knowledge transfer because they recognise its economic and social potential (e.g. Universities Scotland 2006, West Yorkshire Knowledge Exchange 2006). The value of knowledge transfer to those working in health and social care is the improved health and well-being of society (Askew et al 2002, Nuyens and Lansang 2006). There has been some consideration of knowledge transfer in occupational therapy (e.g. Soderback and Frost 1995, Johnson 2005, Loisel et al 2005, MacDermid et al 2006) but the paucity of literature in relation to occupational therapy suggests the concept will be new to many. Although knowledge transfer may be a new concept for many occupational therapists it has a long history (Nuyens and Lansang 2006). It has existed in other guises (for example research utilisation) for a long time (see Caplan and Rich 1975, Weiss 1979 or Brett 1986 for early work on the concept). Whilst knowledge transfer has its roots in research utilisation it is a broader concept that, when used in fields other than health and social care, involves using a wide range of different sources of information, not just research findings.

This chapter will explain what knowledge transfer is, explore why it is relevant to occupational therapists, examine what difference it makes for occupational therapists and their clients in practice, and outline the practical issues that need to be considered in order to determine what occupational therapists can do to facilitate knowledge exchange. Please note that this chapter is an introduction to this topic. There is a lot of literature available, much of which exists outside of occupational therapy, so use the resources suggested (below) to further familiarise yourself with the topic. Whilst it is important to be familiar with the literature, so that we can learn from the experiences of others, you should also not be afraid to just have a go!

What is knowledge transfer?

In health and social care knowledge transfer in the form of research utilisation predates interest in evidence-based practice (see Chapter 14). Research utilisation, i.e. using research findings in practice to improve patient care, is one aspect of evidence-based practice (Bannigan 2004, 2007). That one whole section of a book about *skills for practice* has focused on evidence-based practice confirms that evidence-based practice is now an accepted part of health and social care practice (Canadian Health Services Research Foundation 2004). The emphasis on evidence-based practice ensures that knowledge transfer in health and social care focuses on 'research-based knowledge' as opposed to other sources of information (Canadian Health Services Research Foundation 2004). Evidence-based practice is about clinical decision making in which the decisions made by occupational therapists are made on the basis of patients' values, clinical expertise, a consideration of resources and the best available research evidence (Dawes et al 2005). It is because evidence-based decisions rely on the use of best available research evidence that, in order to be an evidence-based practitioner, an occupational therapist needs to be able to use research findings in their everyday practice (Eakin et al 1997, Ilott and White 2001, COT 2005). The use of research findings to inform practice is an example of 'knowledge transfer', although it would be more accurate to call it research knowledge transfer.

Generally, 'Knowledge transfer is about exchanging good ideas, research results, experiences and skills between universities, other research organisations, business, government, the public sector and the wider community to enable innovative new products, services and policies to be developed' (ESRC 2005a). This means knowledge transfer is a broad concept and in its broadest sense can involve the use of good ideas, experiences, skills and research results. However, when the use of the term knowledge transfer is used in health and social care it refers to the use of research findings, i.e. 'to have knowledge of facts (represented by research results) and to use these facts in their practices, policies and products' (Lomas 2007: 129). The knowledge used in knowledge transfer in health and social care should be research based because we cannot rely on anecdote or experience. After all, '...because patients so often get better on their own, no matter what we do, clinical experience is a poor judge of what does and does not work' (Doust and Del Mar 2004: 474). Although it is emphasised that we use research-based knowledge, occupational therapists as 'health professionals do not apply abstract disembodied scientific research rigidly to the situation around them. Instead they collaborate in discussion, relate the evidence to the context, and engage in work practices that actively interpret and (re)construct its local validity and usefulness' (Dopson and Fitzgerald 2005a: 103). The sorts of activities used in knowledge transfer, include:

- Any form of dissemination, for example a patient information leaflet, conference paper, or paper in an academic journal
- Liaison between academics and policy makers, e.g. health researchers developing national guidelines for practice such as Marion Walker, Professor in Stroke Rehabilitation, who as an occupational therapist was involved in the development of the national guidelines for stroke (Intercollegiate Stroke Working Party 2004)
- Developing an education programme based on research findings, e.g. Enabling Occupation: A Learner-Centred Workbook (Townsend and Wright 1998), and
- Setting up a company to sell the products of research, e.g. Buckingham Healthcare which was set up by Chris Clarke, an occupational therapist, to sell the Buckingham walking frame caddy which she had designed and tested (see http://www.buckinghamhealthcare.co.uk/).

The World Health Organization (2004) defines knowledge transfer as translating knowledge into action to improve health, by bridging the gap between what is known and what is actually done. This means knowledge transfer

- has to go beyond mere dissemination and/or diffusion
- is an on-going and iterative process requiring active and conscious participation of both researchers and research-users, and
- is based on the principles of integration and simplification (International Development Research Centre 2007).

The Canadian Health Services Research Foundation is a leading organisation in the field of knowledge transfer in health care (International Development Research Centre 2007) and it no longer refers to knowledge transfer but now uses the term 'knowledge exchange'. It defines knowledge exchange as collaborative problem-solving between researchers and clinical decision makers (such as occupational therapists) that happens through linkage and exchange (Canadian Health Services Research Foundation 2007a). Effective knowledge exchange involves interaction between the people making the clinical decisions on the ground and researchers who are creating knowledge. It results in mutual learning, for both the occupational therapist and the researcher, through the process of planning, producing, disseminating and applying existing or new research in decision-making (Canadian Health Services Research Foundation 2007a). The shift to using the term knowledge exchange is still relatively recent so knowledge transfer is still the most widely used term. It has also been noted that the following terms, knowledge utilisation, knowledge dissemination, knowledge brokering, knowledge transfer and knowledge exchange, are used interchangeably in the literature (International Development Research Centre 2007). The key features of knowledge exchange are that it

- involves collaboration
- is dependent on interaction
- results in mutual learning, and,
- uses a problem-solving process.

This means it requires the use of the key skills that occupational therapists use in their everyday clinical work.

Knowledge exchange involves collaboration

Knowledge exchange is an area of practice where there is a need for practitioners, researchers, educators and managers to work together. Evidence-based practice involves complex clinical decision-making because it does not just focus on research knowledge but patient characteristics, situations and differences (Jones and Santaguida 2005). This means for knowledge exchange to happen researchers need to work with occupational therapists (Johnson 2005); they cannot work in isolation or just publish their research findings assuming that changes in occupational therapy practice will follow. The need for clinicians and researchers to work together was highlighted in the findings from the Nursing Environments: Knowledge To Action (NEKTA) study. It found that 'In general, the closer participants were to the delivery of care, the less likely they were to have any knowledge of the [research] reports' (Leiter 2006: 1). The recognition of a need for collaboration between clinicians and researchers arises from a shift in understanding about research and clinical decision making. That is, neither activity is a single event or product and there is a need to acknowledge not only the complexity involved in each activity but that this is increased when research is expected to influence clinical decision making (Bannigan 2004, 2007, Lomas 2007). Hence one way to create more research-informed clinical decisions is to focus on better linkage and exchange between the processes that create the facts (research) and the ones that incorporate the values (clinical decision making) (Lomas 2007). Linkage is achieved through the use of collaboration, i.e. practitioners and researchers working together, which means that it is necessary to take into account the context in which people work (Chunharas 2006, Nuyens and Lansang 2006).

Context

Context is an important part of the knowledge exchange process; it has an active role to play and is not just 'a back cloth to action' (Dopson and Fitzgerald 2005a: 102). For example the occupational therapy profession is part of the context in which occupational therapists' work. This means when trying to achieve exchange thought needs to be given to how to secure professional ownership of published research findings (Dopson et al 2005).

234

Every context is different and so the role context will play in achieving knowledge exchange will be different for the findings of each published project. Those engaged in knowledge exchange need to work together to analyse context (Fitzgerald and Dopson 2005). The dynamics of local situations can be difficult to influence from the outside and can produce strong social and cognitive boundaries (Fitzgerald et al 2005). This illustrates the fact that knowledge exchange is a social process; so whilst the research is important, on its own it will not effect knowledge exchange (Fitzgerald et al 2005). This is because, once research findings have been appraised and found to be rigorous (see Chapter 14), the focus of knowledge exchange is the people who will use the research findings and the environments in which they practise (Dopson and Fitzgerald 2005a, Lomas 2007). Although the importance of context is recognised the actual role context plays in achieving change is still not completely understood. Dopson and Fitzgerald (2005a) have suggested that a more sophisticated and active notion of context is needed than is currently found in the literature. Despite this there are things that occupational therapists can do within their environment to create a context in which to facilitate knowledge exchange, i.e.

- use only high-quality research to underpin service development
- stop using ineffective interventions
- provide easy access to information, e.g. desktop access to databases, and library facilities and make sure they are well resourced and well used
- encourage a questioning attitude by adopting a less accepting and more critical approach to service development
- include a responsibility for knowledge exchange in job descriptions and personal appraisal systems
- facilitate the use of journal clubs
- ensure all guidelines, clinical audit and teaching materials are based on evidence
- provide dedicated time for continuing professional development and evidence-based practice
- support all practitioners to develop/maintain their skills in evidence-based practice, and
- develop robust systems for recording and monitoring outcomes (Bannigan and Birleson 2007).

Knowledge exchange in occupational therapy

Beyond the local context occupational therapists also have a role to play in facilitating an evaluative culture so that evidence-based practice can thrive in the profession as a whole. This involves paying attention to infrastructure, including developing incentives for occupational therapists to engage in knowledge exchange. This can be achieved in clinical settings by rewarding the active involvement of occupational therapy teams in using research relevant to service delivery, supporting research and development as part of the profession's activity, ensuring change is driven by research-based knowledge, and including researchers in clinical decision making (Lomas 2007). In higher-education settings practitioners should be included in:

- the research process
- the creation of centres that connect researchers with practitioners, managers and policy makers from health and social care, and
- dissemination of brief research summaries including face-to-face exchanges of information that use plain language (Lomas 2007).

Knowledge exchange is dependent on interaction

Whereas linkage is achieved through collaboration, exchange is achieved through interaction. Lomas (2007) has described '...human interaction as the engine that drives research into practice' (p. 130). The ESRC (2005b) confirmed Lomas's (2007) analysis in their observation that 'At its simplest, knowledge transfer is about starting a conversation' (p. 1). This observation also explains why in Lomas's (1993) schemata of diffusion, dissemination and implementation (see Box 15.1 for explanation of terms) that diffusion and dissemination are unlikely to result in research use. Communication is a two-way process and both diffusion and dissemination involve only one-way communication, i.e. from researcher to occupational therapist, and so do not necessarily encourage the development of a dialogue. Knowledge exchange, like implementation, is contingent on a dialogue being created between researchers and research users, such as occupational therapists (ESRC 2005b). The importance

Box 15.1

A summary of key terms

- **Diffusion** – A passive process of research awareness raising which is largely uncontrolled or unplanned and dependent on the individual seeking out information (Lomas 1993)

- **Diffusion of innovations** – '...a social process in which subjectively perceived information about a new idea is communicated' (Rogers 1983: xix)

- **Dissemination** – A targeted process of raising awareness of research messages (NHS CRD 1999)

- **Implementation** – An active process that aims to change or confirm practice using research findings (Bannigan 2004)

- **Knowledge broker** – An expert who acts as a link between researchers and decision-makers (Gold 2002 cited by Thompson et al 2006)

- **Knowledge brokering** – '...all the activity that links decision makers with researchers, facilitating their interaction so that they are able to better understand each other's goals and professional cultures, influence each other's work, forge new partnerships, and promote the use of research-based evidence in decision-making' (Lomas 2007: 131)

- **Knowledge exchange** – '...collaborative problem-solving between researchers and decision makers that happens through linkage and exchange. Effective knowledge exchange involves interaction between decision makers and researchers and results in mutual learning through the process of planning, producing, disseminating, and applying existing or new research in decision-making' (Canadian Health Services Research Foundation 2007a).

- **Knowledge management** – is a business process that attempts to (a) identify, capture and promote the sharing of knowledge between individuals, (b) use existing knowledge in the creation of new knowledge, and (c) use knowledge to define and improve practice. It supports other processes, such as change management and risk management (Gallagher Financial Systems, Inc. 2007) of interpersonal networks was identified in an ethnographic study by Gabbay and le May (2004) and in a systematic review by Greenhalgh et al (2004). For those trying to facilitate the dialogue needed to achieve knowledge exchange will need to think about how the people involved in change may respond. This is because change is difficult for most people (Bryar and Bannigan 2003). Rogers (2003) identified five types of response to innovations, i.e.

- Innovators, a small group in any team, who are venturesome but may be distrusted by others
- Early adopters who are respected, approachable local opinion leaders
- Early majority who hold traditional values and are capable of change. They often provide the peer pressure to help the late majority
- Late majority who are sceptical about innovation and are reluctant to change
- Laggards who tend to hold traditional values and are generally suspicious of new ideas. They will be the last to embrace change, if at all.

In the light of this analysis any occupational therapists involved in knowledge exchange should try to develop links with early adopters in the first instance.

In interacting with others to facilitate knowledge exchange, as well as thinking about the people involved, it is also important to focus on how the 'actionable messages' from research findings are communicated (Organising Committee 2001, Askew et al 2002). It has been noted that 'In many instances it is possible that the expertise of communicating with [clinical] decision makers is not available within research organisations and therefore researchers may need to use others' (Askew et al 2002: i). The reality is 'The research world favours grant acquisition and academic publication over knowledge synthesis and engagement with the health service' (Lomas 2007: 129). In research grants there may be some support for dissemination plans but this is not always the case. It is often assumed the researcher will disseminate findings because there are a number of career incentives to encourage them to do so. For example, in the UK, the College of Occupational Therapists (2005) code of ethics and professional conduct states 'Occupational therapy personnel undertaking any form of research activity have an obligation to share their findings in order to inform or change practice, e.g. through publication or presentation' (p. 17). Usually the dissemination will just be the passive process of presenting and publishing papers. Yet at the very least multiple audience-specific messages are needed (Lavis et al 2003) to achieve knowledge exchange but this can be time-consuming work and so begs the question whose job is it to do this?

As knowledge exchange involves a two-way process of communication it means that all people in the collaboration need to be open to learning from others as well as sharing their ideas and experiences (ESRC 2005a). This is a significant shift in perspective from the idea of knowledge transfer which implies that knowledge transfers from one group to another and that all parties do not necessarily benefit and learn from each other. It also means knowledge exchange brings groups together who would not normally work together, which results in a better understanding of each other's work (Canadian Health Services Research Foundation 2006, Lomas 2007).

Until recently knowledge exchange has not been anyone's job (Bannigan 2004). In many ways knowledge exchange has fallen between a rock and hard place; researchers have not been funded to do it (Universities Scotland 2006) and equally there have been disincentives for practitioners to engage in this type of activity due to a lack of reward. This means there has been no incentive for occupational therapists to take responsibility for knowledge exchange. Where practitioners have tried to get involved in knowledge exchange the infrastructure was often not in place and their colleagues were not always receptive to these initiatives. Lately universities have set up Research and Enterprise offices and employed people to support this activity, such as Knowledge

Transfer Officers. This is because 'There is increasing recognition that this aspect of higher education is enormously important and universities are being encouraged to do even more of this kind of activity' (Universities Scotland 2006). Whilst knowledge exchange has become increasingly important to universities why should occupational therapists get involved? Is knowledge exchange relevant to the work of occupational therapists?

What is the relevance of knowledge exchange to occupational therapists?

There seems to be a broad agreement about the fact that research evidence rarely has a direct impact on clinical decision making (e.g. Thompson et al 2005). The need for knowledge exchange emerged in response to the gap between the publication of research findings and its use by various stakeholders (Schryer-Roy 2005). It has already been observed that a substantial amount of time and money is invested by health and social services across the world in generating research knowledge but, if this knowledge is not transferred into practice, the benefits for patients do not ensue. In blunt terms it means the investment is a waste of money, which is unacceptable in publicly funded services. As such all professionals working in health and social care, including occupational therapists, have to ask some very serious questions as to why we are continuing to produce these reports if in fact they are not being utilised by policy and clinical decision makers (Juzwishin 2001). This implies that an active process is needed if research findings are to be applied to practice because the mere existence of knowledge is insufficient. In physiotherapy Jones and Santaguida (2005) examined current physiotherapy research programmes and found that a considerable number of them were orientated towards benefiting patients. Despite this they also questioned how much impact these programmes of research have on the broader community. They posed the following questions:

- Do physiotherapists have a clear understanding of the mechanisms of knowledge exchange?
- Do they understand the continuum between research, practice and policy; the nature of the policy process; and the way that organisational goals, values, structures, processes and resources can encourage research projects that are not only relevant and timely for their clinical colleagues, but also for influencing policy-makers?
- Do physiotherapists provide the clinical decision-makers with the information they need and in a format they understand?
- Do physiotherapists have agents of change, who can convince clinical decision-makers to implement their findings? (Jones and Santaguida 2005)

In the light of this analysis they observed '...that physiotherapists must go beyond a circumscribed focus on physiotherapy treatment or publishing research in peer reviewed journals, and must become more attentive to the many factors which drive the policy process' (Jones and Santaguida 2005: 15). They also suggested that physiotherapists will only be able to do this "...if they are familiar with the following:

1. the mechanisms of knowledge transfer
2. the public policy process, and

3. major tools used by political and social scientists to analyse the institutions, ideas and interests that are involved in the design and implementation of policy" (Jones and Santaguida 2005: 15).

While physiotherapy was the focus of Jones and Santaguida's (2005) work it is unlikely that the situation will be any different for occupational therapists who also want to improve the patient experience of and outcomes of their interventions. This means knowledge exchange is as pressing an issue for occupational therapists as it is for physiotherapists.

What difference does knowledge exchange make to occupational therapists and their clients in practice?

Although knowledge exchange as a concept has had limited attention in occupational therapy it does happen (see Vignettes 15.1–15.3). These examples reflect the work of some tenacious researchers in occupational therapy rather than the existence of any formal knowledge exchange processes. In these vignettes it is clear how research-based knowledge can improve patient experience and/or outcomes of occupational therapy interventions.

Vignette 15.1

Example of knowledge exchange: The Mayers' Lifestyle Questionnaire (see www.mayerslsq.org.uk/)

This is an example of how knowledge that was developed by an academic is not only being widely used by occupational therapists in practice settings but is also endorsed by policy makers. The knowledge continues to develop through the dialogue the researcher has with practitioners who use her tool.

The Mayers' Lifestyle Questionnaire (1) was developed by Dr Christine Mayers, Reader in Occupational Therapy at York St John University, for her PhD. It was developed as a tool to enable people with problems related to physical disability or older age to identify and prioritise their quality of life needs before occupational therapy intervention begins. She has subsequently disseminated this work in numerous settings internationally and it is now widely used by occupational therapists in practice. In terms of policy The Mayers' Lifestyle Questionnaire (1) is recommended by the Department of Health for use within the Single Assessment Process (see http://www.dh.gov.uk/prod_consum_dh/idcplg?IdcService=GET_FILE &dID=8338&Rendition=Web). Through working with others it was recognized that different versions of the questionnaire were needed. The Mayers' Lifestyle Questionnaire (2) has been developed for use by people with enduring mental health problems. The development of the Mayers' Lifestyle Questionnaire (3) has now begun. This version has been requested specifically by occupational therapists working with older people. The Mayers' Lifestyle Questionnaires have also been translated into a number of different languages so the knowledge exchange has spread beyond the UK.

239

Vignette 15.2

Example of knowledge exchange: Joint protection (JP)

This is an example of how an occupational therapist's research into rheumatoid arthritis has contributed to the understanding of the work of the occupational therapist and the wider multidisciplinary team.

The current recommendations for JP and education from the Musculoskeletal Specialist Library (See http://www.library.nhs.uk/musculoskeletal/viewResource.aspx?resID=260188&code=c9cc36d3a300b0e37a6b3567c3fcfc9d) are:

1. Occupational therapists who teach JP should make themselves aware of recent developments in JP education and change practice to use behavioural JP methods.
2. Training courses are only the start of the process as time and strategies to change practice need to be factored in to service development.
3. Measures like the S-JPBA could be used clinically pre- and post-JP education to identify if behaviour change has occurred.
4. Client re-education is important. A regular review system would enable therapists to measure knowledge and adherence to JP principles (e.g. using the JPKA and S-JPBA), reinforcing JP education if necessary.
5. JP education should include other members of the multidisciplinary team.

Dr Alison Hammond, Reader at the Centre for Rehabilitation and Human Performance Research, University of Salford, is an occupational therapist with a longstanding research interest in patient education and rehabilitation in musculoskeletal care. She has conducted numerous studies (e.g. Klompenhouwer et al 2000, Hammond & Freeman 2001, Hammond & Freeman 2004), which have been used, alongside other research, to shape guidelines for practice in occupational therapy (College of Occupational Therapists 2003) as well as contributing to more general advice about joint protection and education as seen in the recommendations above. This work has also been incorporated into specialist education programmes for occupational therapists and physiotherapists working in hand therapy.

Vignette 15.3

Example of knowledge exchange: Training occupational therapists in Community Mental Health Team referral prioritisation (see http://www.priscillaharries.com/ email priscillaharries@brunel.ac.uk for passwords). See Chapter 3 for further information.

Dr Priscilla Harries, MSc Occupational Therapy Course Leader at Brunel University, has developed a free-to-access website, based on her PhD findings, to train occupational therapy students and novice occupational therapists to prioritise community mental health team referrals. The prioritisation exercise takes about an hour to use and has been shown to be effective (Harries 2006). It calculates all the statistics in the programme so the user gets their results on how they have performed at the end. The programme involves prioritising a set of referrals, then reading the training information (based on

Vignette 15.3 continued

occupational therapy expert practice), then repeating the prioritisation exercise with a new set of referrals. The user then receives detailed results (which are sent to them by email). It can be used just as an education tool or the user can tick the box to allow their results to be saved for research purposes (its use for research purposes has ethical approval from Brunel University). It is now used by universities as part of the provision of pre-registration occupational therapy education as well as by individual occupational therapists.

The practical issues involved in facilitating knowledge exchange in occupational therapy

To continue to overcome the gaps between publication of research findings and practice practitioners generally need to familiarise themselves with the literature on facilitating knowledge exchange. The difficulty of bringing about change should not be underestimated (Bryar and Bannigan 2003, Dopson et al 2005). The bottom line is there is no guaranteed method of knowledge exchange because of the range of factors that impact on it (Jones and Santaguida 2005). There is wide agreement that passive processes are ineffective and this message has been a consistent over time (Caplan and Rich 1975, Lomas 1991, NHS CRD 1999). The most precise knowledge we have is that interactive engagement (i.e. interpersonal contact) is effective in achieving knowledge exchange (Lavis et al 2003, Thompson et al 2006). The lessons from previous research or evaluations, such as the NEKTA study (Leiter 2006), provide useful insights into the likely challenges. For example the barriers experienced in the NEKTA study were:

* that research reports are too long, too academic and too numerous
* inadequacies in dissemination
* limited access to technology
* filtering of information by managers, and
* vulnerability to political cycles and legal barriers (Leiter 2006).

The likelihood of success was increased by:

* synopses of reports (such as the 'mythbusters' developed by the Canadian Health Services Research Foundation)
* diverse transmission processes
* broad endorsement within environment
* human and financial resources (Leiter 2006).

Therefore practitioners should avoid didactic methods and use the findings from studies, such as the NEKTA study (Leiter 2006), to identify and eliminate barriers and repeat the techniques that contributed to successful knowledge exchange. However, it is important that no one study is assumed to be definitive. The change management literature can also be used to support this process (Bryar and Bannigan 2003) because it is likely to involve changes in behaviour and/or systems. It is important to note that, 'Evidence based healthcare is likely to be imperfectly implemented through uniform approaches within such highly complex and variable settings characteristic of healthcare' (Dopson and Fitzgerald 2005b: 3).

Rogers (2003) proposed a five-stage model for the diffusion of innovations (see Box 15.2) that may be useful for shaping thinking about knowledge exchange in occupational therapy. Again it is important to recognise the model for what it is, i.e. a theoretical model, and not fall into the trap of assuming it is an authoritative method or that it is a rationalistic process (Fitzgerald and Dopson 2005). Even if the model is used to shape thinking there are no precise procedures for each stage. For example in relation to stage one, knowledge (Box 15.2), 'the research literature does not explain how to select the target audience(s) for a message, only that once a target audience is identified, the specific knowledge-transfer strategy should be fine-tuned to the types of decisions clinical decision makers face and the decision making environments in which they live or work' (Lavis et al 2003: 225). A range of sources should be drawn upon (for example Ebener et al 2006, Nuyens and Lansang 2006, Tugwell et al 2006) because there is no one best way to proceed (Fitzgerald and Dopson 2005).

A new role, the knowledge broker, has emerged out of the need for knowledge exchange (Lomas 2007). It has already been highlighted that 'The traditional outputs of research projects, such as final reports and peer reviewed papers, are often inaccessible to the key decision makers, either due to constraints in accessing them or the language in which they are written' (Askew et al 2002: i). In the light of this Askew et al (2002) suggested the need for mediators between information providers and clinical decision makers. Knowledge brokers link '...researchers and decision makers, facilitating their interaction so that they are able to better understand each other's goals and professional cultures, influence each other's work, forge new partnerships, and promote the use of research-based evidence in decision-making' (Canadian Health Services Research Foundation 2007a). Knowledge brokering activities include:

- finding the right people to influence research use in clinical decision-making
- bringing these people together
- creating and helping to sustain relationships among them, and
- helping them to engage in collaborative problem-solving.

As with research utilisation knowledge brokering is not a new concept (Lomas 2007) but it has not been widely used in a health and social care context until recently. This means there is a scarcity of literature about the role of knowledge broker per se. There are other roles that can be identified in the literature, i.e. opinion leader, facilitator, champion, linking agent and change agent, that provide some indication of what is involved in the role of knowledge broker (Thompson et al 2006).

242

Box 15.2

A five-stage model for the diffusion of innovations (Rogers 2003)

- **Knowledge** – learning about and understanding an innovation
- **Persuasion** – becoming convinced of the value of the innovation through discussion and exposure to diverse opinions
- **Decision** – committing to the adoption or rejection of the innovation
- **Implementation** – putting the innovations to use
- **Confirmation** – the ultimate acceptance (or rejection) of the innovation

Ultimately knowledge brokering in health and social care is about increasing the evidence-based decision-making, management and delivery of services in an organisation (Canadian Health Services Research Foundation 2007b). Knowledge brokering can be individually or structurally focused but either way knowledge exchange is achieved through the use of interaction which means it requires a knowledge broker to have a wide range of interpersonal skills (Lomas 2007). 'Knowledge brokering uses a portfolio of resources to make health services research and decision making more accessible to each other' (Lomas 2007: 131). The attributes and skills needed are:

- personal credibility in their own organisation and beyond
- the ability to translate, synthesise and contextualise research for a variety of users
- interpersonal skills to facilitate interaction and collaboration
- tenacity and
- analytical skills (see Fitzgerald et al 2005, Thompson et al 2006, Lomas 2007).

In some countries there are knowledge-brokering services (see Box 15.3). Lomas (2007) is keen to point out that knowledge brokering is not a panacea. While knowledge brokers have a role to play essentially all stakeholders have an obligation to facilitate knowledge exchange and strategies should be developed to accomplish this (Nuyens and Lansang 2006).

Whilst a knowledge broker can be an external facilitator or even be contracted from a specific knowledge-brokering service (Box 15.3) the majority of knowledge brokers that practitioners will come across will be individual occupational therapists who adopt this role as, for example, an opinion leader or facilitators (see Box 15.4), with their organisation or geographical area. Sometimes people will work together, e.g. facilitators and opinion leaders, to increase the effectiveness of a change project (Thompson et al 2006). Ideally knowledge exchange relies on researchers and clinical occupational therapists working together. Although some occupational therapy researchers have been identified who have engaged in knowledge exchange (see Vignettes 15.1–15.3) Stryer et al (2000) found that researchers have not perceived knowledge exchange as part of their role. Whilst knowledge exchange should be fundamental to research work (ESRC 2005a) it is time consuming (Lavis et al 2003). In the light of this researchers should consider working with knowledge brokers, this may be an external agency or a clinician who has adopted the role (Box 15.4). There is also a need for researchers to lobby for the inclusion of knowledge exchange in the research process so that funding for this work is secured; the use of knowledge brokers has cost implications (Bannigan 2004, Nuyens and Lansang 2006).

Box 15.3

Knowledge brokering services in health and social care

- The Sax Institute (2006) in Australia uses a database of available brokers to identify a knowledge broker that best fits the needs of a person requesting the service
- Canadian Health Services Research Foundation in Canada uses knowledge-brokering activities to focus on setting the research agenda, facilitating applied research, disseminating research, and getting research used (see the website in useful resources for more information)

Box 15.4

A summary of the different knowledge broker roles that an occupational therapist can play (based on Thompson et al 2006)

Champion

A person who advocates new ideas, products or projects, which they have personal ownership of. The distinguishing characteristic of a champion is their enthusiasm and vision for the change. However to operate effectively they also have to have the ability to influence others to get them to support the new project. They may be identified by others as a champion but if they are self appointed this should be congruent with others experience of them.

Change agent

This person plays an active role in helping individuals and groups through a process of change. They need to have strong interpersonal skills because they take the lead in a time limited project in which they have to enable others to change their behaviours.

Opinion leader

A person who has credibility and has the ability to persuade others. This person may be a peer or an expert but they are respected because they are seen as authoritative sources of information. As such, because they are trusted, they are a person others will go to for advice. They influence others through word of mouth or face to face communication within their local context because their knowledge is usually context-specific.

Facilitator

A person who is usually appointed and trained to assist others, either an individual or a group, through the process of implementing a change in practice. To be able to do this role they need to have good communication, group work and interpersonal skills. This is because their role is to enable others to achieve their goals rather than their personal goals as a facilitator.

Linking agent

This person brings together two groups, for example researchers and clinical practitioners, to enable collaboration. They are usually trained to do this role and achieve collaboration through creating a network, using a problem solving approach, developing contacts, and sharing information between the groups involved.

Capacity for knowledge exchange in occupational therapy

The lack of research literature in occupational therapy suggests that there may be limited experience of knowledge exchange. A critical mass is needed because knowledge exchange cannot rely solely on a small number of individuals (Bannigan 2004). This suggests there is a need for occupational therapists to develop the skills, structures, processes as well as an organisational culture that allows, encourages and rewards knowledge exchange (Canadian Health Services Research Foundation 2007a).

This may mean developing skills in knowledge exchange by attending a course, getting involved in a project, or shadowing a Knowledge Transfer Officer. Developing skills around knowledge exchange is a challenge because practitioners, whatever sector they work in, are faced with multiple drivers for change and a number of competing agendas. Occupational therapists should try to build on their existing knowledge. This is because they will have some transferable skills and, if these are in evidence-based practice, they will also have developed some of the skills needed for knowledge exchange. Capacity will also be increased if the organisational culture within occupational therapy services encourages knowledge exchange.

Knowledge management

If sharing knowledge and collaboration are key survival skills in today's society, knowledge is not only an asset but is perhaps the most important asset any organisation has (Gallagher Financial System, Inc. 2007). This means that some attention needs to be paid to knowledge management (see Box 15.1) in occupational therapy services. Knowledge management concerns knowledge production and use (Nuyens and Lansang 2006) but knowledge is social in nature because it resides in individuals and is shared through interpersonal networks. Practitioners should think about how knowledge is captured and harnessed to ensure their organisation is operating as effectively as possible (Gallagher Financial System, Inc. 2007). The potential benefits of adopting a knowledge management strategy are numerous and have far-reaching implications for any organisation. The proper use of knowledge management techniques and technology makes an organisation more agile and better able to respond to changes (Gallagher Financial System, Inc. 2007). The sharing of knowledge between knowledge workers increases performance and reduces the amount of training required for new employees (Gallagher Financial System, Inc. 2007). The implementation of a knowledge management strategy will involve paying attention to information technology (as well as personnel) to increase efficiency, flexibility and responsiveness. This 'will require concerted action and facilitation, and time to build and strengthen trust and gradually develop tacit rules' (Fitzgerald et al 2005: 176).

Summary

Knowledge exchange is an important process for improving patient care that requires more attention from occupational therapists. It necessitates recognition that knowledge exchange is as much a social process as a technical process. There is a general trend towards increased interactions between researchers and users, and knowledge exchange strategies increasingly incorporate active processes, interaction and a consideration of context. Every opportunity for knowledge exchange should be approached on its merits. Lessons learnt from previous research and evaluations, as well as other resources, can inform this work. The only certainty is that interactive rather than passive approaches are effective in facilitating knowledge exchange. However the words of Johann Wolfgang von Goethe aptly summates the challenge of knowledge exchange for occupational therapists, 'Knowing is not enough, we must apply; willing is not enough, we must act'.

Useful resources

Canadian Health Services Research Foundation (www.chsrf.ca)

This organization is the leading authority in the world for knowledge exchange in the health

and social care field. It includes KEYS, a guide to implementing effective exchange.

Change here! (www.auditcommission.gov.uk/changehere)

This is a simple (but not simplistic) and accessible resource which should be useful for those involved in leading change.

How can research organizations more effectively transfer research knowledge to decision makers? (Lavis et al 2003)

This is an engaging read that provides a good overview of the subject.

Knowledge to action? Evidence-based health care in context (Dopson and Fitzgerald 2005c)

This book is a serious, but readable, academic text written by researchers with breadth of experience in this field. It is a must read for anyone working in the field and/or charged with developing evidence-based practice/knowledge exchange. It provides good coverage of the topic as well as focusing on the social processes involved in knowledge exchange.

Knowledge Utilisation Studies Program (KUSP) (www.nursing.alberta.ca/kusp/index.html)

This is a research programme devoted to knowledge exchange and so is worth visiting to keep up to date with the latest developments.

References

Askew I, Matthews Z, Partridge R 2002 Going beyond research. University of Southampton, Southampton, UK

Bannigan K 2004 Increasing the use of research findings in four allied health professions (unpublished PhD thesis). School of Nursing, University of Hull, Hull, UK

Bannigan K 2007 Making sense of research utilisation. In: Creek J, Lawson-Porter A (eds) Contemporary Issues in Occupational Therapy: Reasoning and Reflection, 2nd edn., pp. 189–216. John Wiley, Chichester, UK

Bannigan K, Birleson A 2007 Getting to grips with evidence-based practice: the ten commandments. British Journal of Occupational Therapy 70(8): 345–348

Brett JL 1986 Organisational integrative mechanisms and adoption of innovations by nurses (Unpublished PhD thesis). University of Pennsylvania, Pennsylvania, PA

Bryar RM, Bannigan K 2003 The process of change: issues for practice development. In: Bryar RM, Griffiths JM (eds) Practice Development for Community Nurses: Principles and Processes, pp. 57–92. Arnold, London

Canadian Health Services Research Foundation 2006 Knowledge transfer and exchange Online. Available: http://www.chsrf.ca/knowledge_transfer/index_e.php 6th Sept 2006

Canadian Health Services Research Foundation 2004 What counts? Interpreting evidence-based decision-making for management and policy Report of the 6th CHSRF Annual Invitational Workshop Vancouver, British Columbia March 11. Canadian Health Services Research Foundation, Ottawa

Canadian Health Services Research Foundation 2007a Glossary of knowledge exchange terms as used by the foundation Online. Available: http://www.chsrf.ca/keys/glossary_e.php 2nd Feb 2007

Canadian Health Services Research Foundation 2007b Knowledge Brokering Online. Available: http://www.chsrf.ca/brokering/index_e.php 2nd Feb 2007

Caplan N, Rich RF 1975 The use of social science knowledge in policy decisions at the national level. Institute for Social Research, University of Michigan, Ann Arbor, MI

Chunharas S 2006 An interactive integrative approach to translating knowledge and building a "learning organization" in health service management. Bulletin of the World Health Organization 84(8): 652–657

College of Occupational Therapists 2003 National Association of Rheumatology Occupational Therapy Clinical Guidelines for the management of rheumatoid arthritis. College of Occupational Therapists, London

College of Occupational Therapists 2005 College of occupational therapists code of ethics and professional conduct. College of Occupational Therapists, London

Dawes M, Summerskill W, Glasziou et al 2005 Sicily statement on evidence-based practice BMC Medical Education. 5: 1 doi: 10.1186/1472-6920-5-1 Online. Available: http://www.biomedcentral.com/1472-6920/5/1 18th Feb 2005

Dopson S, Fitzgerald L 2005a The active role of context In: Dopson S, Fitzgerald L (eds) Knowledge to Action? Evidence-based Health Care in Context, pp. 79–103. Oxford University Press, Oxford, UK

Dopson S, Fitzgerald L 2005b Introduction In: Dopson S, Fitzgerald L (eds) Knowledge to Action? Evidence-based Health Care in Context, pp. 1–7. Oxford University Press, Oxford, UK

Dopson S, Fitzgerald L (eds) 2005c Knowledge to Action? Evidence-based Health Care in Context. Oxford University Press, Oxford, UK

Dopson S, Locock L, Gabbay J et al 2005 Evidence based healthcare and the implementation gap In: Dopson S, Fitzgerald L (eds) Knowledge to Action? Evidence-based Health Care in Context, pp. 28–47. Oxford University Press, Oxford, UK

Doust and Del Mar 2004 Why do doctors use treatment that do not work? British Medical Journal 328: 474–475

Eakin P, Ballinger C, Nicol M et al 1997 College of Occupational Therapists: Research and Development Strategy. British Journal of Occupational Therapy 60(11): 484–486

Ebener S, Khan A, Shademani R et al 2006 Knowledge mapping as a technique to support knowledge translation. Bulletin of the World Health Organization 84(8): 636–642

Economic and Social Research Council 2005a What is knowledge transfer? Online. Available: http://www.esrc.ac.uk/ESRCInfoCentre/Support/knowledge_transfer/about/what_is_KT/index.aspx?ComponentId=8766&SourcePageId=8852#0 2nd Feb 2007

Economic and Social Research Council 2005b Introduction to knowledge transfer. Online. Available: http://www.esrc.ac.uk/ESRCinfocentre/support/knowledge-transfer/ 2nd Feb 2007

Estabrooks CA 1997 Research utilisation in nursing: an examination of formal structure and influencing factors (Unpublished PhD thesis). University of Alberta, Edmonton, Alberta

Fitzgerald L, Dopson S 2005 Professional boundaries and the diffusion of innovation In: Dopson S, Fitzgerald L (eds) Knowledge to Action? Evidence-based Health Care in Context, pp. 104–131. Oxford University Press, Oxford, UK

Fitzgerald L, Dopson S, Ferlie E et al 2005 Knowledge in action In: Dopson S, Fitzgerald L (eds) Knowledge to Action? Evidence-based Health Care in Context, pp. 155–181. Oxford University Press, Oxford, UK

Gabbay J, le May A 2004 Evidence based guidelines or collectively constructed 'mindlines?' Ethnographic study of knowledge management in primary care. British Medical Journal 329: 1013–1017

Gallagher Financial System, Inc. 2007 Knowledge Management and Knowledge Automation Systems Online. Available at: http://hosteddocs.ittoolbox.com/gallagher052307.pdf 27 May 2007

Gold I 2002 Knowledge brokers. Online. Available: http://www.nursing.ualberta.ca/knowledgetransfer/news.html 2 Apr 2003

Greenhalgh T, Robert G, Macfarlane F et al 2004 Diffusion of innovations in service organisation: systematic review and recommendations. Milbank Quarterly 82: 581–629

Hammond A, Freeman K 2001 One-year outcomes of a randomised controlled trial of an educational-behavioural joint protection programme for people with rheumatoid arthritis. Rheumatology 40: 1044–1051

Hammond A, Freeman K 2004 The long term outcomes from a randomised controlled trial of an educational-behavioural joint protection programme for people with rheumatoid arthritis. Clinical Rehabilitation 18: 520–528.

Harries P 2006 The development of a web-based tool for training referral prioritization skills. International Journal of Therapy and Rehabilitation 13(6): 244

Ilott I, White E 2001 College of Occupational Therapists' strategic vision and action plan. British Journal of Occupational Therapy 64(6): 270–277

Intercollegiate Stroke Working Party 2004 National clinical guidelines for stroke, 2nd edn. Clinical Effectiveness & Evaluation Unit. Royal College of Physicians of London, London

International Development Research Centre 2007 Knowledge Translation: Basic Theories, Approaches and Applications. Online. Available: http://www.idrc.ca/en/ev-90105-201-1-DO_TOPIC.html 2nd Feb 2007

Johnson LS 2005 Developing expert practice. From knowledge transfer to knowledge translation: applying research to practice. Occupational Therapy Now 7(4): 11–14

Jones RJE, Santaguida P 2005 Evidence based practice and health policy development: the link between knowledge and action. Physiotherapy 91: 14–21

Juzwishin D 2001 The challenge of bringing EBDM to the diffusion of health technology. In: Alberta Heritage Foundation for Medical Research Proceedings of the conference on evidence based decision making: how to keep score? HTA Initiative #3. Alberta Heritage Foundation for Medical Research, Alberta, pp. 7–9

Klompenhouwer P, Lysack C, Dijkers M et al 2000 The Joint Protection Behaviour Assessment: a reliability study. American Journal of Occupational Therapy 54: 516–524

Knexa 2005 knexa knowledge shared Online. Available: http://www.knexa.com/ 2nd Feb 2007

Lavis JN, Robertson D, Woodside JM et al Knowledge Transfer Study Group 2003 How can research organisations more effectively transfer research knowledge to decision makers? The Milbank Quarterly 81(2): 221–248

247

Leiter MP 2006 Nursing environments: Knowledge to action Final report submitted to Health Canada, Health Policy Research Program: Quality workplaces for health professionals, Acadia University, Wolfville, NS

Loisel P, Falardeau M, Baril R et al 2005 The values underlying team decision-making in work rehabilitation for musculoskeletal disorders. Disability and Rehabilitation 27(10): 561–569

Lomas J 1991 Words without action? The production, dissemination, and impact of consensus recommendations. Annual Review of Public Health 12: 41–65

Lomas J 1993 Diffusion, dissemination, and implementation: who should do what? Annals of the New York Academy of Sciences 703: 226–237

Lomas J 2007 The in-between world of knowledge brokering. British Medical Journal 334: 129–130

MacDermid JC, Solomon P, Law M et al 2006 Defining the effect and mediators of two knowledge translation strategies designed to alter knowledge, intent and clinical utilization of rehabilitation outcome measures: a study protocol [NCT00298727] Implementation Science 1: 14 doi:10.1186/1748-5908-1-14 Online. Available: http://www.implementationscience.com/content/1/1/14 17th Aug 2006

NHS CRD 1999 Getting evidence into practice. Effective Health Care 5(1) Royal Society of Medicine Press, London

Nuyens Y, Lansang MAD 2006 Knowledge translation: linking the past to the future (editorial). Bulletin of the World Health Organization 84(8): 590

Organising Committee 2001 Knowledge transfer: Looking beyond health A report on the conference held in Toronto, October 26-27, 2000 Organising committee for Knowledge Transfer: Looking beyond health, Canada

Rogers EM 1983 Diffusion of Innovations, 3rd edn. The Free Press, New York

Rogers EM 2003 Diffusion of Innovations, 5th edn. The Free Press, New York

The Sax Institute 2006 Knowledge Brokering Online. Available:http://www.saxinstitute.org.au/policyresearchexchange/KnowledgeBrokering.cfm?objid=542 2nd Feb 2007

Schryer-Roy A 2005 Knowledge translation Basic theories, approaches and applications. Online. Available: http://www.idrc.ca/uploads/user-S/11473620631Knowledge_Translation_Basic_Theories,_Approaches_and_Applications_-_May_2006.pdf 2nd Feb 2007

Soderback I, Frost D 1995 The transfer of knowledge in occupational therapy: the case of work ability assessment. Work 5(3): 157–165

Strang D, Meyer J 1993 Institutional conditions for diffusion. Theory and Society 22: 487–511

Stryer D, Tunis S, Hubbard H, Clancy C (2000) The outcome of outcomes and effectiveness research: impacts and lessons from the first decade. Health Services Research 35(5): 980–993

Thompson C, McCaughan D, Cullum N et al 2005 Barriers to evidence based practice in primary care nursing – viewing decision-making as context is helpful. Journal of Advanced Nursing 52(4): 432–444.

Thompson GN, Estabrooks CA, Degner LF 2006 Clarifying the concepts in knowledge transfer: a literature review. Journal of Advanced Nursing 53(6): 691–701

Townsend E, Wright WA 1998 Enabling Occupation: A Learner-Centred Workbook. Canadian Occupational Therapy Association, Canada

Tugwell P, Robinson V, Grimshaw J et al 2006 Systematic reviews and knowledge translation. Bulletin of the World Health Organization 84(8): 643–651

Universities Scotland 2006 What is knowledge transfer? Online. Available: www.universities-scotland.ac.uk/Facts%20and%20Figures/knowledge.pdf 17th Aug 2006

Weiss CH 1979 The many meanings of research utilisation. Public Administration Review 39(5): 426–431

West Yorkshire Knowledge Exchange 2006 Who are we Online. Available: http://www.ke-westyorkshire.ac.uk/modules/MrContent/index.php?id=2 17th Aug 2006

World Health Organization 2004 World Report on Knowledge for Better Health. World Health Organization, Geneva

Clinical effectiveness skills in practice

16

Jenny Miller

Highlight box

- Being clinically effective does not mean that you have to be skilled in every aspect of the clinical effectiveness process.
- Implementation of effective practice requires a range of skills; change management skills are core to the process.
- Everyone can undertake effective practice.
- Making small changes which are evaluated, reviewed and monitored can lead to sustainable service improvement.
- Service user involvement should remain at the centre of effective practice.

Introduction

Keeping professional knowledge and skills up to date and ensuring best practice by monitoring and reviewing the ongoing effect of our activity, making changes accordingly (Health Professions Council 2005) is easier said than done.

The challenge is not so much about finding the right evidence to do the right practice at the right time in the right place; it is about being the right person to deliver the practice, about feeling enabled to implement new practice and having the resources to keep up to date with all the new evidence being generated.

Being clinically effective is non-negotiable. So how can effective practice become the norm and something that all practitioners feel able to engage with? This chapter explores the core components of clinical effectiveness, highlights the barriers to engagement and provides tools to assist practitioners to contribute to the clinical effectiveness agenda in their workplace. Effective practice is not just about clinical practice though, it is about all practice; it includes managers, educationalists, researchers, clinicians, care providers and service users. Clinical effectiveness interlinks with several other skills for practice and this chapter should therefore be read and used in conjunction with other chapters within this book, as many of them discuss and present particular aspects of effective practice. Clinical effectiveness doesn't just happen. It requires reflection of planning and action.

This chapter, however, is not an academic appraisal or 'how to' guide to clinical effectiveness. It is an introduction to the topic and reference point for further reading with direct links to everyday occupational therapy practice.

Context

Policy, both in the UK (NHS Executive 1998, NHS Wales 1998, Scottish Executive 1998, College of Occupational Therapists 1999) and internationally, has seen an increasing emphasis on the quality of health service provision and the drive for evidence-based interventions over the last 20 years. Within the UK this is set in a backdrop of high-profile cases where serious malpractice has injured the credibility of health-care practitioners (Department of Health 2002a, 2002b, 2004) and led to the rise of a process by which every part of the health service was able to quality assure its decisions. More recently there has been progress from a measuring and assuring process to a more mature approach to developing and improving services which involves working in partnership across organisations and with services users and their carers. This transparency is promoting a culture of improvement that is driven by learning from and with partners (NHS Plan 2000, Scottish Executive 2005).

Clinical effectiveness is a tool or a group of tools that can be used to improve individual practice and whole services. There are many available resources that assist in overcoming barriers and developing practitioners' clinical effectiveness skills, and ensure that they become part and parcel of everyday practice (see Tables 16.1, 16.2).

Frequently practitioners are involved in clinical effectiveness activities of some shape and form but do not always label it as such. Prior to commencing an allied health professions clinical effectiveness network project in Scotland, allied health professionals were questioned about their involvement and confidence with clinical effectiveness. The responses highlighted that specific clinical effectiveness activities were patchy with a large number of respondents stating that they needed assistance to undertake such projects. A limited number of respondents highlighted that they were already implementing guidelines within their practice (Holdsworth et al 2005). The barriers to engaging with clinical effectiveness are highlighted later in this chapter but many of the issues that stopped practitioners in this study from practising clinical effectiveness activities related to their confidence.

What is clinical effectiveness?

Various definitions of clinical effectiveness exist:

> *The extent to which specific clinical interventions, when deployed in the field for a particular patient or population, do what they are intended to do - that is, maintain and improve health and secure the greatest possible health gain from available resources (NHS Executive 1996). There are a significant number of issues and methodologies concerned with the quality of clinical care, for example clinical audit, R&D, education and training, continuous quality improvement, integrated care pathways, clinical guidelines. The real world definition and application of these terms varies, sometimes for organisational or historical reasons .... The umbrella term 'clinical effectiveness' refers to activities that have as their focus the measuring, monitoring and improvement of clinical care. Clinical Effectiveness is a component of Clinical Governance (Scottish Executive 1999).*

The Chartered Society for Physiotherapists' definition of clinical effectiveness has been widely used and states that it is, 'the right person (you) doing: the right thing (evidence based practice) in the right way (skills and competence) at the right time (providing

Table 16.1 Overcoming Barriers to Implementing Clinical Effectiveness

Barriers	Possible solutions
Lack of theoretical and practical clinical effectiveness skills	Consult colleagues with good current clinical effectiveness skills: for example new graduates, research practitioners. Involve your local clinical effectiveness departments who will support development of skills through education. Join or form a journal club where skills can be developed and practised.
Access to resources/ information	Many electronic databases are now available and easily accessible from your department, local hospital or community library. Get involved in specific practice networks. For example special interest groups and local, national and international practice development networks.
Support – local, organisational	Develop links with peers. Use or create coffee break support groups, join formal and informal networks, managed clinical networks, etc. Find out about local clinical effectiveness departments and their agendas. Highlight significant areas within your organisation's plan which support your clinical effectiveness work and present this to managers and peers. Ensure that there are clinical effectiveness objectives within your personal development plans.
Time	There is no easy answer to this but consider how you use your time. Use or negotiate CPD sessions – at least ½ session per month is recommended.
Authority to act	Clarify this via supervision. Ensure your work fits with your organisation's strategic plan. Establish links with your clinical effectiveness departments/ organisational development or change and innovation departments. Seek out champions who are both credible and influential within the practice context and/or who will support/champion your work within their area.
Resources	Use electronic resources. Make links with higher education institutes. There are a number of grants that can be accessed both nationally and locally. Check your professional body, local clinical effectiveness departments, and government health departments. Think small change.
Colleagues' apathy	The model for improvement can show colleagues the possibilities.
Motivation	Buddy systems. Coffee break CE groups.

treatment/services when the patient needs them), in the right place (location of treatment/services), with the right result (clinical effectiveness/maximising health gain)' (Chartered Society of Physiotherapists 2007).

The NHS Scotland online education resource states that clinical effectiveness has been actively used to improve the quality of treatments and services since the late 1980s. Health professionals are involved in audits and improvement projects as an integral part of promoting good clinical practice. Clinical effectiveness is reliant on the wealth of expertise, knowledge and skill of those who work with patients and who have an insight and understanding as to how the service works and how it could be improved (NHS Scotland 2007).

All these definitions highlight that clinical effectiveness is about practitioners continually assessing and analysing what they do, in context of the evidence that is available to improve care and practice. Clinical effectiveness is a cycle that entails a series of steps. These can at times seem onerous, until you realize the resources that are available for each step (see Figure 16.1 and Table 16.2).

'A successful clinical effectiveness initiative not only identifies the best information about those interventions which work but also makes that information available in an accessible and understandable format and ensures that it is used in practice' (McClarey and Duff 1997). But in reality how does all this work? Vignette 16.1 provides one example.

Vignette 16.1

In 2002 a group of occupational therapists within a NHS Board in Scotland set out to ensure that the records they were keeping met the standards set by the College of Occupational Therapists (2002, 2005). The relevance of this standard in the context of clinical effectiveness has been further highlighted more recently by the Department of Health. It states:

'Records are a valuable resource because of the information they contain. High quality information underpins the delivery of high quality evidence based health care.... Information is of greatest value when it is accurate, up to date and accessible. An effective records management service ensures that information is properly managed and is available when needed:

- To support patient care and continuity of care;

- To support day to day business which underpins delivery of care;

- To support evidence based clinical practice;

- To support sound administrative and managerial decision making, as part of the knowledge base for NHS services;

- To meet legal requirements, including requests from patients under subject access legislation;

- To assist clinical and other audit

- To support improvements in clinical effectiveness through research and also support archival functions by taking account of the historical importance of material and the needs of future research;

- Whenever, and wherever there is a justified need for information, and in whatever media it is required.'

(Department of Health 2006, section 2)

Vignette 16.1 continued

What is the clinical question?

The occupational therapists asked the question 'Do our records meet the required standard as stated within the College of Occupational Therapists Code of Ethics and Professional Conduct (2005) and the record keeping core standard (2000)?'

What is the best evidence for good practice?

The group undertook a literature review on record keeping using Medline and CINAHL electronic databases and identified 98 relevant articles. They also included a letter in OT News that attracted interest and information from as far afield as Hong Kong.

Is the evidence applicable for our area of practice?

The available literature was read and appraised. A retrospective audit tool was designed which differed from the COT tool in the fact that it had additional responses. The tool was piloted in four different geographical areas and across three different specialisms. This highlighted areas for amendment and the need for a guidance sheet to be developed in order to ensure uniformity of interpretation.

Is there local evidence of implementing good practice in relation to record keeping?

There were no local examples of auditing occupational therapy record keeping within this health board area so there was no sound evidence of good practice. The audit tool and guidance notes were distributed across the region and services were audited retrospectively against the standards.

Did the audit confirm that the OT service was providing good practice?

The audit was returned by 78% of occupational therapists and was analysed anonymously by the audit resource department within the health Board. The results showed that the audit tool was successful in identifying both good practice and areas requiring improvement.

Is a change in practice required?

The audit identified areas requiring change. These and other areas of good practice were fed back to the services via the heads of department. Offers of facilitation to develop and implement local action plans ahead of the second cycle were also given.

Impact on service

A second cycle was developed and implemented and improvements had occurred. The additional benefits were also highlighted by the group.

Dissemination and sharing of practice

The learning from this project was not only shared locally amongst occupational therapists but also within the local health board record keeping group set up by the clinical governance department. Nationally it was presented at a conference and submitted to the Clinical Improvements (CLIP) database (www.eguidelines.co.uk) A poster was made and has been presented at a variety of conferences. The tool has been disseminated internationally (Gibson et al 2004).

253

Room for improvement?

Looking at this piece of work (Vignette 16.1) several years on it is clear that there is a missing component in the process – the engagement and involvement of service users. The project team highlighted this in their conclusions. If this tool was examined today one would expect to find that it also supported service users, both in the development of the audit tool and in reporting their involvement with their clinical records. This could take the form of a questionnaire regarding their involvement with the treatment process particularly asking for evidence of collaborative goal setting, or ease of access to their occupational therapy notes when requested. It may also include a question on service users ease of access to local standards of record keeping.

Figure 16.1 The clinical effectiveness process (Adams C 1999a)

Questioning

• Whether the service/treatment/intervention that you are giving is having the desired result
• Asking an answerable question

Find the available evidence to answer your question

This may include evidence from:

• Research, usually found in journals or from databases such as Medline, OVID, PRODIGY etc.
• Systematic reviews (e.g. Cochrane reviews). These are often the best sources of summary information about primary research studies and frequently make recommendations on the outcome of the review.
• Consulting with colleagues – using clinical networks, special interest groups etc. This may then highlight the 'grey evidence' that is in the making or unpublished.

It should be noted that there are now some excellent search bodies that have already done this step for you (e.g. OTSeeker) references to these can be found at the back of this chapter

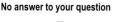

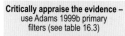

No answer to your question

Evidence available

There is no evidence

Should this be researched?
If yes this will take a different route
(see chapter on research in practice).
Ask – what is it you should be trying
to achieve?
Agree with peers/service users
local benchmarks or
performance measures.

Critically appraise the evidence –
use Adams 1999b primary
filters (see table 16.3)

Critical appraisal

Newman and Roberts (2002) divide critical
appraisal into three related parts:
• Is the quality of the study good enough for
me to use the results?
• Is the study design appropriate to the question?
• What do the results mean to my practice?

Validity of the evidence within your service context

Ascertain appropriateness of evidence for the service users that you work with/ the context
in which you are working

Are there already vehicles to put this new evidence into practice?

Find out if there are:
• National standards e.g. those produced by professional bodies such as the College of Occupational
Therapists. The American Occupational Therapy Association, or other national bodies.
• Clinical guidelines - these may be national (for example those produced by NICE (National Institute for
Health and Clinical Excellence) or SIGN, Scottish Intercollegiate Guidelines Network) or Clinical
Resource Efficiency Support Team (CREST - Northern Ireland) or profession specific.

Review your current practice in light of the evidence

Identify what improvements need to happen and/or what you are doing right
Conduct first audit cycle.

Figure 16.1—Cont'd

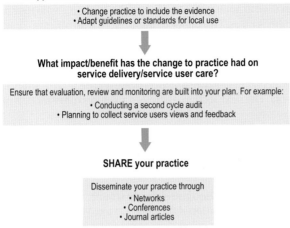

The ingredients for success

There were obviously a number of factors that contributed to the success of the record-keeping project.

Success factors

- **National policy** – Clinical governance was a key national driver that supported this type of project and provided evidence for how departments were meeting the national agenda. At that time there was the introduction of a national requirement to produce evidence of an annual audit of medical records. This was later backed up with the Laming enquiry into the death of Victoria Climbie that highlighted further the need for evidence-based care records (Department of Health 2003).
- **Local support and expertise** – the NHS Board had a very active clinical governance department that was closely linked to the clinical effectiveness team who assisted with the design of the audit tool and the project process. This gave the project instant credibility as well as an objective partner.
- **Peer/team approach** – there was a small group of committed practitioners who carried out the project providing support for each aspect.
- **Commitment from leaders and local champions** – the heads of service all signed up to the project and the service manager in the pilot area was a particular champion. Evidence, although divided in opinion, suggests that opinion leaders can influence the practice of others. This project supported the research that highlights the use of opinion leaders to influence the practice of others (Lomas et al 1991, Armstrong et al 1996, Doumit et al 2006) (see Chapter 20 for more information on Leadership Skills in Practice):-
- **Credibility** – The project leaders were well respected amongst their peers and colleagues.
- **Time** – This was specifically allocated and authorised by management in order to develop, implement, evaluate and disseminate the project.
- **Positive encouragement** – was given to staff undertaking the project from both management and clinical effectiveness departments.

- **Project team commitment and attention to detail** – Examples of this included heads of service briefings, training and support for sites in carrying out the audit, facilitation to develop action plans, and involvement of all staff including support staff.
- **Buddy system** used to audit notes. Staff were able to choose who they teamed up with to audit each other's notes. This allowed staff to work with other occupational therapists that they felt comfortable with, which in turn developed a positive learning environment.

The above list is not exhaustive but these elements form some of the important aspects that are key to the success of effective practice. However this level of support and influence is not always available. The next section, therefore, explores other models of participation.

'But I don't have the time to do that'

The record-keeping project, although relatively simple, was complex in its involvement of a whole health board occupational therapy service. What could you have done if you did not have the support of your colleagues or manager, a major barrier to implementing effective practice?

The literature search and review

Could you link with higher education establishments and request to work with undergraduate students as a possible project? Could this be carried out within monthly clinical professional development sessions? Could you form a journal club; reviewing with peers may also have the desired effect of motivating others to take part.

Development of the audit tool

In the UK most health and social care establishments have clinical effectiveness, clinical governance or quality departments. These resources can be invaluable as they provide tools to use in the workplace but they are also a very useful resource to support practitioners' skills in audit and practice development. In the original project the team collaborated with their local clinical effectiveness department to develop their record-keeping audit tool. This is a sound method of undertaking a high-quality piece of work and also ensures that local clinical effectiveness departments are engaged in the programme.

Start small

Having considered the evidence – start small. Practitioners should look at their own practice and record keeping and find out if they are achieving the standards. Working with another colleague enables the audit of each other's notes, highlighting any issues and developing an action plan.

Change management

Making changes within a service can be very difficult, especially when this is trying to be achieved alone. Change management skills are crucial within clinical effectiveness projects. There is an extensive evidence-base that suggests practitioners should take a multi-faceted approach to changing practice (Grol 1997, Glanville et al 1998, West et al 2001). Grol (1997) specifically highlights that practitioners need to identify their barriers to change before they begin. Another useful change management model (the model for improvement) was developed by Langley et al (1992). The benefits of this approach are that it looks at very small and manageable changes.

The model for improvement

The model was developed by Langley et al (1992) and is now being used extensively within organisations. It works on a series of small change cycles that can grow into fairly substantive improvements. Because it takes a change cycle at a time it is less intrusive and less risky than implementing major change. It allows practitioners to test their work as they go along to ensure that it is really making an improvement to the service they are delivering.

The model has two parts – thinking and doing.

Thinking Ask three fundamental questions:

- **Question 1: What am I/are we trying to accomplish?**
  Being clear about the desired improvement is essential. What needs to be different?
- **Question 2: How will I/we know that a change is an improvement?**
  Measurement is crucial in order to ascertain improvement. What data need to be collected that will tell you the service has improved or the system has changed?
- **Question 3: What changes can I/we make that can lead to an improvement?**
  Decide what changes need to be made to improve the service/systems. Look for evidence or ideas from elsewhere or discuss with colleagues and other members of the team. Practitioners have the knowledge and experience of their own service. Keep your vision clear (question 1) and some really innovative ideas will follow. These ideas and questions lead to the next stage: **doing.**

Doing: Plan, Do, Study, Act (The PDSA cycle) The PDSA process allows practitioners to test out their ideas about the changes that they believe are required to make an improvement (**Plan**), working on one idea at a time. The secret of success is to focus on very small-scale changes (**Do**). This means that there is very little altered and it is easy to revert back to the original way of working if something is unsuccessful. It also means that changes can be made and feedback received very quickly – how motivating is that! If it does work and information supports the change it can go ahead and be fully implemented within the service.

The '**Study**' part of the cycle gives space to reflect on and learn from what happened.

The '**Act**' part allows practitioners to question whether they re-run the same cycle again to gather more evidence, adapt what they have done following reflection, or develop further cycles to move the project forward.

In relation to record keeping (Vignette 16.1; see Chapter 13) it might be that an organisation wants to ensure that service users are involved in their own goal planning and that this is easily identifiable within their occupational therapy notes. Trying this out with one service user allows the approach to be easily and speedily tested.

It can be helpful to use this model to examine a hunch about something that might make a difference. Once the PDSA cycle is complete it will be clear if the hunch was correct. One example of this is when a team of practitioners decided to introduce a two-page assessment which they thought would assist with the implementation of a low back pain guideline. When they took this to the multidisciplinary team there were concerns that it would lengthen the initial assessment. It was agreed that two clinics would trial this assessment. The results of these trials highlighted that the assessment form had in fact speeded up the initial assessment process and was easy to use. The rest of the team then adopted this new process. The PDSA approach supported the practitioners' initial hunch but was tested before full-scale adoption, a far less risky approach. It is useful to record your PDSA reasoning at each stage as this supports the rationale for change which can then be more easily shared with colleagues as in the example above.

The barriers – reality laced with possible solutions

There is a massive volume of literature out there – it really is no wonder that many practitioners feel overwhelmed and paralysed. The reality is that evidence-based practice is not yet part and parcel of everyday practice (Holdsworth et al 2005) and although there has been progress there are still a large number of practitioners who are practising without a sound basis of evidence. That does not always mean that what they are doing is wrong but practitioners are not in a strong position to justify its existence if they do not make any attempt to prove its validity and value. There are of course practitioners who do consciously develop clinical effectiveness strategies and these are highly valued (see Vignette 16.2).

Vignette 16.2

During a 3-year project to set up allied health professions clinical effectiveness networks many clinicians were adamant that they were not involved in clinical effectiveness but when questioned further were in fact doing some really innovative work. One group of senior practitioners had begun to meet informally on a regular basis for coffee and peer support. The support was very much welcomed and as staff got to know each other they began to speak about wider issues like new treatment approaches and interesting journal articles. When the Scottish Intercollegiate Guidelines Network (SIGN) guidelines for stroke came out they found themselves discussing the implications for their area of practice. The next session one of them brought an occupational therapy journal article on implementing guidelines that they read and discussed. A couple of them admitted feeling rusty on critical appraisal and so the following coffee break meeting they had a practical review session and from that session on they became a clinical effectiveness group for neurology. The group evolved from a basis of mutual respect and trust where all participants felt safe to explore practice. This foundation has grown confident practitioners who run monthly journal clubs, implement professional guidelines and have presented their work at conferences. One member of the group has become a regional practice development network representative.

Much has been written on the barriers to implementing clinical effectiveness and evidence-based practice (Groll 1997, Haynes et al 1998, Nolan et al 1998, SIGN 2008). Local, national and international resources have been established to assist clinicians in overcoming these barriers (Glanville et al 1998, West et al 2001, Holdsworth et al 2005). Table 16.1 highlights some of these barriers and outlines possible solutions which are detailed further in the resources listed in Table 16.3 in the Resources Section.

A common barrier in this lack of engagement is time. And despite many clinical effectiveness initiatives this issue does not seem to be going away; so how do we get around it? Consider a meeting where a senior health board executive told the audience that the key components of effective practice were:

- WILL
- IDEAS
- EXECUTION.

His advice was to forget the IDEAS, as the organisation 'is awash with ideas'. What was needed, the audience were informed, was the WILL to change and the EXECUTION of the agreed health board priorities.

Whilst an initial feeling of indignation may appear justified (after all, clinicians and service users surely need to contribute their expertise, knowledge and skill to generate IDEAS too) it may be he was not completely wrong and may have had a point! Perhaps the best way to overcome the barriers listed above is to have the WILL to work in partnership; teaming up people with different skills and the tenacity to EXECUTE the ideas together.

There are some really good examples of how partnerships have worked in this way – senior clinicians working with undergraduates to look at the evidence underpinning certain aspects of their everyday work; new graduates being encouraged to use their research and critical appraisal skills (Table 16.2) from the moment they graduate so that the skills are not lost and their organisation fully uses the strengths of its workforce; managers using their skills in change management to bring on the implementation of effective practice; and in some dynamic practices the teaming up with an often underestimated partner, the service users and carers themselves. When it comes to change management and influencing skills the power of a personal narrative can really change hearts and minds.

Table 16.2 Critical appraisal Primary filters (Adams 1999b)

- Is the evidence relevant to your practice?
- Was the research based on a systematic review?
- Has the research been chosen for inclusion in a secondary source of research?
- Where was the article published?
- Was the evidence peer reviewed before being published? This does not mean that evidence that does not pass through this should be written off as there is some excellent practical descriptive evidence that may greatly assist your practice question. However proving that this evidence is valid is often harder to do. Conversely, just because a paper has been published one should not assume that this is a guarantor of high-quality evidence. Critical appraisal of research articles becomes easier with experience.

In summary you will be following these questions:
- Is the evidence from a reliable source?
- Is the research reliable – who did it, is it a leader in the field of practice and where is it published? This will often determine the quality and level of evidence.
- What is it about – does the title or the abstract highlight the content? And if so is it related to your area of practice?
- Is the research question clear and are there specific aims?
- Is there a transparent methodology which should allow you to determine bias?
- Are you able to ascertain how the data was analysed and are the results/findings clear and understandable?
- Were there any ethical issues and were these and the strengths and weaknesses of the study highlighted?
- Did the findings answer the research question and were these discussed in context of service improvement?
- Were further recommendations made?
- Would service user care be improved if the findings were implemented?

259

Practice development

There is an increasing interest in the concept of practice development which addresses the complex arenas in which practitioners work. It recognises that clinical effectiveness requires additional scope so that practice can be examined and valued even when the same effect is not regularly produced. It has been suggested that practice development is a prerequisite to clinical effectiveness (Manley 2000).

The broad approach that practice development adopts is perhaps closer to what many practitioners feel they are involved in. Described as,

> 'a continuous process of improvement towards increased effectiveness in person-centred care... brought about by helping health care teams to develop their knowledge and skills and to transform the culture and context of care. It is enabled and supported by facilitators committed to systematic, rigorous continuous processes of emancipatory change that reflect the perspectives of service users' (Garbett and McCormack 2002: 88).

Practice development was initially a nursing concept but there is growing interest from other professionals.

Page (2002) describes practice development as

- Focusing upon the improvement of patient care
- Incorporating a range of approaches
- Taking place in real practice settings
- Being underpinned by the development and active engagement of practitioners
- Being collaborative and interprofessional
- Being evolutionary
- Being transferrable rather than generalisable.

This approach is frequently viewed as both motivating and acceptable by practitioners. It identifies with commonly held values and practices and allows practitioners to feel that they have something to offer in the development of effective practice. Becoming part of a practice development network enables practitioners to meet with others working in the same field to discuss approaches, identify underpinning research which may be influencing ways of working and even begin to develop some rigorous multisited research projects. McCormack et al (2004) is an excellent resource for practitioners interested in developing their understanding of practice development.

Resources

Table 16.3 Resources to support clinical effectiveness

Clinical effectiveness and research information pack http://www.dh.gov.uk/ prod_consum_dh/groups/dh_ digitalassets/@dh/@en/documents/ digitalasset/dh_4042462.pdf	Achieving effective practice – a clinical effectiveness and research information pack for nurses, midwives and health visitors
Clinical Effectiveness Support Unit (CESU) http://www.cesu.wales.nhs.uk/	Clinical Effectiveness Support Unit (CESU) for Wales supporting the Welsh Office Clinical Effectiveness Initiative and implementation of clinical governance

Clinical Governance – Educational resource http://www.clinicalgovernance.scot.nhs.uk/section2/introduction.asp	This website aims to help you use clinical governance and risk management quality improvement methods in your work. The website can be used in 3 ways as a: Programme of learning Reference source Training resource
Cochrane Collaboration www.cochrane.org	The Cochrane Collaboration produces core content for The Cochrane Library, including the Cochrane Database of Systematic Reviews
Clinical Governance Support Team (CGST) http://www.cgsupport.nhs.uk/	This site has been developed for healthcare professionals, and is a central resource for clinical governance. It provides information, guidance to assist organisations in understanding and successfully implementing clinical governance
Clinical Resource Efficiency Support Team (CREST) http://www.crestni.org.uk/	The Clinical Resource Efficiency Support Team (CREST) group comprises 19 health care professionals from the health service in Northern Ireland with an active interest in promoting clinical efficiency
The Critical Appraisal Skills Programme (CASP) http://www.phru.nhs.uk/casp/critical_appraisal_tools.htm	This programme helps to develop the skills to find and make sense of research evidence
Centre for evidence-based medicine http://www.cebm.net/critical_appraisal.asp	Provides information on how to find and appraise evidence
Crombie (1996) The pocket guide to critical appraisal	A pocket guide which provides a basic introduction to the principles underlying critical appraisal and details the process of appraisal, identifying the types of questions to be asked of each paper
Effectiveness Matters www.york.ac.uk/inst/crd/pdf/em51.pdf	Volume (5, Issue 1) of this regular publication from the NHS Centre for Reviews and Dissemination, University of York provides information on how to access and interpret clinical effectiveness resources efficiently
E-library (although Scottish based is available online worldwide) www.elib.scot.nhs.uk	Huge resource of electronic information, databases, library facilities. Also houses the following:
Communities of practice	Communities of Practice are 'groups of people who share a concern, a set of problems, or a passion about a topic, and who deepen their knowledge and expertise by interacting on an ongoing basis'. (Wenger et al: Cultivating Communities of Practice: Harvard Business School Press, 2002) Communities of Practice reflect the fact that much of the knowledge within the health service lies in the heads of its staff, rather than in databases. Communities are therefore a natural place to seek out and access specialised knowledge

(Continued)

261

Table 16.3 Resources to support clinical effectiveness—Cont'd

The knowledge exchange	The knowledge exchange service provides a virtual workspace which Communities of Practice are invited to use in a way that integrates knowledge support with their day to day practice and service modernisation
Managed Knowledge Networks MKN – elibrary	The name given to large groups of healthcare staff who need to access, share and apply knowledge in a common broad area of interest – e.g., cancer, coronary heart disease, mental health, diabetes, stroke, healthcare associated infections. Overall aim of developing MKNs is to ensure that knowledge is managed effectively across boundaries of discipline, organisation and sector to support patient care and delivery of health services
Evidenced-Based Occupational Therapy Web-portal http://www.otevidence.info/	This Evidence-Based Occupational Therapy Web-portal has been designed to provide strategies, knowledge and resources to aid occupational therapists in finding out about and using evidence
Health Exec TV www.healthexectv.tv	An online television channel for managers and professionals across the NHS. Using best practice case studies, high profile interviews, expert panel discussions and field reports to examine the latest developments in health-care management
The Joanna Briggs Institute (JBI) www.joannabriggs.edu.au	An international collaboration involving nursing, medical and AHP researchers, clinicians, academics and quality managers across 40 countries. The role is to improve the feasibility, appropriateness, meaningfulness and effectiveness of health-care practices and health care outcomes by facilitating international collaboration between collaborating centres, groups, expert researchers and clinicians throughout the world
The Model for Improvement Langley, Nolan et al	Tried and tested approach to achieving successful change
NHS Quality Improvement Scotland (NHS QIS) www.nhshealthquality.org	The role of NHS QIS is to lead on improving quality of care and treatment delivered by the health service
Practice Development Unit http://www.nhshealthquality.org/nhsqis/1977.html	A dedicated unit within NHS QIS works to promote a consistent and cohesive approach to health care by: issuing Best Practice Statements organising Practice Development programmes supporting networking for nurses, midwives and allied health professionals encouraging the sharing of best practice
The Practice Development Network for Allied Health Professions	The network is made up of uniprofessional networks. You can access information about the occupational therapy network via the NHS QIS website

National Institute for Health and Clinical Excellence (NICE) www.nice.org	The National Institute for Health and Clinical Excellence (NICE) is the independent organisation responsible for providing national guidance on the promotion of good health and the prevention and treatment of ill health
National Library for Health http://www.library.nhs.uk	Includes: Evidence based reviews, Bandolier, Cochrane Library etc Guidance – NICE, care pathways etc Specialist libraries Evidence updates NICE/Published clinical guidelines
OT Seeker http://www.otseeker.com/	OTseeker is a database that contains abstracts of systematic reviews and randomised controlled trials relevant to occupational therapy
Social Care Institute for Excellence (SCIE) www.scie.org.uk	SCIE's aim is to improve the experience of people who use social care by developing and promoting knowledge about good practice in the sector. Using knowledge gathered from diverse sources and a broad range of people and organisations

Conclusions

This chapter has provided an introduction and overview of clinical effectiveness in practice. The references and resources provided in this chapter are an opportunity to examine your own practice and recognise areas where you are already developing effective practice and others where more can still be achieved. However, these resources are merely tools and in themselves cannot make the necessary changes. At the end of the day the key to clinically effective practice is you.

Acknowledgements

Thanks to Fiona Duncan, Sue Young and Michael Sykes for allowing me to use the case study highlighted in Vignette 16.1.

References

Adams C 1999a Clinical effectiveness: Part two. Finding the best evidence. Community Practitioner 72(7): 205–207

Adams C 1999b Clinical effectiveness: Part three. Interpreting your evidence. Community Practitioner 72(9): 289–292

Armstrong D, Jones R, Reyburn H 1996 A Study of general practitioners' reasons for changing their prescribing behaviour. British Medical Journal 312: 949–952

Chartered Society of Physiotherapists Clinical Effectiveness. http://www.csp.org.uk/director/effectivepractice/clinicaleffectiveness.cfm Accessed on 3 November 2007

College of Occupational Therapists 1999 Position Statement on Clinical Governance. College of Occupational Therapists, London

College of Occupational Therapists 2000 Occupational therapy record keeping core standard. Standards for practice

(SP002). College of Occupational Therapists, London

College of Occupational Therapists 2005 College of occupational therapists code of ethics and professional conduct. College of Occupational Therapists, London

Crombie IK 1996 The pocket guide to critical appraisal. BMJ Books, London

Department of Health 2002a The Shipman inquiry Safeguarding Patients: Lessons from the Past – Proposals for the Future. The Stationery Office, London

Department of Health 2002b Learning from Bristol: the Department of Health's Response to the Report of the Public Inquiry into Children's Heart Surgery at the Bristol Royal Infirmary 1984–1995. Command Paper CM 5363. The Stationery Office, London

Department of Health 2004 The Shipman Inquiry Fifth Report Safeguarding Patients: Lessons from the Past – Proposals for the Future, Command paper. The Stationery Office, London

Department of Health 2006 Records Management: NHS Code of Practice. Part 1, section 2. 14, page 5

Department of Health and Social Services in Northern Ireland Fit for the Future – a new approach. The Stationery Office, London

Doumit G, Gattellari M, Grimshaw J et al 2006 Local opinion leaders: effects on professional practice and health care outcomes. Cochrane Database of Systematic Reviews Issue 3. Art. No.: CD000125. DOI: 10.1002/14651858. CD000125, pub 3

Garbett R, McCormack B 2002 A concept analysis of practice development. Journal of Research in Nursing 7(2): 87–100

Gibson F, Sykes M, Young S 2004 Record Keeping in Occupational Therapy: Are we meeting the standards set by the College of Occupational Therapists? British Journal of Occupational Therapy December 67(12): 547–550

Glamville J, Haines M, Auston I 1998 Getting research findings into practice. Finding information on clinical effectiveness. British Medical Journal 317: 200–203

Grol R 1997 Beliefs and Evidence in Changing Clinical Practice. British Medical Journal 315: 418–421

Haynes B, Haines A 1998 Getting research findings into practice. Barriers and bridges to evidence based clinical practice. British Medical Journal 317: 273–276

Health Professions Council 2005 Standards of Proficiency for Occupational Therapy. Health Professions Council, London

Holdsworth L, Blair A, Miller J 2005 The Scottish physiotherapy clinical effectiveness network: Supporting clinical effectiveness activity? Clinical Governance: An International Journal 10(2): 148–164

Langley GJ, Nolan KM, Norman CL et al 1992 The Improvement Guide: A Practical Approach to Enhancing Organisational Performance. Jossey-Bass, San Francisco, CA

Lomas J, Enkin M, Anderson G 1991 Opinion leaders versus audit and feedback to implement practice guidelines. Journal of the American Medical Association 266(9): 1217

Laming Lord 2003 The Victoria Climbie Inquiry – Report of an inquiry. HMSO, London

Manley K 1997 Operationalising an advanced practice/consultant nurse role: an action research study. Journal of Clinical Nursing 6:179–190

Manley K 2000 Organisational culture and consultant nurse outcomes: part 1. Organisational culture. Nursing Standard 14(36): 34–38

McClarey M, Duff L 1997 Clinical effectiveness and evidence-based practice. Nursing Standard 11(51): 31–35

McCormack B, Manley K, Garbett R 2004 Practice Development in Nursing. Blackwell Publishing Ltd, Oxford, UK

Newman M, Roberts T 2002 Critical Appraisal 1: is the quality of the study good enough for you to use the findings? In: JV Craig, RL Smyth (eds) The Evidence-based Practice Manual for Nurses. Churchill Livingstone, Edinburgh, UK

Nolan M, Morgan L, Curran M et al 1998 Evidence-based care: can we overcome the barriers? British Journal of Nursing 7(20): 1273–1278

NHS Executive 1996 Promoting Clinical Effectiveness – A framework for action in and through the NHS. Department of Health, London

NHS Executive 1998 A first class service; Quality in the new NHS. HMSO, London

NHS Executive 2000 NHS Plan. HMSO, London

NHS Scotland 2007 Educational Resource: Clinical Governance http://www. clinicalgovernance.scot.nhs.uk/section2/ introduction.asp Accessed on 3 November 2007

NHS Wales 1998 Putting Patients First. The Stationary Office, London

Page S 2002 The role of practice development in modernising the NHS. Nursing Times 98(11): 34–36

Scottish Executive 1998 Designed to Care –
Renewing the National Health Service in
Scotland. Scottish Executive Health Department,
Edinburgh, UK

Scottish Executive 1999 Goals for Clinical
Effectiveness MEL. Scottish Executive Health
Department, Edinburgh, UK

Scottish Executive 2005 Building a Service Fit for
the Future – A national framework for service
change in the NHS Scotland. Scottish Executive
Health Department, Edinburgh, UK

Scottish Intercollegiate Guidelines Network 2001
SIGN 50: A guideline developers' handbook
http://www.sign.ac.uk/guidelines/fulltext/50/
index.html Accessed on 3 November 2007

Scottish Intercollegiate Guidelines Network 2008
SIGN 50: A guideline developers' handbook.
SIGN Executive, Edinburgh, UK

Wenger E, McDermott R, Snyder W 2002
Cultivating Communities of Practice: A guide to
managing knowledge. Harvard Business School
Press, Boston

West BJM, Wimpenny P, Duff L et al 2001
An educational initiative to promote the use
of clinical guidelines in nursing practice.
The Centre for Nurse Practice Research and
Development, Aberdeen, UK

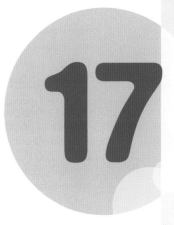

Developing research in practice

Edward A.S. Duncan

Highlight box

- People have various reasons for wanting to 'do' research in practice.
- There are increasing opportunities to actively participate in research in practice.
- Research career opportunities are now beginning to unfold. These require a structured and comprehensive research training.
- Deciding what to research requires careful consideration.
- Research collaborations vary in form, but are essential for most practice-based research. These require careful consideration in order that you find the best collaborator(s) and clearly articulate your expectations of the collaboration.

Introduction

The emphasis on research is probably the biggest development in occupational therapy practice in recent years. Whilst research once appeared a very remote issue to most practitioners – today it is central to the reality of their everyday working lives. Developing research in practice however is not simple. If it were then there would not be such a dearth of evidence. Doing research is challenging, whether you are a busy practitioner or a full-time researcher. There are many issues and options to consider if you wish to conduct meaningful studies that can impact on practice.

This chapter is neither a 'how to' guide to the research process or to specific research methods; there are a myriad of books that already cover this, some of which are written from an occupational therapy perspective and give relevant examples (Depoy and Gitlin 1998, Kielhofner 2006). Instead, this chapter addresses the 'why', 'what' and 'how' questions that practitioners should initially consider when they wish to conduct research in practice. It describes various rationales that people may have for conducting research (the 'why'), explores potential areas of research (the 'what') and latterly examines different models of conducting research in practice (the 'how'). Once these questions have been answered then practitioners can more meaningfully explore the research process and specific research methods.

The challenge of research

On the whole, occupational therapy continues to lack a substantial evidence base to support its practice in a wide variety of areas. However it is important to note that this situation is not substantially different from many other professions (Scottish Executive 2002, 2004). And there have been some excellent examples of occupational therapy research in various areas including falls, stroke rehabilitation, and dementia amongst others (Clark et al 1997, Walker 1999, Graff et al 2006).

Of course generating robust evidence to support practice is challenging. Much of practice is difficult to predict and uncertainty appears to abound in all occupational therapy practice.

Uncertainty

It is true that uncertainty is not all bad. Life would be very boring indeed (and potentially very stressful), if we were able to predict exactly how our day, our career, our family or our life would unfold. Sometimes it is good not to know what lies ahead in life. And in most situations, uncertainty cannot be completely excluded from decisions practitioners make in practice; even in a robust multi-centre clinical trial there is still a (low) chance that the crucial finding was due to luck and not causally related to the intervention. But as health-care professionals, occupational therapists have an implicit contract with clients to select and guide them to interventions or recommendations that (in general) have a higher chance of being successful or beneficial than not. If this were not the case then clients would have no reason to see an occupational therapist and would be as well consulting their next door neighbour instead! Therefore the reality of uncertainty must not stop us from working to limit it in clinical practice. This requires good-quality research to develop a strong evidence base. For some, the difficulty in generating evidence of the effectiveness of occupation for health has led to the conclusion that it is impossible to achieve, not least due to the complex nature of occupational therapy interventions (Cook 2003, Creek et al 2005). That it is difficult is unquestionable, but it is not impossible (Duncan et al 2007, Sweetland 2007, Wade 2007), and the previous examples of high-quality controlled trials in occupational therapy clearly evidence this.

The quest to limit or accept unpredictability through research, has often polarised the profession, with one camp championing the cause of randomised controlled trials and measurement in general, and the other camp not only rejecting such a position and embracing constructivist epistemologies as an equally valid form of 'evidence', but also suggesting that an embracement of measurement is a betrayal of the profession's core values. Such polarisation of views is unhelpful. Frequently studies would benefit from a mixed methods approach (Pope and Mays 2000) which draw on both quantitative and qualitative methods to answer a study's questions. Moreover, a third epistemological stance exists, is increasingly recognised as being of value in health-care research, and has much to offer occupational therapy: subtle realism (Kirk and Miller 1986, Hammersley 1992, Duncan and Nicol 2004).

Subtle realism

Subtle realists recognise that all research involves subjective perceptions and concede that different research methods will produce different pictures; however this perspective is not taken to the same extent as constructivists. The aim of research from a subtle realist perspective is to, '...search for knowledge about which one can be reasonably confident' (Murphy et al 1998: 69). To some this may appear as epistemological fence sitting.

Yet it does bridge the yawning gap between researchers and practitioners who recognise the importance of measurement with others who reject measurement and embrace personal narratives or other qualitative approaches. Subtle realism recognises the reality of uncertainty, but upholds that, whilst it can never be completely controlled, it can be and should be significantly diminished. Surely this position is the most useful perspective for occupational therapy research today?

It is vital that all practitioners are consumers of research; but we are also asked, and have an ethical obligation (COT 2000, Bannigan and Hughes 2007) to be research active as well. That is to generate new knowledge about what works (and what doesn't!) with the clients with whom we have the privilege to meet. Other chapters in this section have addressed 'using research' (see Chapters 14–16). This chapter focuses on 'doing research' in practice.

Why conduct research?

Whilst the importance of undertaking good-quality research, that answers clinically relevant questions, has been gathering momentum for several years the opportunities have arguably never been greater than they currently are. Yet relatively few practitioners undertake research. There are many reasons that may motivate someone to undertake research in practice. This chapter considers three (personal curiosity, project-based research and a research career), but these are neither exclusive nor exhaustive.

Personal curiosity

Curiosity, or a naturally inquisitive nature, is arguably the most essential capacity for a person to have if they wish to undertake a research study. Everyone can learn the necessary skills and knowledge of 'how' to do research. Without possessing an inquisitive nature practitioners will lack the internal motivation that frequently underlies 'why' they do it. There are, of course, other reasons for doing research but for some it relates to personal curiosity alone. Often this arises after a practitioner has worked in an area for some time and notices something about their practice, an intervention or a process, which makes them question why it happens. There may be little or no external pressure to do research, but such a practitioner wishes to do it anyway in order to answer their unanswered question.

Vignette 17.1

Angela was a senior practitioner in a busy social work department where she had worked for the last 7 years. A core part of her job was the assessment of adults' needs at home after they had been discharged from hospital. Usually she assessed her client's needs over one or two visits and then made specific recommendations for adaptive equipment and, if required, environmental alterations (which required more frequent visits). Following this, her service's usual practice was for technical services and support staff to deliver the equipment and carry out the alterations. Angela would then visit her clients at a later date to see how the clients were getting on.

Over the years, Angela had noted that many of the pieces of adaptive equipment she had initially ordered were not being used by her clients when she visited them several weeks after their delivery. As these were usually relatively straightforward appliances Angela felt that their lack of use was not related to a lack of knowledge about how to use them, but wasn't sure why this occurred.

Vignette 17.1 continued

As a first stage, Angela decided to conduct a longitudinal audit of equipment usage by clients throughout her local authority over time. This audit indicated a marked decline in equipment usage by a large percentage of clients over a 6-month period. As a next stage, Angela decided to conduct a series of semi-structured interviews with ten clients who had received equipment 6 months previously to enquire about their perceptions of the initial assessment and intervention process. She applied for and received appropriate ethical and managerial approval for the study. Following this, Angela decided to pilot a shared decision-making intervention (Montori et al 2006) (see Chapter 4) with a cohort of clients. This intervention focused on developing partnership working and the development of trust and mutual respect between the therapist and client; explicitly exchanging information about the technical options, social and personal contexts, and values and preferences; deliberating on options by considering both the pros and cons of certain pieces of equipment for a client; and on-going partnership working in deciding and acting upon the decision reached together, so that the decisions can be re-visited if circumstances change. Whilst these were all aspects of therapy that Angela had previously thought she and her colleagues carried out routinely it had become apparent, through her audit and qualitative groundwork, that the service's clients did not feel this occurred in practice. Angela wondered whether this more explicit strategy of shared decision making would affect the number of adaptive appliances ordered (with a potential cost saving for equipment that had previously been inappropriately placed in clients' homes), and improve outcomes by increasing the usage of equipment ordered for clients over time.

Project-based research

Another reason that a practitioner decides to undertake a research project may be related to a specific personal or collective project. An example of this is the practitioner who decides to undertake a postgraduate degree such as a Masters. Masters degrees can be taught (e.g. MA or MSc) or research based (MPhil), but both contain a research thesis or dissertation of some description. These options are excellent opportunities for a practitioner who wishes to start conducting research but feels they do not have the required skills or confidence to do so alone and would like to gain some form of formal qualification for their newly acquired knowledge.

A different type of project-based research is to participate in a research study that is led by someone else. Participation may take the form of being a research worker, collecting data, or a clinical collaborator providing the link between the practice and academic settings. Such opportunities are not currently numerous in occupational therapy, but they do exist and will become more common with the increasing development of research in practice.

Research career

Despite the challenges of an unclear career pathway for an occupational therapy researcher (Bannigan 2001) undertaking a research career is now a real possibility. Recent history illustrates how occupational therapists previously had to leave the profession if they wished to pursue a research career. Fay Fransella published what was perhaps the first controlled trial of occupational therapy (Fransella 1960) and was later lauded as a ground-breaking researcher (Creek 2001, Ilott and White 2001). However an analysis of her career illustrates that whilst she was groundbreaking, there was no research pathway, at that time, for her to follow and she was left with a choice. Fransella explains it in her own words, 'I was at the top of my profession in my early thirties both in status and in financial terms. The choice was to stay put and know more and more about less and less or do something radical...I chose the latter' (Fransella 1989: 119–120). Dr Fransella

Vignette 17.2

I worked as a clinical collaborator and data collector whilst working in a high-security psychiatric hospital in Scotland. The department where I was based had formed a collaboration with the United Kingdom Centre for Outcomes Research and Evaluation (UKCORE). Part of this collaboration included collecting data for international validation studies of standardised assessments (specifically the Model of Human Occupation Screening Tool MOHOST (Forsyth et al submitted)) and developing new versions of existing assessments (specifically the Occupational Circumstances Assessment Interview and Rating Scale OCAIRS (Forsyth et al 2005)). These projects provided excellent opportunities to develop my research skills and expertise; collaborate with an international research group; and participate in large international studies. It was more than I could have ever managed to achieve on my own at that stage in my research career. Skills developed during this project included developing successful research study outlines for the hospital research and development committee, completing and submitting relevant ethics committee documentation, developing local study information leaflets, informing and consenting patients to participate in the study, negotiating with colleagues to act as fellow data collectors and anonymising, cleaning (the process through which you check all the data are there and have been entered correctly) and collating data to be sent back to the study centre in Chicago.

went on to study personal construct psychology and became an international leader in her field (Duncan 2001)! Undertaking research as a career pathway in occupational therapy is certainly now more achievable; however this doesn't necessarily make it straight forward or well defined.

Whilst personal curiosity and project-based research can be excellent introductions to doing research, developing a research career demands undertaking a more structured and comprehensive research training. The aim of this training is to prepare a practitioner to undertake larger-scale funded research as a principal investigator. This aim is best met by undertaking a doctorate (i.e. a PhD or clinical doctorate) followed by post-doctoral studies (Scottish Executive 2005). Undertaking a PhD or post-doctoral research programme is a demanding (but highly rewarding) challenge. Whilst only a few may wish to pursue this option, if you do want to develop a research career it is important to get off to the right start. A helpful position is to consider three factors: you, the research, and the available support (Scottish Executive and NES Scotland 2005).

You

Consider the following. Are you:

- An experienced practitioner? Not essential, but it certainly helps.
- Innovative? You will need to problem solve and spend a lot of your time finding ways around potential hurdles.
- Able to work in a team? Whilst some research may be carried out in isolation, the majority of larger-scale studies require teamwork.
- Focused on improving services? The most pressing research is that which is service focused. Do you want to improve the services in your area of specialism through research?
- Committed? Developing a research career is no mean feat and there will be plenty of hurdles and obstacles that will need to be overcome. Many individuals undertake a series of temporary appointments before finally being given a

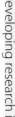

permanent research position. And those who remain in practice have the challenge of balancing their clinical duties with their research role.

- Thick-skinned? Are you ready to face up to the highs and lows of applying for, undertaking and disseminating research? Being a researcher is a real rollercoaster of a professional career. The 'ups' of being award grants, undertaking research and disseminating findings are excellent, but the 'lows' of grant and paper rejections and the struggles to complete some studies can be very challenging and off putting for some.

Your research

- Is your research relevant to practice?
- Does it fit with the needs of the people with whom you work, and where the research will be based?

Support

- Are your family and friends supportive of what you want to do? A research career is very demanding and will inevitably impact on your family and social life.
- Do you have support from your employer? Make sure they understand the rationale and consequences of what you want to do.
- Do you have access to advice from experienced researchers, statisticians, etc. (see below)?

What to research?

Fundamentally this is up to you and the subject of your research may have been what spurred you on in the first place. However there are several issues that you would do well to consider before taking your research plans much further (Scottish Executive, NHS Education for Scotland 2005):

- Focus your question on an issue, question, or challenge you are faced with in your everyday professional activity.
- Decide exactly what you want to find out and why it is important to do so.
- Examine the literature to see what is already known about your subject.
- Consult the clients with whom you work to see if they agree your subject area is of interest.
- Talk to other people (fellow practitioners and potential collaborators) about your research idea and refine your research question.
- Begin to consider what research method(s) you may use.
- Share or present your ideas in front of an experienced group of researchers and practitioners.
- Consider whether your study requires funding. If yes, how much? Where could you apply for funding for your study?

How to research?

Once you have considered why you wish to undertake a research study, it is also important to consider how you wish to conduct the research. Whilst the principal investigator of a study carries the burden of responsibility, and often the work, research is rarely carried out in isolation, and collaboration is the name of the game in the vast majority of successful research projects.

Issues of scale

Of course the degree of collaboration will largely be dependent on the scale of the research being undertaken. A small research project undertaken in a single site, with low participant numbers is likely to need considerably less collaboration than a larger-scale multisite randomised control trial (RCT) or cluster randomised control trial (CRCT).

Going it alone

With small research projects there is always the option of going it alone and foregoing collaboration with others. However, even when it is feasible to do so, it is rarely desirable; especially when you have had little experience of conducting research before. The research process is like many things in life: relatively straightforward if you know what you are doing, but can cause real headaches if you don't! Working together with others allows you to learn from their previous experience and knowledge and can save you considerable energy that may otherwise be wasted.

Personal research collaborations

Personal research collaborations are partnerships between a practitioner and one or more experienced researchers. Frequently, though not necessarily, the experienced researcher is based in an academic department of a university. The importance of

Vignette 17.3

Paul had been qualified for 3 years and was employed in a learning disability community day service. He was very interested to learn more about the time use of the clients he worked with and decided to independently carry out a relatively small study exploring the perceptions of ten clients regarding their time use and then record their actual time use through client self report. Though the study seemed straightforward, Paul struggled to get his research ethics application approved by the research ethics committee, who repeatedly raised concerns regarding the content of the study information leaflet and the manner in which Paul intended to gain consent. When he eventually managed to negotiate these issues and gained ethical committee approval he then struggled to recruit clients to his study: he hadn't previously discussed the project with the staff of the day service and they did not share Paul's enthusiasm for the importance of the topic he had chosen. This meant that some of the staff were less than enthusiastic in supporting clients to participate. Eventually Paul managed to interview five clients, three of whom returned their time use data a week later. Though disappointed by this, Paul wrote up the study and submitted it to his national peer-reviewed journal, only for it to be rejected by the peer reviewers who cited the low participant numbers, relative lack of meaningful data and poor academic presentation of the submitted paper as their reasons. One reviewer suggested that the author (Paul) should consider collaborating with a more experienced researcher/author when next submitting a paper to the journal. Despondently, Paul vowed never to undertake a research project again!

Each of the challenges faced by Paul could have either been avoided or overcome more efficiently and effectively if he had collaborated with a more experienced researcher.

selecting the right people to collaborate with cannot be underestimated. Often practitioners seek collaborations with academics who had previously lectured them as students and with whom they already have an existing relationship, or alternatively with lecturers in a local university from which they take students on practice placement. Obviously the ease of geographical proximity and previously established relationships are strong bonuses worth considering when looking to forming research collaborations. But they may not be the most essential criteria. And in the current age of electronic communication (email, internet, Skype, etc.) the necessity of geographical proximity has become much less important. Instead, first consider the skills you require from your collaborator, then look for who best fits the criteria. It is important to consider what it is that you are looking for from research collaboration before you look for the best individual(s) to collaborate with; and then to negotiate expectations and roles with your collaborators before you agree to work together.

Considering a research collaboration

Research collaborations are excellent, and you will often find willing and able individuals with whom you could work. There are, however, some issues worth considering *before* you make contact with any potential collaborators. These include:

- At the most basic level – what do you need from your research collaborator(s)? Is it experience of completing ethics applications, navigating the R&D process, writing research grant applications, methodological expertise, statistical know how, or something else?
- If you want to be the principal investigator or are you willing to hand that over to your collaborator?
- If you are writing a grant application, consider where you want the research funds to be based? There may be good reasons for the funding to be based in your institution, or in the institution of your research collaborator(s).
- What you are willing to offer in return for a potential collaboration? Some people may be happy to collaborate without any *quid pro quo* or on the basis of negotiated inclusion on a grant proposal and/or research outputs such as publications (see below). Others may ask for you to undertake some visiting lecturing, or to take a student of theirs for a practice placement in return for their input.

Individual collaborations Finding such individuals can be challenging, but you may know of someone's specific interest and expertise through their published work, or from hearing them at conferences. Some professional bodies (for example the College of Occupational Therapists) hold registers for researchers that can be searched for specific criteria. It is also worth considering placing a request on an email discussion list, if one exists for the area you wish to research. These are becoming increasingly popular methods of networking and gaining helpful research collaborations. Potentially relevant e-discussion groups include the European Cooperation in Occupational Therapy Research and Occupational Science ECOTROS (http://www.uniklinik-freiburg.de/ecotros/live/index.html), the Model of Human Occupation Listserv (an international e-discussion group for all things pertaining to MOHO http://www.moho.uic.edu/listserv.html) or the Forensic Occupational Therapy e-discussion group (an international network of over 500 practitioners working, researching, or lecturing about forensic occupational therapy – http://uk.groups.yahoo.com/group/forensic_occupational_therapy/).

Research units As well as looking for individuals, it may also be worthwhile to look for established research units that are interested in the topic you wish to research. Such units are often very keen to engage with clinical collaborators, as without them they find it very challenging to conduct their research. Research units have a variety of different interests and funding sources, each of which will influence the type and focus of research they conduct. Some research units are interdisciplinary (for example Scotland's national Nursing, Midwifery and Allied Health Professions Research Unit (NMAHP RU), or its sister units: the Health Services Research Unit (HSRU) and the Health Economics Research Unit (HERU)). Others, such as the Centre for Outcomes Research (CORE) in the United States or its United Kingdom counterpart the United Kingdom Centre for Outcomes Research and Evaluation (UKCORE) have a profession-specific focus. An advantage of collaborating with a well-established research unit is that they often have their own excellent networks and can link you up with experts in specific fields of interest such as statistics or economic evaluation.

Negotiating collaboration

When developing research collaborations, it is important that you negotiate each others roles and expectations at an early stage. Time spent doing this at the beginning avoids unnecessary confusion, frustration and conflict when the research has progressed further down the line. One clear example of where early negotiation pays benefits is in the development of a publication agreement. That is a document that outlines what papers (and other outputs) will be developed from the research, to where they will be submitted (you may have a prioritised list of options here), who will be authors on each publication and where their name will be listed in each paper. Normally collaborators form part of the author list for papers that are published from their research and contribute to the paper(s) development. The position of each individual's name on each paper requires to be agreed; this usually depends on their contribution; both to the research and writing of the paper. Some journals require authors to specify each of their contribution to a submitted paper. If there is more than one paper coming from a study then negotiation may centre on who is leading on the development of each paper? It can seem a bit strange, and at times awkward, to have such a frank discussion about something that has not yet been completed; however experience has demonstrated that spending time and effort considering this avoids what can be difficult moments and conflicts at a later stage when you discover that you have different ideas about who will be first author, etc. More developed research units and academic departments already have established protocols for developing publishing agreements for precisely this reason.

275

Service collaboration

Some services recognise the importance of doing research as part of their professional duties and form specific service collaborations with experienced researchers. These collaborations are therefore at a different organisational level to individual collaborations. Service collaborations take different forms, but there are broadly three types: 1:1, project based, and total service models.

1:1

In this type of service model, whilst the collaboration is at a service level, the experienced researcher engages with individual members of staff on specific individual projects to meet their specific needs. The advantages of this model are that each practitioner is able to receive individual support depending on their need. In one service, where this model successfully functioned, the role of the experienced researcher varied from helping support staff to construct meaningful clinical notes following sessions with clients to supervising a senior member of staff who was undertaking his PhD part-time whilst based in practice. Staff appreciate this tailored approach to research collaboration, but there are challenges to this approach too.

The nature of individualised research collaborations means that research outcomes tend to be relatively small scale, to develop in a relatively ad hoc fashion and according to practitioners' interests rather than clinical need (Duncan 2008). Another interesting challenge that can arise from a 1:1 service model is the perception that such research activities need to be undertaken over and above a practitioner's clinical role. Frequently this can mean that such activities are not given due priority by staff – even when they have direct management support to do so.

Project-based service collaboration

This form of service model typifies the sort of project-based research that academics are on occasion called in to support departments in practice settings. The difference between this model of service collaboration and the following model (total service models) are to do with the time frame and the extent of the collaboration. Project-based service collaborations tend to be of a shorter duration than total service models and are also more focused in nature.

Total service models

An alternative service collaboration approach is for the experienced researcher to collaborate with the service as a whole, not solely individual practitioners and over a prolonged period of time. One successful model which exemplifies this approach is known as 'The Scholarship of Practice' (Kielhofner 2005). Hammel et al (2001) outline the key components of the Scholarship of Practice as follows:

- Being committed to carrying out research that directly contributes and impacts on practice
- Working in partnership with individuals and organisations outwith academic settings
- Developing synergies that practice and scholarship simultaneously.

An advantage of this approach is that the aims of the research collaboration are central to the practice of individual clinicians and the service as a whole. This means that research activities are more easily integrated into everyday activities and become more relevant to practice. Further, as such collaborations are at a service level the scale of the research that can be undertaken is significantly increased. Of course these benefits are not without cost, and some practitioners may prefer the individual collaboration and flexibility that is more clearly tangible in a 1:1 model (Duncan 2008). A case study presenting a UK example of a service research collaboration model has already been published elsewhere (Forsyth et al 2005); and several other examples of service collaborations have been published in the same special edition of *Occupational Therapy in Health Care*.

Summary

The opportunities and expectations for occupational therapists to undertake research are greater now than they have ever been. Practitioners conduct research for a variety of reasons, but these can be broadly summarised as personal curiosity, project-based research and the development of a research career. Whatever an individual's motivation for doing research is, it is unlikely to be carried out alone and close consideration should be given to the type of collaboration which is most suitable for the research and desired by the principal investigator. Forming research collaborations brings together a range of research expertise and can greatly assist in the smooth planning, execution and dissemination of a research study.

References

Bannigan K 2001 Is research valued as a legitimate career pathway in occupational therapy? The British Journal of Occupational Therapy 64(9): 425

Bannigan K, Duncan EAS 2001 A survey of post-registration research students in occupational therapy. The British Journal of Occupational Therapy 64(6): 278–284

Bannigan K, Hughes S 2007 Research is now every occupational therapist's business. The British Journal of Occupational Therapy 70(3): 95

Clark F, Azen SP, Zemke R et al 1997 Occupational therapy for independent-living older adults. A randomized controlled trial. Journal of the American Medical Association 278(16): 1321–1326

College of Occupational Therapists 2000 Code of ethics and professional conduct for occupational therapists. The College of Occupational Therapists, London

Cook S 2003 What interventions produced the evidence of positive outcomes? Mental Health Occupational Therapy 8(1): 20–23

Creek J 2001 Occupational science as a selected research priority – response [letter]. The British Journal of Occupational Therapy 64(8): 420–421

Creek J, Illott I, Cook S et al 2005 Valuing occupational therapy as a complex intervention. British Journal of Occupational Therapy 68(6): 281–284

Depoy E, Gitlin LN 1998 Introduction to Research: understanding and applying multiple research strategies, 2nd edn. Mosby, St. Louis, MO

Duncan EAS 2001 Is research valued as a career pathway? The British Journal of Occupational Therapy 10(64): 517–518

Duncan E 2008 Twist and turns: The development of a clinical academic partnership: In: McKay EA, Craik C, Lim KH et al (eds) Advancing Occupational Therapy in Mental Health Practice. Blackwell Publishing, Oxford, UK

Duncan EAS, Nicol M 2004 Subtle reasoning and occupational therapy: An alternative approach to knowledge generation and evaluation. The British Journal of Occupational Therapy 67(10): 453–456

Forsyth K, Parkinson S, Kielhofner G et al submitted The measurement properties of the Model of Human Occupation Screening Tool (MOHOST). The British Journal of Occupational Therapy

Forsyth K, Walker K, Duncan EAS 2005 Forensic Occupational Circumstances Assessment Interview and Rating Scale. In: K Forsyth, S Deshpande, G Kielhofner et al (2005) The Occupational Circumstances Assessment Interview and Rating Scale (OCAIRS)©. University of Illinois, Chicago, IL

Fransella F 1960 The treatment of chronic schizophrenia: intensive occupational therapy with and without chlorpromazine. Occupational Therapy 23(9): 31–34

Fransella F 1989 A fight for freedom. In: W Dryden, L Spurling (eds) On Becoming a Psychotherapist, pp. 119–120. Routledge, London

Graff MJ, Vernooji-Dasses MJM, Thijsseen M et al 2006 Community based occupational therapy for patients with dementia and their care givers: randomised controlled trial. British Medical Journal 333: 1196

Hammel J, Finlayson M, Kielhofner G et al 2001 Educating scholars of practice: An approach to preparing tomorrow's researchers. Occupational Therapy in Health Care 15(1/2): 157–176

Hammersley M 1992 What's wrong with ethnography? Routledge, London

Ilott I, White E 2001 College of Occupational Therapist's Research and Development Strategic Vision and Action Plan. The British Journal of Occupational Therapy 64(6): 270–277

Kielhofner G 2005 A scholarship of practice: Creating discourse between theory, research and practice. Occupational Therapy in Healthcare 19(1/2): 7–16

Kielhofner G 2006 Research in Occupational Therapy: Methods of Inquiry for Enhancing Practice. F. A. Davis, Philadelphia

Kirk J, Miller M 1986 Reliability and validity in qualitative research. Sage, Newbury Park, NJ

Montori VM, Gafni A, Charles C 2006 A shared treatment decision-making approach between patients with chronic conditions and their clinicians: the case of diabetes. Health Expectations 9(1): 25–36

Murphy E, Dingwall R, Greatbatch D et al 1998 Qualitative research methods in health technology assessment: a review of the literature. Health Technology Assessment 2(16)

Pope C, Mays N 2000 Qualitative methods in health research. In: C Pope, N Mays (eds) Qualitative Research in Health Care, 2nd edn. British Medical Journal Publishing Group, London

Scottish Executive Health Department 2002 Choices and Challenges: the strategy for research and development in nursing and midwifery in Scotland. Scottish Executive Health Department, Edinburgh, UK

Scottish Executive Health Department 2004 Allied Health Professions Research and Development Action Plan. Scottish Executive Health Department, Edinburgh, UK

Scottish Executive, NHS Education for Scotland 2005 Making Choices Facing Challenges: Developing your research career in nursing, midwifery and the allied health professions. Scottish Executive, NHS Education for Scotland, Edinburgh, UK

Sweetland J 2007 Guidance in a research journey. The British Journal of Occupational Therapy 70(10): 453

Wade D 2007 Complexity and research. The British Journal of Occupational Therapy 70(6): 269

Walker MF, Gladman JR, Lincoln NB et al 1999 Occupational therapy for stroke patients not admitted to hospital: a randomised controlled trial. Lancet 354: 278–280

Presentation and publication skills

Alister Landrock
Ann Landrock
and Edward A.S. Duncan

Highlight box

- Being able to share your work (that is in writing, presenting and publishing) is an essential skill for occupational therapists today.
- Be clear in what you want to say.
- Always follow the guidance you are given.
- Seek out a critical friend who can give you honest feedback.
- Don't be disheartened if your first attempts are unsuccessful; effective dissemination is a skill that requires to be developed. Persistence pays dividends.

Introduction

Occupational therapists are routinely being called upon to share and disseminate their work. University degree programmes now require students to develop good writing skills, design posters and prepare presentations, and yet many are still fearful of broadcasting information more widely when they graduate and start working. And others did not receive such education during their training. This chapter aims to highlight key skills and issues to help students and therapists overcome the fear factor and/or enhance their existent skills.

Knowledge of publication and presentation skills is essential for all occupational therapists. There are various reasons for this. An understanding of how to communicate in a variety of ways is crucial when developing treatment literature or designing information leaflets for patients and their relatives, colleagues or students (see Chapter 9), producing health-promotional publications, composing scientific posters, presenting at work or at professional conferences and submitting your work for publication in a magazine or journal. This chapter focuses on the key skills you require to be successful in disseminating your work.

Writing an abstract

Most formal presentations, be they poster or oral in format, will initially be developed and submitted for consideration as an abstract: that is a summary of what the presentation is about. Abstracts are usually submitted to conference organisers who use this information to judge firstly whether or not to accept your presentation and secondly in which format (e.g. oral presentation, poster, workshop or seminar). It is vital, therefore, that the content and presentation of an abstract is accurate, succinct and appealing. Abstracts are potential presenters' main opportunity to sell their idea initially to conference abstract reviewers and latterly, if they are successful at that stage, to participants of the conference – who will often decide whether or not to attend a presentation on the basis of the abstract which will be published in the conference programme (Bannigan 2005).

Written guidance

Many people find writing an abstract challenging. Yet most 'call for papers' (where organisations request people to submit abstracts for presentations) contain detailed information about the length of the title, the length of the abstract, a rough format of desired content, whether references are desired and if so how many and in what format, and adherence to conference theme, etc. Some 'call for papers' go as far as publishing the marking schedule and this gives a fairly detailed idea of the amount of information that is being looked for by reviewers. The first and most important piece of advice that can be given in writing an abstract is to follow the conference organiser's guidance! Failure to do so in a conference that receives a surfeit of abstracts is a sure way to have yours rejected. Reviewers will be looking for easy ways to whittle down the number of abstracts they have to consider and not following the defined format for an abstract is commonly used by reviewers as being the first and easiest criteria for rejection.

What to present

It is often tempting to submit an abstract for a piece of work that is not yet completed, but you expect will be by the time the conference will be held. This is a dangerous strategy (Haigh 2006), which is best avoided where at all possible. Whilst you may plan for your research to go smoothly, a variety of factors may not be within your control resulting in delays and an inability to present the paper you have described in your paper; this is not popular with either conference organisers who have worked hard to develop the programme, or delegates who may have made a difficult choice between sessions only to be disappointed when they attend your session. Further advantages to submitting abstracts on completed work is that you are then able to include interesting statistics from your study, or key theoretical proposals from more conceptual work (Haigh 2006). Doing so is likely to increase your chances of success further.

Having reinforced the central importance of following the organisers' written guidance and submitting abstracts on completed work, other factors should also be considered in order to develop an attractive and successful abstract submission: consideration of your target audience and clarity of your message (Bannigan 2005).

Think about your audience

Both reviewers and conference delegates are frequently faced with a huge number of abstracts to read and consider when making judgements of whether they should either accept the abstract, or attend your session. You may consider your paper or poster to be fascinating and of vital importance, but if you are not able to communicate this very early on in the abstract (preferably in the title), then you are likely to lose the interest of your reader. So carefully consider your audience. Use words and phrases that are likely to be meaningful to them, and avoid unnecessary jargon. Carefully considering the language you use is important in developing your abstract. Organisations such as the Plain English Campaign and marketing and communication companies exist to help people to communicate well (Bannigan 2005) but these are likely to be expensive and inappropriate for most practitioners' needs. Instead, it can be very helpful to find yourself one or more critical friends, preferably people who have had abstracts accepted for similar events. Asking for their honest feedback and appraisal of your draft abstract can be extremely useful and help create a significantly stronger final work than if you had written it alone. Of course asking for and receiving honest and critical feedback is not always easy, even when it is given in a constructive manner as one would hope it would be. Here however, lies the necessity to develop another subtle yet vital 'skill' for any practitioners who wish to disseminate their work: the development of a thick skin (Meshack 2004)! Honest feedback from your critical friends is likely to be at least slightly difficult to accept; after all if you didn't think it was good you wouldn't have written it like that would you! However, it is pointless to ignore their comments as you would be as well not soliciting them in the first place if you did that. Therefore, careful consideration should be given to all feedback. Even if you do not take on board their suggestions, you should think about ways in which to improve the section(s) they found difficult as you obviously weren't managing to communicate your message there as well as you had hoped. The most helpful attitudes to cultivate when you receive constructive criticism are ones of gratefulness and humility (Meshack 2004), though this is much easier to suggest than to embrace!

Clarity of your message

By their very nature, abstracts are concise; often only 150–200 words in length. Use your words wisely and make full use of the number of words you have available (Haigh 2006). Clear and simple explanations are vital if the abstract is to read well. In order to achieve this, you first have to have a very good idea of what you want to say – if you don't know, how will you be able to clearly tell other people (Bannigan 2005)? Ensure that you make your abstract of as wide an interest and relevance as possible. Experience of sitting on the scientific committee of various conferences' organising committees has highlighted that one of the questions that (rightly or wrongly) strongly influences reviewers' opinions of an abstract can be summed up as follows, 'Do I give a damn?' Even with the clearest of scoring schedules, if the topic does not grab the reviewer's attention it stands much less chance of acceptance.

Creating written presentations

Although it is important to carefully deliberate over the content within a written document, such as a poster, it is also necessary to be aware of its typographical layout. The way that it is composed will add or detract from the reader's understanding. Without order on the page there is chaos and an awareness of design principles will help organise your information. Papanek (1985: 4) stated that, '...design was the conscious and intuitive effort to impose meaningful order'; a colleague, Innes (1988) adapted this quote to read, 'Design is the conscious and intuitive effort to arrange elements'. The elements being arranged would depend on the design work being undertaken but generally speaking in graphic design these are words, blocks of text, photographs, illustrations, lines, space, etc. If you give careful consideration to layout as well as content, your work will be further enhanced.

All layout is based on the legibility of the message to aid or ease the communication between the written word and the human eye. Anything that impedes this is poor layout. The eye, and to a large extent the mind, is habit formed and layout is as much to do about what the eye expects to find as with what is easy to read. The eye demands a certain amount of border around a design or a page: too much space tends to compete with and dwarf the work, too little does not allow the work to sit comfortably on the page. Wheildon (1996) stated, 'Typography is the art of designing a communication by using the printed word. Typography must be clear. At its very best it is virtually invisible' (p. 23). When the eye is exposed to any image the brain tries to make sense of it if it is not readily accessible. You will probably be aware of the perceptual illusion drawing of the vase and the faces. Viewed one way you will see a vase, viewed another and you will see the profile of two faces. The eye is trying to make sense of the ambiguity of the image. This same ambiguity can also occur on the printed page when the unconsidered positioning of type, lines, spaces, etc. can draw unintended attention away from the message (Figure 18.1).

The remit of this chapter does not extend to discussing at length the variety of computer programs available to produce finished copy or how to use them. It is enough to state that there are various desktop publishing, word processing and multimedia (PowerPoint) software packages which can be used to create a variety of documents. As it would also take too long to discuss how to create the variety of publications that you are likely to produce this section will focus on designing a scientific poster. Many of the principles for designing a poster also apply to the design of leaflets, newsletters, fact sheets, etc.

Scientific posters

Over recent years there has been a great upsurge in the demand for scientific posters at occupational therapy conferences. This is a healthy sign as it indicates that there are now many involved in research that want to share their knowledge. A scientific poster can be

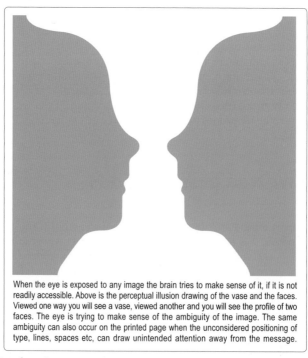

When the eye is exposed to any image the brain tries to make sense of it, if it is not readily accessible. Above is the perceptual illusion drawing of the vase and the faces. Viewed one way you will see a vase, viewed another and you will see the profile of two faces. The eye is trying to make sense of the ambiguity of the image. The same ambiguity can also occur on the printed page when the unconsidered positioning of type, lines, spaces etc, can draw unintended attention away from the message.

Figure 18.1 Two faces in conversation

defined as a recent display of research or educational material on a vertical panel that usually requires the presence of the author to discuss his or her work. It is important to read a conference's poster presentation instructions before embarking on your design as protocols differ from one conference to the next. It is crucial to know exactly what size the end product should be and understand the explicit layout instructions. Simmonds (1984) suggested that the following questions written by Sir Austin Bradford should be addressed when writing about your research:

- Why did you start?
- What did you do?
- What answers did you get?
- What does it mean?

These answers should then be supported with Dr Stephen Locks' criteria (see Simmonds 1984):

- Choose the correct word
- Choose the familiar rather than the obscure word
- Prefer the single word to the several
- Prefer the concrete to the abstract
- Prefer the short to the long
- Prefer the word of the Saxon to that of the Roman
- Write with nouns and verbs not adjectives or adverbs.

For the purposes of presentation the poster can be divided into three main areas, the title, the text or copy and visual imagery.

The title

The title is usually written across the top of your poster and is generally the first element that will be read, therefore it should be eye catching, enticing and perhaps even controversial, to engage the passer by. Many of the conference delegates who will visit your poster will have read your abstract beforehand and will be sympathetic to your topic. It is imperative that you also try to attract those who may not be particularly interested in your subject matter. One way to do this is to write a short statement or questions that will encourage a wider audience to view your work. We have much to learn from the tabloid press when looking for the short snappy headline that will attract attention. Some conferences will clearly specify the number of words that can be used in the title but if a limit is not stated, no more than ten words would be a good guide to follow. The shorter the title the larger the type that can be used, ensuring it can be read at a greater distance.

The text

The vast majority of people prefer reading sitting down and because posters are generally read standing up it is essential to keep posters as visual and concise as possible. A short historical summary followed by the aims of the present study should introduce your content. Simmonds (1984) suggests that one should describe the logical basis for experimentation and mention any limiting factors. Illustrate changes and trends by displaying simplified tables and graphs. Standard deviation, standard errors of mean and other details can be given on a handout. Finally discuss the relevance of your work. Transmit a sense of excitement to the observer; state how the results will alter the course of your practice and mention any developments planned for the future. Try to convey all of this in 500 words. You will not be able to present all the data you have collected, so choose the major points you feel communicate the essence of your subject matter. Your contact details will allow those who want to have more information to communicate with you. The text should be written using easily read fonts and only three, at the most, should be used in your poster; remember that type style (normal, bold, etc.) and point size can alter the appearance of a typeface. Avoid script, calligraphic or decorative fonts, as these can be difficult to read. Recommended typefaces include Times Roman, New Century Schoolbook or Palatino which are serif typefaces or Arial, Helvetica or Futura that are sans-serif typefaces. Serifs are lines or curves projecting from the end of a letterform. Sans-serif typefaces are also referred to as Gothic and do not have these finishing strokes. A contrasting typeface might be used for actual quotations or within tables but do assess the overall impact of this before producing the final poster.

Type size

Harms (1995) advocates the use of a simple calculation which can help determine the varying point sizes of type to be used throughout the poster:

$$\frac{\text{Viewing distance in mm}}{200} = \text{height of type in mm}$$

$$\frac{2000 \text{ mm (2 metres)}}{200} = 10 \text{ mm high type}$$

Type is measured in points (pts), an old imperial measurement with 72 pts equalling an inch or 25.4 mm. The point size of a typeface is determined by measuring from the top of an ascender to the base of a descender. Typefaces that have the same point size will not necessarily have the same height; invariably serif typefaces appear smaller than sans-serif typefaces when the same point size is chosen (see Figure 18.2).

Three sizes of type might be used for the title, headings and the text. The title should be at least 72 pts, the section headings 20–30 pts and text 18–24 pts; this would depend on the typeface, the type style you employ and the space available; for example bold type might be used for all the headings.

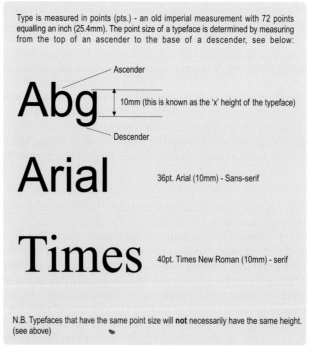

Figure 18.2 Type measurement

Type style

There are various type styles that that can be adopted to enhance the text:

Normal **Bold** *Italic* <u>Underline</u> ⬛Outline Shadow

Arguably the most easily read of these are 'normal' and 'bold' but experiment with the typeface styles which are available to you. Use 'bold' as a contrast to 'normal' type; reading large passages of bold text can be tiring on the eye.

Uppercase (or capital letters)

When reading a line of type the eye recognises letters by the shape, specifically of their upper halves. With lower case letters this is easier because the upper halves of lower case letters are generally distinctive, framed by white space that surrounds them permitting easy recognition. We also recognise words by their overall shape. If one only uses upper case letters words appear as a series of rectangles and recognising them becomes a task instead of a natural process (Wheildon 1996). Figure 18.3 provides some examples.

Use colour to interest the reader within graphs, tables, photographs, etc. Coloured lines or bullet points can be added to the poster to enhance a mainly black on white page. Only use one or two colours of print within your poster and ensure they do not clash with colours in photographs or illustrations. A contrast between the type and the background is essential and white or pastel colours are most appropriate. Coloured backgrounds often compete with the various elements in the poster and should be used with care.

Avoid the use of long lines of text as these are tiring to read. The most efficient to read line length in English is 36–40 characters long and the RNIB (1995) suggest a line should be between 50–65 characters long. The best way to achieve this is to use a number of columns to organise your work. Justified line lengths alter the spaces between words to ensure two straight edges to the block of text. This results in larger than usual spaces between the words which can compromise your writing. Although there is far from universal agreement, evidence suggests that readers find the consistent word spacing found in align left/ragged right text easier to read.

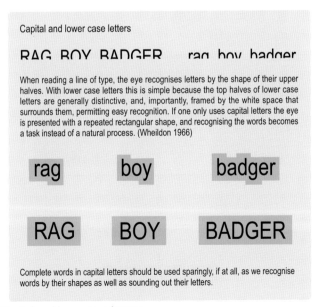

Figure 18.3 Capital and lower case letters

Visual imagery should be positioned in the top half of the poster aligned to the column width. Select your illustration or photographs with care; one good image is much better than three that do not precisely reflect your topic. If using coloured imagery ensure that colour is reflected in the type, lines, etc. used elsewhere in the poster.

Posters should attract, interest and inform. To do this hours must be spent on the typographical layout; the end result will often belie the time and effort expended on the final product (see Figure 18.4).

Visual presentations

Taking time to address the following guidelines can often further enhance artwork created by clients. The 'rules' governing the presentation of artwork are the same as those for presenting any two-dimensional piece of work. When necessary, the work for display should be neatly and accurately trimmed using a rotary trimmer or craft knife. A neutral background (black, white or grey) will be most useful for displaying coloured pieces of artwork to advantage. A coloured mount or background behind a colourful piece of artwork will influence what the viewer will be attracted to. When mounting a single piece of work the borders on the top and sides of the artwork should be equal. For visual effect the border below the artwork should be a little deeper. When displaying several pieces of work on the same mount either make the top or bottom edges level, also keep the edges of work parallel to the mount, avoid if possible a diagonal arrangement of artwork as this tends to take the eye away from the individual pieces of work. The spaces between the artwork

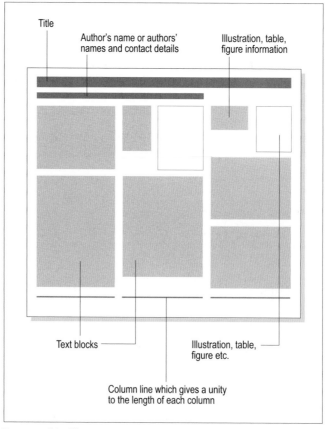

Figure 18.4 Typographical layout

should be the same; this will bring harmony to the overall arrangement. When displaying circular or irregularly shaped artwork consideration should be given to the spacing and balance of the arrangement. Peculiarly shaped spaces created between the pieces of work can compete with the artwork for the eyes' attention. Irregularly shaped work can be most effectively displayed by positioning them on to a rectangular-shaped mount before adding them to the overall arrangement. As far as possible keep the background unobtrusive so that all the attention will be focused on the artwork.

For the purposes of this chapter the content is not of direct relevance; what is of interest is the author's use of fonts, placement of material.

Oral presentations

Delivering an oral presentation to an audience requires many of the skills used by an actor. Your audience want to know the detail of your presentation, but to a certain extent they also want to be entertained or at least to find it pleasurable and enjoyable to listen to what you have to say. The presentation needs to be prepared, structured and rehearsed to guarantee a successful performance.

Before embarking on your presentation clearly identify:

- What is the purpose of the presentation?
- What facilities will be available to you?
- How much time do you have?
- Who will be in the audience?

The ability to answer the questions above will enable you to select an appropriate style of delivery and give structure of your work. The purpose of the presentation will dictate whether a formal or informal approach is chosen. Conferences are usually formal affairs where a chairperson will introduce a speaker, ensure that the time schedule is kept and oversee the question and answer session at the end of your talk. On these occasions formal dress and a formal posture should be considered. For an informal presentation a more flexible approach can be assumed and a more relaxed posture and dress code selected.

Introduce yourself and your topic to establish credibility with the audience. Then follow the three golden rules of any presentation:

- Say what you are going to say
- Say it
- Say what you have just said.

It is also important to remember that an audience's concentration is high at the start, flagging in the middle and can be distracted towards the end so use a variety of sensory techniques to keep them alert. Kinder (1973: 39) said that people remember:

- 10% of what they read
- 20% of what they hear
- 30% of what they see
- but 50% of what they hear and see.

Therefore a combination of visual images with both oral and written communication will aid the transference of knowledge. The use of visual imagery will also communicate an idea more quickly than words and it could be argued will remain longer in the memory than spoken or written words. Photographs, illustrations and video will all enhance your presentation but choose the correct image; be cautious especially when using clipart as these computer-generated pictures are often overused and lose their impact when shown repeatedly. Visual aids will also help to engage an audience but ensure these are positioned or held for all to see.

Presenting

Most people find presenting at least a little nerve wracking. Some will go to great lengths to avoid having to do it. However the skill of being able to stand up and present your work is invaluable and the benefits it can bring to you, your service, or your profession are significant. So do not be put off by performance anxiety, stick your neck above the parapet and begin to present your work: initially where you feel most comfortable and then move on to what you may consider to be a more challenging audience.

Nowadays developing presentational skills is a central component to all undergraduate degrees, but the target audience is generally the same – tutorial group, year group, lecturers, etc. As a practitioner, you may be required to present work in a variety of different settings, to large or small groups, to people you do know (such as your clinical team) or do not know (such as at a conference). Each of these different settings requires slightly different skills.

The American psychologist Albert Mehrabian is perhaps best known for his work on nonverbal communication and body language. Mehrabian (1971) examined the impact of the content, voice intonation and body language on communication and coined the 7%, 35%, 55% rule. That is we are more likely to like and accept the presenter if they manage to convey positive messages with their words, tone of voice and body language; the respective impact of each being 7%, 35% and 55%. The importance of having positive body language is therefore clear.

Body language

Eye contact establishes and maintains rapport with your audience, it will also help you detect if they understand or are interested in what you are saying. Make eye contact with all the audience so that they all feel included. If you are in a standing position place both feet firmly on the floor, about the same width as your shoulders, and avoid the temptation of trying to balance on one leg! If you are sitting keep your legs still and refrain from swinging or twisting your legs as this can be distracting. Gestures should be used in moderation. The use of deliberate hand and arm movements can make you appear more confident and relaxed. Keep hand gestures above waist height so that all the audience can see what you are doing and avoid repetitive hand or arm movement for no apparent reason as this can suggest insecurity or anxiety.

Often we can be unaware of our own idiosyncratic body language when we present. Perhaps you perch on one foot like a stork, or rock back and forth like a Weeble ('Weebles wobble but they don't fall down!'). Alternatively you may use hand gestures more appropriate for conducting the last night of the proms! Whatever it is (and you are likely to have at least some subtle habits) it is quite possible you are unaware of them. Ask colleagues who have seen you present to give you feedback on your body language. Ideally get yourself videoed whilst delivering a presentation and then closely analyse your body language. Few people are completely comfortable watching themselves 'perform', but it can be an invaluable method of getting feedback and altering your performance.

Using your voice

Most presenters get at least a little nervous and your voice can be one of the tell-tale signs of your nerves to your audience. Anxious presenters often speak much faster than necessary; a kind of, 'lets get this over and done with as soon as possible' principle.

Unsurprisingly this does not lead to a good presentation. So watch the pace that you speak at. If you know that you get nervous then it can be helpful to consciously slow down what you are saying. However your presentation should flow and not drag; vary the pace of your presentation and slow down further for important points. Alter the pitch of your voice by using the full range of high and low tones throughout your presentation, to avoid your voice becoming monotonous. Use volume to suit the environment and be prepared to ask the audience if they can all hear you; not only will this ensure that you are speaking loud enough it will also mean that you are seen as being a considerate speaker. Common sense should prevail however; if the last three speakers have asked the audience if they can hear them then don't repeat it – people just find this tiresome.

The final word on using your voice must be given not to what you say, but to what you don't: silence and pauses. Pausing, for short periods, during your presentation can be used to excellent effect. It can emphasise a point you have just made, or enable your audience to assimilate what you have just said before you move on to your next point.

Structuring your presentation

Think of your presentation like a story. You need to have a beginning, middle and end. As your audience's concentration is high at the start of your talk, you should try to give an excellent introduction: lose them here and you will have lost them for good (or at least for the rest of your presentation). So start off strong, introduce yourself, grab their attention with some sort of statement or reflection as to why your presentation is important and outline what you are going to be talking about.

The middle phase of your presentation is where the majority of your presentation will take place. In effect this is where you tell your 'story', present your research, etc. Make sure it flows well. For research presentations this is easier as there are tried and tested structures to follow (e.g. background, method, results, discussion), for more discursive presentations there are less traditions and careful consideration needs to be given to whether what you are saying makes sense and is easy to follow; here too is an opportunity to use your 'critical friend'.

The last phase of your presentation is the conclusion. This should tie up your presentation, summarising what you have said and neatly bring your audience to realise that you have finished. As your introduction is an excellent opportunity to come in with a 'high', your conclusion is an excellent opportunity to go out on a 'high'. Leave your audience in no doubt as to the main messages or key points of your presentation. And finally remember to thank your audience for their attention. It is a simple courtesy, and is always well received.

Visual aids

Your choice and use of overhead transparencies, PowerPoint, etc. or a combination of these will be governed by the facilities available to you. Make yourself familiar with whatever you select to use and do not expect technical help to be present on the day. It is always a good idea to bring a back up of your presentation too, whether on a different disk, or in differing formats (i.e. one copy on PowerPoint and another on transparency).

Overall the key to a good presentation is preparation and rehearsal.

Writing for presentation

Writing for publication is another method of disseminating your work. It is an excellent way to share your research or practice. The advantage of having your work published is that it lasts longer and will almost certainly be more widely accessed than if you present your work at a conference. Whilst writing for publication is undoubtedly challenging, it can also be hugely rewarding.

Where to submit?

The first task is to consider where best to submit your work. Think about who you want to read what you publish: what journals or magazines does your desired audience peruse? Could your potential paper fit the format used in one of these publications? Do you want to submit your work to a magazine, where its inclusion will be accepted or rejected by the editor alone? Or is your work more scholarly or research based and would be suitable to be submitted to a peer-reviewed journal, where it would be independently scrutinised by at least two 'experts' who would make recommendations to the editor for acceptance or rejection? Such questions will help you make decisions about where to submit your work. Other factors that can be important (typically in considering where to submit a peer-reviewed paper) include whether or not a journal is indexed in relevant databases (e.g. CINHAL, PsychInfo, Medline) and whether it has an impact factor.

Impact factors

Impact factors are published in Journal Citation Reports by Thomson Scientific (www.isiwebofknowledge.com). An Impact Factor is a score assigned to a journal based on the number of times that articles that were published in one year were cited in indexed journals the following year, divided by the number of citable items (letters, editorials and obituaries are not typically counted in this calculation). Much controversy exists about the worth and value of impact factors. It is certainly not a perfect system, however it is the internationally accepted academic measure of a journal's quality. At present very few occupational therapy journals have a published impact factor, however most major peer-reviewed occupational therapy journals are now working towards achieving this (Editorial Board 2005, Fricke 2006, Swedlove 2006). Potential authors should consider the quality of the journal they wish to publish in, remembering that the ideal one may not be a profession-specific journal and that other journal titles often contain a wider readership and may have great quality recognition (as indicated by their impact factor rating). Some authors, however, may not be so concerned with a journal's impact factor and may be happy to submit a paper based on the target audience alone. And remember, you may be able to submit more than one paper from your work, so there may be opportunities to do both.

Developing papers

Writing for publication is a skill that people develop over time. If you have not written before, and especially if you are aiming to submit a paper to a peer-reviewed publication, then get an experienced author to co-author your paper. Their skills and experience will be invaluable for you as a novice author, and could avoid some heartache if your papers are rejected fundamentally through lack of writing experience more than anything else. It is important to note at this stage, however, that an experienced co-author is certainly no guarantee of acceptance! The experience of rejection or major article revision is a common experience; and normally one that, if you can get over it and take on board the reviewers' recommendations, will help you to develop as a writer.

Journals or magazines normally have advice or author's guidelines, for potential authors. As with submitting abstracts careful attention must be paid to this advice. Failure to comply with it will lead to your paper being rejected. Often the guidance will outline various different categories of submission (e.g. original research, opinion piece, letters to the editor, etc...). If you are not sure which would be best then consider what you are planning to write and have a look through the journal to see if there are any similar publications.

Whether writing with an experienced author, or alone, it is vital to consider the structure of your paper. Here too it is worth closely examining the guidelines for authors of a journal or magazine, as well as papers that deal with a similar subject or method area. These will often give you an idea of a structure to follow.

Last minute checks…

So you have written your paper and chosen a publication to submit it to. You have probably spent long hours planning, writing and revising the text, either alone or with your co-author(s). By now quite frankly you may be getting a bit sick of it and just want to send it off! Stop. Before you do, it is wise to spend a little more time checking it and getting someone completely neutral (perhaps your critical friend) to read it and give you comments.

Giving your paper to someone for feedback is an excellent way to find out how readable it is. If the paper is unclear to your friend, then it will most likely be unclear to the editor or reviewers. Time spent revising your paper now may significantly enhance its chance of acceptance. Dixon (2001) recommends asking your friend to write down the four or five most important points that they understood from reading your paper; if they are not the same as yours, or are in a different order then you need to give consideration to the structure and flow of your work. Further checks worth carrying out before you submit your paper include:

- Checking (again) that you have followed the author's guidelines
- That any statistics included are appropriately presented
- And that (where appropriate) you have included a statement about the ethical issues of your work and, if required, that formal ethical approval was gained.

Summary

Competition for the ever-shrinking attention of people living in a world filled with an endless number of communications is fierce. Understanding when, where and what to publish or present is important and knowledge of how to publish or present well is paramount. As Whieldon (1996) states typography at its best is virtually invisible this could also be said about any good communicator who does not impede the message. The good poster, oral and visual presentation or paper often belies the time and effort spent on the development, arrangement and revision undertaken to achieve its perfect result.

References

Bannigan K 2005 Disseminating Research Results. Mental Health Occupational Therapy

Dixon N 2001 Writing for publication – a guide for new authors. International Journal for Quality in Health Care 13(5): 417–421

Editorial Board 2005 Internationalisation and impact factors: A communication from the editorial board. British Journal of Occupational Therapy 68: 97–98

Fricke J 2006 On impacts and other factors. Australian Occupational Therapy Journal 53: 1–2

Haigh CA 2006 The Art of the Abstract. Nurse Education Today 26(5): 355–337

Harms M 1995 How to …Prepare a Poster Presentation. Physiotherapy 81(5): 276–277

Innes G 1988 Unpublished lecture notes. Queen Margaret College, Edinburgh, UK

Kinder JS 1973 Using Instructional Media. D van Nostrand Co., New York

Mehrabian A 1971 Silent Messages. Wadsworth, Belmont, CA

Meshack BL 2004 Developing a Thick Skin: How to Accept Criticism. Vision: A Resource for Writers. http://fmwriters.com/Visionback/Vision24/developingthickskin.htm Accessed on 22 August 2007

Papanek V 1985 Design for the real world, 2nd edn. Academy Chicago Publishers, Chicago, IL

RNIB 1995 'See It Right' Clear Print Guidelines. RNIB Publications, London

Simmonds D 1984 How to...produce a good poster. Medical Teacher 6(1): 10–13

Swedlove F 2006 Implications of the impact factor. Canadian Journal of Occupational Therapy 73: 3–6

Wheildon C 1996 Type and Layout: How Typography and Design Can Get Your Message Across-Or Get in the Way. Strathmoor Press, Berkley, CA

SECTION 4

Leadership, supervision and management skills for practice

293

Management of self

19

Katrina Bannigan

Highlight box

- In an ever-changing work environment self care has become an essential component of good performance at work.
- Resilience involves the ability to bounce back from difficult experiences; it is not an innate ability and can be developed by anyone through the use of self management strategies.
- Self management strategies involve taking a proactive stance towards self care.
- Incorporating good habits into everyday work life, such as taking regular breaks, can increase resilience.
- If we have specific issues, such as an inability to say no, using specific techniques, such as assertiveness training, may be required to increase personal effectiveness.

Overview

The ever-changing nature of modern health and social care settings means it is necessary for occupational therapists to think about resilience. Resilience is the capacity an individual has to bounce back from stressful events and situations. It is not an innate quality or attribute, i.e. it is not one of those things like intelligence that you either have or not, which means it can be learned. Developing resilience can help in the prevention of problems occupational therapists may experience in the workplace, such as burnout. Burnout is a serious problem with a number of features, e.g. fatigue, exhaustion and the inability to concentrate. It involves a loss of interest in work coupled with a sense going through the motions. There are other less serious challenges experienced at work that can also make life uncomfortable, such as work–life imbalance. This means individual occupational therapists need to take personal responsibility for their self care by developing self-management strategies. In terms of self management there are some general principles, such as developing good habits, which can be applied to working life as well as specific techniques, such as mentoring, which occupational therapists can use to improve their self management.

Background

Occupational therapists extol the virtue of work–life balance and promote it through occupational balance (Backman 2004). Much of the everyday work we do as occupational therapists is dependent on us as people, i.e. our therapeutic use of self (see Chapter 9). There has been a focus in occupational therapy literature on the need to avoid burnout (e.g. Hume and Joice 2002). Yet how many of us really look after ourselves? It is very easy for people in caring roles to neglect caring for themselves hence the aphorism 'physician heal thy self', which has been expanded to 'healer heal thyself, or you won't be any good at healing your patients' (Chacksfield 2002a: 5). We are a precious resource and, as we are the main tool we have to do our work, if we do not care for ourselves we will become prone to burnout and so undermine our ability to be occupational therapists.

Although focus on burnout is still relevant today (and burnout will be discussed in more detail in this chapter) we need to rethink the issue of looking after ourselves. This is because the delivery of modern health and social care services places a wider range of challenges and demands on us. We work in an ever-changing environment focused on improvement, reform and modernisation of services. This requires occupational therapists to be able to act-into-the-situation and reflect on their experience in order to make a positive contribution. We also need to be able to change practice as required, using patient experience and working to challenge the conventions that no longer meet expectations of patients or organisations. This, in turn, means occupational therapists need not just to avoid burnout but also to develop resilience, which involves taking a more proactive approach. The bottom line is self care has become essential to good performance at work. It is something we can address and, in the light of this, this chapter will explore:

- what is meant by resilience
- the challenges occupational therapists are likely to face in the workplace
- the concepts of self care and self management, and
- strategies occupational therapists can use for self management.

The chapter has been written in the expectation that you will make links between this chapter and the chapters on clinical supervision (Chapter 22) and leadership (Chapter 20) because each informs and supports the other. The overall aim of this chapter is to stimulate thought about how we, as occupational therapists, can perform at our best in our work by thinking about the measures we can take to care for ourselves.

What is resilience?

Before considering self care and the need for self management it is necessary to be clear about why this topic is important. Self management is increasingly becoming part of an occupational therapist's working life because we need to seek a balance between our professional development needs and the needs of the present and future health and social care system within which we work. In health and social care, as with other areas of employment, the landscape of work has changed. In essence organisations can no longer be defined as clearly as they once were as they have had to adapt to the changing environments in which they operate (Lee and King 2001). The key features of organisations today include:

- a focus on the customer rather than hierarchies
- less emphasis on jobs and more emphasis on tasks and assignments
- shift in the location of work (fewer people work in the same place every day of the week)
- generational shifts (for example the Net generation, i.e. those who have never known life without the internet, have very different expectations of work to the baby boomer generation) (Tapscott 1994, Lee and King 2001).

This means occupational therapists can no longer expect cradle-to-grave job security and there is a need to take personal responsibility for developing the skills needed to function in today's organisations. In the absence of structures we all need to learn how to be innovative, flexible, responsive and comfortable with ambiguity and change (Lee and King 2001). This involves developing an awareness of the strategic direction of health and social care, and identifying ways to read ourselves into it. An individual practitioner cannot rely on others to do this for them because with flatter structures there are fewer managers – and they often have a broader portfolio of responsibilities. More often than not there will be no direct professional line management (i.e. by an occupational therapist); so it cannot always be assumed that your manager will understand the contribution occupational therapy can make to new agendas. This shift in expectations means resilience is now a quality that employers look for when recruiting new employees (Contu 2003).

Resilience is valued by employers because it is the means by which many people face and overcome challenges in the workplace. It has been defined as '...the process of adapting well in the face of adversity, trauma, tragedy, threats, or even significant sources of stress – such as family and relationship problems, serious health problems, or workplace and financial stressors. It entails the capacity to bounce back from difficult experiences' (APA Help Center 2004a). It 'involves maintaining flexibility and balance in your life as you deal with stressful circumstances and traumatic events' (APA Help Center 2004b: 5). It is essentially about hardiness (Contu 2003) and becomes '...a reflex, a way of facing and understanding the world, that is deeply etched into a person's mind and soul. Resilient people and [organisations] face reality with staunchness, make meaning of hardship instead of crying out in despair, and improvise solutions from thin air' (Contu 2003: 17–18). In a climate of constant change in the workplace the ability to adapt and be flexible consistently over time is a valuable skill. As occupational therapists, regardless of whether this is something our employers want to see us demonstrating, it should also be a skill we want to nurture because it will help us to function optimally. This chapter generally focuses on the use of resilience in the workplace. It is inevitable, however, that anything an individual does to develop resilience in order to help them cope with the challenges they face at work is also likely to have benefits in other aspects of their life.

Resilience is a skill not a trait

If you are feeling overwhelmed by change in your place of work (or study) and do not feel particularly resilient remember that you can do something about it. The literature identifies that 'Resilience is not a trait that people either have or do not have. It involves behaviours, thoughts and actions that can be learned and developed in anyone' (APA Help Center 2004b: 1). By understanding the characteristics of resilient people you can assess where your personal weaknesses lie and develop strategies to overcome them. However, as with most things in life, this will require effort and commitment. It is not a one-off task that can be ticked off a 'to-do' list. The APA Help Center (2004b) has identified a combination of factors as contributing to resilience, i.e.

- caring and supportive relationships within and outside the family
- the capacity to make realistic plans and take steps to carry them out
- a positive view of yourself and confidence in your strengths and abilities
- skill in communication and problem solving, and
- the capacity to manage strong feelings and impulses.

Of these the primary factor is having caring and supportive relationships within and outside the family. 'Relationships that create love and trust, provide role models and offer encouragement and reassurance [to] help bolster a person's resilience' (The APA Help Center 2004b: 2). Therefore if you do not have good social networks you need to develop them to increase your resilience. This example clearly shows why developing resilience involves a long-term commitment; building caring and supportive relationships calls for considerable time and effort. Contu (2003) has outlined that there are three qualities needed for resilience, i.e. the capacity to accept and face reality, the ability to find meaning in some aspects of life, and the ability to improvise (Contu 2003).

The capacity to accept and face reality

It may be thought that a positive attitude, or optimism, is a prerequisite for personal development and/or change and that resilience stems from an optimistic nature. Whilst a positive attitude and/or optimism can be useful in the face of adversity or trying circumstances it is not enough. It is only useful in so far as it does not distort a person's view of reality (Contu 2003). The reason for this is '...for bigger challenges a cool, almost pessimistic, sense of reality is far more important' (Contu 2003: 7). Some people use 'denial' as a coping mechanism. This is a psychological process by which human beings protect themselves from things which threaten them by blocking knowledge of those things from their awareness (Community Alcohol Information Program 1997). It is a defence mechanism which distorts reality; it keeps us from feeling the pain and uncomfortable truth about things we do not want to face (Community Alcohol Information Program 1997). Denial or an overly positive or optimistic attitude in the face of difficult circumstances, e.g. the death of a colleague or redundancies, does not promote resilience. In fact it may be regarded as wholly inappropriate by others sharing the same experience (Dutton et al 2003). Being positive or overly optimistic can also stop an individual facing the reality of their situation. 'The fact is, when we truly stare down reality, we prepare ourselves to act in ways that allow us to endure and survive extraordinary hardship' (Contu 2003: 9). Accepting and facing up to a situation also calls for us to demonstrate our humanity and to be compassionate; having resilience does not mean that an individual is devoid of emotion or that they leave their emotions at the door when they are in work (Dutton et al 2003). In fact it may be that a compassionate response that allows people to make sense of a situation is a more effective response than one in which a situation is ignored because it is regarded as inappropriate to be emotional at work (Dutton et al 2003). This links with Contu's (2003) second characteristic of resilience, i.e. the ability to find meaning in some aspects of life.

The ability to find meaning in some aspects of life

In difficult circumstances many of us take on a victim role revealed in the question 'Why is this happening to me?' The question can equally be posed 'Why not me?' Contu (2003) contends 'resilient people devise constructs about their suffering to create some sort of meaning for themselves and others' (p. 10). In this situation, meaning making becomes a coping mechanism, i.e. we cope by making sense of a situation for ourselves by setting it in a context. For example, we set the situation in the context of our life, future or past events or our faith (if we have one). Frankl (1984), a Jew who survived the German concentration camps in the Second World War, wrote 'We must never forget that we may also find meaning in life even when confronted with a hopeless situation, when facing a fate that cannot be changed...In some way, suffering ceases to be suffering at the moment it finds a meaning' (p. 135). However, it is emphasised that 'Resilience is neither ethically good nor bad. It is merely the *skill* [my emphasis] and the capacity to be robust under conditions of enormous stress and change' (Contu 2003: 12).

The ability to improvise

The third characteristic, improvisation, links to flexibility and can be defined as 'a kind of inventiveness, an ability to improvise a solution to a problem without proper or obvious tools or materials' (Contu 2003: 14). It involves the ability to make do with whatever is at hand and organisations that survive regard improvisation as a core skill (Contu 2003). For example UPS supports its drivers to do whatever it takes to get its deliveries done on time but improvisation, as practised by UPS, 'is a far cry from unbridled creativity' (Contu 2003: 16). UPS also works within rules and regulations. It is recognised that improvisation has not been widely encouraged in health and social care services but it does highlight how individuals will sometimes have to take the initiative rather than rely on or expect existing hierarchies or systems to provide the solutions. This is not dissimilar to what Bennis and Thomas (2003) call adaptive capacity, that is an ability to transcend adversity and emerge stronger than before. These three attributes show how we need resilience to enable us to adapt to life-changing situations and stressful conditions. Therefore it is a useful skill for practitioners to develop to cope with the challenges they face at work.

Challenges faced by occupational therapists in the workplace

For many occupational therapists it is not just that they face a challenge at work, it's the sheer number and range of challenges presented by day-to-day work that can be wearing. Therefore it is important to be able to identify the warning signs and then do something to ameliorate the situation if problems arise. The most serious consequence of not being resilient is burnout but, whilst burnout is the worst-case scenario, there are other less serious problems that can also undermine our ability to do our job properly. These include a lack of work–life balance, being unable to keep abreast of technology, and succumbing to impostor syndrome.

The worst-case scenario – burnout

Burnout is a serious issue in health and social care settings. Taylor (2005) has contended that allowing ourselves to burnout 'is tantamount to negligence as burnout is next to impossible to treat once it is established' (p. 220). It is not without its warning signs. There are three main symptoms – feeling emotional, loss of rapport and achievement. The danger signs of burnout include:

- Your energy is being used up quicker on a daily basis than you recover it
- Being out of control of demands at work
- Trying to be a hero at work
- Lacking the assertiveness skills to say no, and
- Being young ('It takes two years (on average), if the conditions are right, from starting clinical work to burnout') (Taylor 2005: 220).

People experiencing burnout have described themselves as feeling used up, emotionally exhausted, seeing their patients as problems rather than as people and feeling that all the energy they are putting into their job is not achieving much (Taylor 2005). Other symptoms include fatigue, exhaustion, inability to concentrate, depression, anxiety, insomnia, irritability, increased use of alcohol or drugs, a loss of interest in one's work or personal life, and a feeling of 'just going through the motions' (Gundersen 2001). Burnout is a complex problem that is not caused by any one factor so it makes more sense to prevent rather than treat it (Grosch and Olsen 1994). In trying to prevent burnout there are no simplistic formulas; it is not just about substituting a leisure activity with some of the time you spent at work. Grosch and Olsen (1994) have developed an approach to preventing burnout based on a theory of family origin. However it is possible to delineate steps to prevent burnout that stand alone from this theoretical perspective (see below).

Ongoing self assessment

By assessing ourselves regularly we can determine the difference between normal tiredness and early signs of burnout.

Understanding our patterns of behaviour

Recognise what the issues are that are contributing to burnout, e.g. perfectionism.

Breaking behaviour patterns

Taking action to resolve issues identified, e.g. if taking on too many responsibilities is an issue you may need to learn to say no and set firm boundaries.

Emotional intelligence

Developing our capacity to manage strong feelings and impulses in the face of stress and anxiety-provoking situations.

A lack of work–life balance

'Overwork is the curse of our time. Working long hours has become a badge of honor among professional people, whose complaints about overwork are often mixed with a sense of pride in their dedication and importance' (Grosch and Olsen 1994: 101). Overwork is perpetuated through a need for chronic busyness and is prevalent in the helping professions (Grosch and Olsen 1994). By contrast work–life balance is about achieving the right balance of focus, energy and time between your work and the other important areas of your life (Lee and King 2001). It is not easy to achieve because there is no prescription and everyone has to work it out for themselves but it is also not about being perfect in all aspects of your life (Lee and King 2001). Work–life balance helps us to be more effective at work because, for example, single-minded devotion to work is correlated with poor performance (Lee and King 2001). As has already been suggested in the discussion about resilience (above) the benefits of achieving work–life balance will not just be experienced in the work arena but in our personal lives as well. Lee and King (2001) suggest there are five strategies for achieving balance, i.e.:

- Integrating. Counter intuitively instead of trying to keep work and life separate through having clear boundaries between the two we should allow boundaries to be more flexible and allow overlap.
- Narrowing. This involves recognising that there is only so much any one individual can do and so we need to make only those commitments we can keep.
- Moderating. This builds on the maxim 'everything in moderation' and means spending the right amount of time in each area of your life, not overdoing things.

- Sequencing. Recognising that we cannot do everything at once so we need to plan and have priorities, concomitantly some activities may have to fall by the wayside.
- Adding resources. Use additional resources where we can to enable us to get more done.

Being unable to keep abreast of technological developments

The need to keep abreast of technological developments can cause anxiety as well as feelings of being out of control at work. There is no doubt that technology in health and social care will continue to need a wider community of practitioners to test technology solutions with the user/carer. A positive critical use of technology can optimise the care and rehabilitation experience. This demands a group of people who understand and are able to use technology in rehabilitation practice. Whilst there has always been new technology to keep abreast of this is an example of how generational shifts have an impact on work. 'The technologies available as a generation matures influence their behaviors, attitudes, and expectations. People internalize the technologies that shape information access and use, as well as the ways they communicate. Matures (born 1946–1964) were exposed to large vacuum-tube radios, mechanical calculators, 78 rpm records, dial telephones, and party lines. Baby Boomers grew up with transistor radios, mainframe computers, $33\frac{1}{3}$ and 45 rpm records, and the touch-tone telephone. Gen-Xers matured in the era of CDs, personal computers, and electronic mail. For the Net Generation, the prevailing technologies are MP3s, cell phones, and PDAs; they communicate via instant messaging, text messaging, and blogs. For each successive generation "technology is only technology if it was invented after they were born"' (Hartman et al 2005). This means for those of us who are not part of the Net generation we need to work not only towards fluency in information technology but also understand how it has influenced the mindset and behaviour of society (Moore et al 2005). Keeping abreast of technological developments requires:

- **An awareness of the Net generation's approach to technology.** We do not just need to know about what the new technologies are but also how they are used and how they influence lifestyle; computer technology has changed how people live and work.
- **Professional development.** To develop the skills needed to use technology alongside other knowledge, such as facilitating meaningful occupations.
- **Ongoing professional development.** As technology and practice change so rapidly we have to have an on-going plan of development (Moore et al 2005).

Succumbing to impostor syndrome

Impostor syndrome is the phrase used to describe people who feel like a fraud in their professional lives. These are people who play down their successes because they believe that they have only achieved what they have achieved through good fortune and it is likely that this will be exposed at any time. It used to be a phenomenon observed in the university sector but Bhargava (2007) has noted that 'Researchers say that these vague feelings of self doubt, intellectual fraudulence and anxiety are so common among people, it's almost an epidemic. The 'impostor syndrome' strikes people everywhere especially high achievers. It makes them discount their success attributing it to luck, not real ability. Along with it comes the fear that anytime they could be found out' (p. 1–2). As the experience of impostor syndrome involves an inability to internalise success, strategies for overcoming it are linked to the need to internalise success.

- **Challenging the thinking that allows impostor syndrome to flourish.**
  Thoughts such as I have only got here by luck need to be questioned.
- **Developing benchmarks for success.** Using benchmarks for success that not only
  look at future goals but that also acknowledge how far we have come can be used as
  reality check (Caltech Student Counseling Center 2007).
- **Focus on positive achievement.** Developing a highlights list can help us focus on
  our positive achievements and keep them at the forefront of our minds.

Self care and self management

Having considered what resilience is, and some of the challenges occupational therapists
may face in performing well at work, the next step is to think about what we can actually
do to develop or increase our resilience. Burnout has been identified as the worst-case
scenario but it is avoidable. Taylor (2005) has emphasised that 'Burnout is extremely
difficult to recover from once well established. There is no pharmaceutical solution and
too little internal energy to fight it effectively...Just as a bankrupt business cannot easily
revive itself, so you will not have the resources to bounce back. And no one can do this for
you. Prevention is our own personal responsibility, however 'selfish' the steps we need to
take' (p. 220). If this analysis is accepted it means preventing burnout is not an option but
essential to good performance at work. In combating burnout Taylor (2005) identified
that there are two fundamental points to consider:

- Recognise there is risk of burnout if we do not take care of ourselves, and
- Ask ourselves the question 'Do we care enough about ourselves to actively avoid
  burnout?'

This demonstrates that 'self care' is the foundation to developing resilience.

The concept of self care

As with most things in life self care means different things to different people. Generally
self care involves taking personal responsibility for ensuring the maintenance of health
and well-being. Patients are increasing expected to take more responsibility for their own
care, for example 'Self care was highlighted in the NHS Plan as one of the key building
blocks for a patient-centred health service. More recently self care featured as a component of the model for supporting people with long term conditions' (DH 2005: 1). The
NHS recognises that there are benefits for patients and services by supporting self care
and so is committed to developing and supporting a range of initiatives to facilitate this
(DH 2005). However, if there is an expectation that patients will increasingly take responsibility for their own health perhaps occupational therapists also need to practise what
they preach? However, as Taylor (2003) highlighted whilst we may recognise there is risk
of burnout if we do not take care of ourselves, we can often feel like we are being selfish
if we put ourselves and our needs high on our agenda. So it is not just about recognising
that we need to put our self first but we also have to actively take steps to care for ourselves
however selfish we may feel that is.

Caring for ourselves

Caring for yourself literally means '...you must look after yourself as well as you possibly
can...When you look after your own needs as much as you look after those of others you
become better able to do your work' (Kersley 2004: 64). However, how we care for ourselves will depend to a certain extent on our personal interests, needs and circumstances.

For example someone working full time with young children may have different needs in relation to work–life balance to another person who is under-stimulated by their work and feels the need to be stretched more. As each individual's needs are different and change over time we need to monitor ourselves. Self care is not something that we can address once in our careers and assume all will be well for the duration; we need to revisit the issue every so often to ensure that the measures we put in place are still relevant to our needs. It may be a question we pose for ourselves annually, perhaps at the time of our appraisal, even if it is not a question on the official forms that we have to complete.

An overarching issue for all occupational therapists is the need to maintain health. Chacksfield (2002b) has outlined 12 strategies for maintaining good mental health (see Box 19.1) and although he was discussing mental health he also mentioned exercise. It is very difficult for any of us to have escaped the message that exercise has an essential role to play in maintaining good health and that it benefits our physical and mental health. However, how many of us integrate exercise into our everyday routines and habits? A quick win in terms of exercise can come through the use of a pedometer – 'people with pedometers do more steps than people without' (Hebert 2005: 221). Another issue in terms of health and burnout is that many of us come to work when we are ill. We know we should not do it but many do. This type of behaviour can play a role in developing burnout because when we go to work ill this is not caring for ourselves. Although maintaining health is required to actively prevent burnout, other issues, such as time management and the control we feel we have over our work, are also relevant. This is why self management, built on the premise of the need for self care, has a role to play in developing resilience.

Self management and self management strategies

Self-management refers to methods, skills and strategies by which individuals can effectively direct their own activities. Whilst employers have a responsibility to support their employees by providing a safe environment in which to work, in order to build resilience

Box 19.1

Twelve strategies for maintaining good mental health

1. Exercise helps mental fitness as well
2. Find people to share your stress with
3. Practise what you preach – listen to those relaxation tapes
4. Say 'no' when you need to
5. Ask for help when things get too difficult – use supervision
6. You do not have to tackle problems alone – work together
7. Make your goals achievable
8. Stop when you feel you are doing too much – it does not matter if everything is not done immediately
9. Concentration, done properly, does not require effort – only focus
10. Stick to your own remit – despite pressure from others (or yourself) to do more
11. Think what it is like to realise that life is not perfect
12. Laugh as much as possible (Chacksfield 2002b: 5)

we also have to take responsibility for engaging in activities to promote our effectiveness at work. It has already been identified that occupational therapists are all different and so will have different needs and that these change over time. This means there is no 'off the shelf' self management plan because there is no one-size-fits-all solution. However there are a number of things we can do to help ourselves. As well as the specific suggestions for preventing burnout, developing work–life balance, keeping abreast of technological advances and overcoming impostor syndrome (see above) there are other tactics available. These can be summarised under two headings, i.e. general principles to develop good habits and specific techniques. The remainder of this chapter will present a range of ideas under these headings which you can use to experiment and explore what will work best for you. In the vignettes (below) I have used my own experiences to illustrate how I have tried to develop/apply self management strategies to myself. However, the ideas presented here only provide a flavour of the available literature. There is a lot of information available and there may be particular issues or ideas that you want to explore in more detail (a number of useful resources have been provided as a starting point for further exploration of these topics).

Self support strategies: general principles to develop good habits

In Box 19.2 some simple, but effective, good ideas have been listed. Each of these ideas is relatively easy to implement but does require the person involved to act. After all actions only become habits when they become an integral part of what we do without conscious thought or attention. This usually occurs through repetition. We need to be proactive about developing good habits because 'We often get so busy "sawing" (producing results) that we forget to "sharpen the saw" (maintain or increase our capacity to produce results in the future)' (Covey et al 1994: 85). Covey (1989) calls the habit of taking time out to re-energise and renew 'sharpening the saw'. You may find it helpful to reflect on the list of good ideas (Box 19.2) to see if there are any you could adopt to change your current behaviours around work. Even if you are quite good at caring for yourself are there other things you could incorporate into your life to increase your effectiveness? Whatever you decide to do set yourself a realistic goal and set a date to review this, perhaps as part of your appraisal?

Self management strategies: specific techniques

The general principles are inexpensive, relatively easy strategies to adopt. There are other more specific techniques that occupational therapists can use as part of their self management. These are more likely to require a higher investment of either time or money or both. You may be supported by your employer to use these techniques but whether you are supported or not, you may still decide that the investment is worthwhile because of the increase in your performance and effectiveness at work and other important areas of your life.

Vignette 19.1

Scholarly activity meeting

I am a part of an informal meeting with a group of colleagues who get together to support each other with continuing professional development. We each set goals annually and then use them to monitor our activity over the year. We have set-up a reminder system with an administrator who sends us a personal reminder to remind us what work we had agreed to complete by the next meeting. Although there is no obligation to attend the meeting all members are committed because we have found that by committing to goals, discussing progress and encouraging each other all of us have increased our productivity.

Box 19.2

Examples of good habits that promote self care and will enhance your resilience

Develop outside interests

'If you are to avoid the overworking trap you need to meet as many of your needs as possible by life outside work…think of enjoyable and creative ways to meet your needs outside work' (Work life balance centre 2007)

If you need help, ask for it

Use structures that are in place (see, for example, Chapter 22 on clinical supervision), make use of the leadership literature (see the Chapter 20) and seek support from others.

Introduce variety

Vary your daily routine but also vary your career (Taylor 2005). After all, variety is the spice of life!

Learn to say no (without feeling guilty)

'Our patients have needs, but so do we. Balance them' (Taylor 2005: 220)

Take breaks

Take small, frequent breaks. Avoid competitive negativity, i.e. the state of trying to 'out busy' everyone else you speak to (Work life balance centre 2007)

Watch your language

Sometimes our use of language reinforces our sense of being busy and/or out of control.

Do not be constrained by others

Only be limited by 'your' imagination. Do not let other people shape your views of what is possible.

Learn from stories

Reading about the experiences of others can help to inspire us (e.g. Glicken 2006).

Develop positive outlook

This does not mean tolerating the intolerable.

Value serendipity

Make the best use of opportunities that come along.

The working environment

Does the culture in your department promote or militate against work–life balance? Are there behaviours, practices or ideas that need to change in your department to promote the health and well-being of the people who work in it?

Head for work each day with one single priority

Do not confuse your reminder list with your list of priorities and make sure whatever else crops up you make significant progress on that task that day.

- **Assertiveness training.** Not feeling like you have any control over your work can be very stressful and this type of stress can lead to work spilling into home life and upsetting your work life balance. If you feel out of control at work, particularly if you find it difficult to say no, assertiveness training may be needed (see also the article by Wolverson (2006)).
- **Career development planning.** As one of the features of modern health and social services is that there are flatter management structures it means that the processes for career development are not so clear cut. The changes in organisations encourage varied and portfolio careers. This means we may have to develop alternative strategies to manage our careers. To plan in this context it may be helpful to work with a life coach or an occupational psychologist.
- **Coaching.** Coaching is usually focused on a task or skills and performance. The role of the coach is to pass on skills and knowledge so your line manager could adopt this role. The agenda is set by the coach and tends to be more directive and short term than mentoring.
- **Mentoring.** Mentoring is often used when the normal support/developmental structures are not available to individuals. Although you can engage in peer-mentoring (see Vignette 19.2), it is usually a one-to one relationship with someone who inspires you or an experienced/trusted adviser. Mentoring is used to help and support people to manage their learning in order to maximise their potential, develop their skills and improve their performance. Although the roles of mentor and mentee are clearly defined mentorship is regarded as a reciprocal relationship from which both benefit (see Vignette 19.3). A mentor can fulfil a number of roles (see Box 19.3).
- **Networking.** A network is a group of people with whom you can exchange information, contacts and experiences for professional (or social) purposes. Networking operates on several levels and in different ways but is essentially about managing your career. The benefits include information sharing, increasing self-confidence, mutual support, discussion, increased knowledge and personal development (Conroy 1997). The types of activities that can be used for networking are business meetings, email, breakfast meetings, conferences, journeys, events that happen around meetings/conferences (e.g. coffee breaks, workshops and lunch), letter writing and telephone calls. Notice that most of these are social type gatherings and the predominant skills you need are communication skills. Once you have initiated communication with someone you would like to network with make sure that you have follow-up strategies in place to establish regular communication.
- **Time management.** There are numerous courses, books and articles available on time management skills (see for example Boyes 2006). Covey et al (1994) encourage

Vignette 19.2

Peer mentoring

In the past I wanted to be more focused and felt I had lost some clarity about my work. Following a discussion with a colleague who had similar concerns we decided to set up peer mentoring to support each other. The publication of 'The 8th habit' (Covey 2004) coincided with this discussion and we decided to use the chapters from this book to structure our discussions. We committed to meeting once a month and to reflect on the reading we had done from the book and current issues from our work. Having a colleague to work with, who was equally committed to continuing professional development, was a privilege. However I am not sure if the sessions would have been as effective without the reading to structure it. The reading kept us focused on our task and both of us had a clearer sense of focus about our work and lives by the end of the year.

Vignette 19.3

Being mentored

My organisation participates in the 'Yorkshire Accord Mentoring Scheme', a partnership between public sector organisations in York. The scheme aims to provide individuals with personal and professional development, support and challenges by offering them the opportunity to work one-to-one with another individual in a mentoring relationship. Following a promotion, having come across the scheme by accident, I applied for a place. I hoped it would help me focus on meeting the expectations of my new role. Being accepted as a mentee provided me with an extremely useful experience. I was matched with a senior manager from another organisation who was more experienced and knowledgeable than me. The meetings with my mentor not only focused on my needs but also provided me with an opportunity to reflect on my progress with someone outside of my organisation. This is an example of how serendipity, the faculty of making happy and unexpected discoveries by accident, can provide us with excellent opportunities within the workplace that we should try to take advantage of if we can.

Box 19.3

Roles and skills of a mentor

The roles of the mentor can involve any combination of these:

- advising
- guiding
- teaching (this may be by example through being a role model)
- opening doors for
- empathising
- challenging
- encouraging
- promoting
- explaining the politics and the subtleties of the job
- helping their mentee succeed
- being a resource
- prompting
- supporting (including emotional support)
- mediating
- facilitating and
- advocating

Skills of a mentor

1. Mentor as critical friend
   - helps the mentee clarify their situation, set goals and explore options
   - encourages mentee to find solutions

(Continued)

Box 19.3—Cont'd

- looks for opportunities to practise new skills
- provides feedback
- plans action

2. Mentor as a sounding board
   - suspends judgement
   - keeps one's own counsel (listening more than talking)
   - helps the individual understand his/her own motivations and feelings
   - helps the individual focus on the real problem
   - moves the discussion from the problem to searching for alternative solutions

3. Mentor as facilitator
   - helps mentee get to know relevant parts of their network
   - helps mentee map and make better use of their existing networks
   - coaches the mentee in how to approach contacts and in the skills of networking

others to think about time management in terms of self management. This approach acknowledges that time management is a misnomer because the challenge is not to manage time but to manage ourselves. The key to effective self-management is priorities. What are the three or four things that truly matter most to you? Are these things receiving the care, emphasis and time you really want to give them? 'Top performers are ruthless about their priorities. They are crystal clear about what they want and, somehow or other, they manage to give them a lot more time' (Scott 1992: 23) (Vignette 19.4).

Vignette 19.4

Time management

I subscribe to a weekly alert from BMJ Careers and many of the articles provide useful reflections on the different challenges we face in our working lives. A recent article (Hobbs 2007) helped me to revisit my time management skills. It provided a series of three exercises that I used to explore how I use my time

Exercise 1 Exploring the sense of control I have over my time

Exercise 2 Being a more effective planner and

Exercise 3 Planning for the unexpected (Hobbs 2007)

(There is also a website www.hobbspartnership.co.uk with additional exercises that can be used without charge.) These sorts of exercises provide a quick check on skills that can contribute to self management without having to take time out to go on a course. Often when I have read or completed the exercises I am reassured that I am working well but on other occasions it provides an early warning that I am not on top of my game and I need to invest some time in reviewing my habits.

Box 19.4

Steps towards self management

1. Recognise that you need to care for yourself
2. Take active steps towards caring for yourself
3. Self assessment through reflecting on your own needs, systems and procedures
4. Identify whether you have any issues impeding your effectiveness at work? Are you resilient?
5. If you could be more effective or resilient, identify what needs to change. Develop solutions tailored to your needs for doing a better job in the future (including seeking additional support if necessary)
6. Implement the strategies
7. Monitor the impact that the strategies are having on your effectiveness and resilience. If they are having limited impact go back to step six and look for alternative solutions

Summary

In this chapter a process for self management has emerged (see Box 19.4). Although the need for self management is indicative of how organisations have changed, and that the work arena presents more challenges, it also means we can have more control over our careers. One of the exciting aspects of working in health and social care today is that we can truly have the careers we want to have. It is now possible for occupational therapists to enjoy 20 years of experience rather than having one year's experience 20 times (Hollis and Clark 1993). However if we are to rise to the challenges and enjoy the diverse range of experiences on offer we need to be more resilient than previous generations.

Useful resources

BMJ Careers (www.bmjcareers.com). Whilst this publication has been developed for medics it has a range of useful resources related to self management. A lot of excellent writers in this field have written articles for BMJ careers and they are all archived on the site.

Center for Creative Leadership (www.ccl.org). This website has a number of useful resources particularly if you currently hold a leadership position but will be of use to anybody interested in personal leadership.

OT Coach website (www.otcoach.com/). This website has been developed by a company providing personal and professional development services for occupational therapists. It has a number of free resources as well as a monthly newsletter you can sign up to.

Productivity under pressure: how do you cope? (Broadhurst and Keyes 2003). This article suggests a number of tasks to facilitate improvements in personal effectiveness.

The Road to Resilience (www.apahelpcenter. org/dl/the_road_to_resilience.pdf). This workbook is concisely written and so provides a good introduction to the subject of resilience. It can also be used as a starting point for looking at how to develop resilience.

Work Life Balance Centre (www. worklifebalancecentre.org/). This centre researches work and its impact on people's lives. It also has resources about how to overcome work–life imbalance issues.

Work Life Research centre (www.workliferesearch. org/). This centre undertakes research into the relationships between employment, care, family, leisure and community. An example of their work includes the Work-life manual; a practical tool for employers offering a step-by-step approach to implementing a work–life strategy.

References

APA Help Center 2004a What Is Resilience? Online. Available: http://www.apahelpcenter.org/featuredtopics/feature.php?id=6&ch=2 6th June 2007

APA Help Center 2004b The Road to Resilience Online. Available: http://www.apahelpcenter.org/dl/the_road_to_resilience.pdf 6th June 2007

Backman CL 2004 Muriel Driver Memorial Lecture Occupational balance: Exploring the relationships among daily occupations and their influence on well-being. Canadian Journal of Occupational Therapy 71(4): 202–209

Bennis WG, Thomas RJ 2003 Crucibles of leadership. In: Harvard Business Review, ed. Building personal and organisational resilience, pp. 39–58. Harvard Business Services Publishing, Boston, MA

Bhargava S 2007 The Imposter Syndrome: Feeling like a fraud Online Available http://fecolumnists.expressindia.com/full_column.php?content_id=32033 29th March 2007

Boyes C 2006 Time management. Therapy Weekly 32(37): 7–9

Broadhurst J, Keyes S 2003 Productivity under pressure: how do you cope? Therapy Weekly November 13: 10–13

Caltech Student Counseling Center 2007 Introduction of the Imposter Syndrome Online Available: http://www.counseling.caltech.edu/articles/The%20Imposter%20Syndrome.htm 29 Mar 2007

Chacksfield J 2002a Be your own therapist. Therapy Weekly 29(19): 5

Chacksfield J 2002b Healer, you must first heal yourself. Therapy Weekly October 17

Community Alcohol Information Program 1997 Denial Online Available: http://www.nh-dwi.com/caip-202.htm 8 Oct 2007

Conroy C 1997 'Why are you doing that?' A project to look for evidence of efficacy within occupational therapy. British Journal of Occupational Therapy 60(11): 487–490

Contu DL 2003 How resilience works. In: Harvard Business Review, ed. Building personal and organisational resilience, pp. 1–18. Harvard Business Services Publishing, Boston, MA

Covey SR 1989 Seven Habits of Highly Effective People. Simon & Schuster, London

Covey SR 2004 The 8th habit. Simon & Schuster, Australia

Covey SR, Merrill RA, Merrill RR 1994 First Things First. Simon & Schuster, New York

Department of Health 2005 Self care – A real choice self care support – A practical option. Online. Available: http://www.dh.gov.uk/PublicationsAndStatistics/Publications/PublicationsPolicyAndGuidance/PublicationsPolicyAndGuidanceArticle/fs/en?CONTENT_ID=4100717&chk=Khgu1l 16 Mar 2006

Dutton JE, Frost PJ, Worline MC et al 2003 Leading in times of trauma. In: Harvard Business Review, ed. Building personal and organisational resilience, pp. 19–38. Harvard Business Services Publishing, Boston, MA

Frankl VE 1984 Man's search for meaning. Beacon Press, Boston, MA

Glicken MD 2006 Learning from resilient people. Sage Publications, CA

Grosch WN, Olsen DC 1994 When helping starts to hurt. WW Norton, New York

Gundersen L 2001 Physician burnout. Annals of Internal Medicine 135(2): 145–148

Hartman J, Moskal P, Dziuban C 2005 Preparing the Academy of Today for the Learner of Tomorrow. In: Oblinger DG, Oblinger JL(eds) Educating the Net Generation Online Available http://www.educause.edu/educatingthenetgen 17 Oct 2007

Hebert K 2005 How to be a healthy doctor without trying too hard – update. BMJ Careers 19 November: 221

Hobbs P 2007 I haven't got time. BMJ Careers 27 January: 29–30

Hollis V, Clark CR 1993 Core Skills and Competencies: Part 3, Excellence made Explicit. British Journal of Occupational Therapy 60(7): 290–294

Hume C, Joice A 2002 Rehabilitation. In: Creek J, ed. Occupational Therapy and Mental Health, 3rd edn., pp. 353–369. Churchill Livingstone, Edinburgh, UK

Kersley S 2004 The ABC of change: S, T, U. BMJ Careers 18 October: 164

Lee RJ, King SN 2001 Discovering the Leader in You. A Guide to Realising your Personal Leadership Potential. Jossey-Bass, San Francisco, CA

Moore AH, Moore JF, Fowler SB 2005 Faculty Development for the Net Generation. In: Oblinger DG, Oblinger JL(eds) Educating the Net Generation Online Available http://www.educause.edu/educatingthenetgen 17 Oct 2007

Scott M 1992 Time Management. BCA, London

Tapscott D 1998 Growing up digital. The rise of the Net Generation. Mc-Graw-Hill, New York

Taylor F 2005 Will you burn out? BMJ Careers 19 November: 220

Wolverson C 2006 Assertiveness in the workplace. Therapy Weekly 32(35): 9–11

Work Life Balance Centre 2007 A brief guide to active living and workload management. Online. Available http://www.worklifebalancecentre.org/briefguide.php 31st July 2007

Leadership skills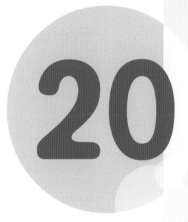

Charles Christiansen

Highlight box

- In order to thrive, all groups require some form of leadership.
- Leadership involves influencing people in particular directions.
- Management differs from leadership. It determines *how* people will work.
- There are four levels or types of leadership skills, beginning with the self.
- Servant leadership is characterised by cooperation, trust and the development of people.

Overview

Leadership in occupational therapy requires the same skills as in any other endeavour. In this chapter, important skills for leadership are discussed. The chapter begins with a consideration of how and why people in groups learned to organise to achieve common purposes and how such organisation led to the need for leaders. A definition of leadership is then proposed based on this evolutionary theme, illustrating that the idea of leadership with an orientation toward serving groups (or servant leadership) is centuries old.

The characteristics and skills associated with effective leadership are identified and discussed, based on the idea of increasing circles of influence, beginning with the self. Specific skill requirements associated with ever-widening circles of influence are then identified, including group leadership, communication skills, coaching and mentoring, and building a sense of community based on trust. It is argued that servant leadership is well suited to occupational therapy settings because of the congruence of principles and values between servant leadership and client-centred practice, including collaboration, trust, ethical practices and empathy. Strategic skills necessary for leading larger groups are also identified, including visioning, planning and motivating. Because a vital part of servant leadership involves self-awareness and growth on the part of the leader, the chapter describes strategies for leadership performance appraisal, including the '360 degree feedback process'. The chapter concludes with the identification of additional resources for pursuing leadership development drawing from contemporary authorities on leadership in organisations.

Evolutionary and Historical Context

People live and work in groups. Ethnologists contend that these arrangements are key to the evolution of the human species. Humans evolved as social animals who learned to cooperate in order to assure their collective safety, survival and mutual advantage (Dawkins 1989). Robert Trivers proposes that ancestral humans learned cooperative and helping behaviours based on an expectation that kind acts would be reciprocated, leading to future reward (Trivers 1971). The idea of groups of people working together for shared benefit and common purpose is key to the idea of organisation. In fact, an appropriate definition of an *organisation* is 'a group of people intentionally organised to accomplish an overall, common goal or set of goals' (McNamara 2006).

As societies have evolved, groups have become larger and more complex. The division of labour in society, where specific roles are assigned to group members based on tasks necessary to accomplish different purposes, has become commonplace. Specialised groups within larger groups have evolved. Nowadays, these larger groups, or organisations, may have hundreds or thousands of members, with highly sophisticated structures consisting of many smaller workgroups organised within a larger group. The purposes of these organisations may range from serving the needs of communities to producing goods and services on a global scale.

Why Leadership?

Regardless of the size or structure of an organised group, however, each has in common a need for leadership, whether it requires one person or a group of people. Leadership is necessary to determine the common purposes that will be pursued by the group and the means or processes for accomplishing those purposes.

Defining Leadership

Leadership has been defined in many ways. Simply put, leadership is setting directions and influencing the people in a group to work in pursuit of those directions. The overall direction of an organisation may be spelled out in a mission statement. For example, the mission statement of Google ™, Inc., defined by its leadership, is 'to organise the world's information and make it universally accessible and useful' (Google™ 2006). One can easily imagine that each of the smaller workgroups within Google is organised to help achieve that overall purpose. Thus, Google must have workgroups that specialise in collecting information, others that find ways to make it more easy to find, and still others that devote their attention to understanding how and why people seek information in order to make information more useful to them.

While typically, in a large corporation such as Google™, a group of people (the board of directors), determines its direction, there is typically one person charged to assume responsibility for carrying out or executing the actions necessary to attain the mission. This leader, or chief executive officer, is at the top of the leadership hierarchy. As organisations or groups become larger, their hierarchies become more complex. These leadership hierarchies are usually depicted graphically in organisational charts.

Even group-living animals other than humans have a clear hierarchy of leadership. In the animal kingdom, this position in the group is typically determined by strength or power. For example, the pecking order of birds and dominance among primates is established through aggression and demonstrations of strength (Baer and McEachran 1982).

In humans, while the idea of attaining leadership by power, force or family lineage is still alive and well in various parts of the world, in most cases leadership roles in organisations are assumed by people who are appointed or elected based on their leadership capabilities or attributes. The extent to which leadership is effective depends on a complex array of factors, as we shall see in the following section.

What Makes An Effective Leader?

There is a popular cartoon depicting a group of men being whipped by a man expressing a sentiment similar to 'the floggings will stop when morale improves'. Clearly, we all agree that the use of force or power might be an effective way of motivating people to accomplish a task in the short term, but in the longer term it is unlikely to achieve the desired results. What then, are the characteristics of an effective leader, and how can those attributes and skills be learned or developed?

Because effective leadership typically involves attributes other than size or strength, it is important to consider it along its many other dimensions. As considered below, these dimensions pertain to a leader's skills, traits and values.

Leadership Skills, Traits and Value Orientations

The skills necessary for effective leadership vary by situation. Stephen Covey, in his book *Principle Centered Leadership* (Covey 1990) notes that leaders have circles of influence. The first circle of influence is the self. Leaders must have the skills necessary to influence individuals immediately around them in positive ways. This is the second circle.

As groups become larger, different skills are needed, since it is difficult to have one-to-one, regular contact with more than a handful of people. Thus, a third important set of skills (and the third circle of influence) pertains to being able to organise people, lead meetings, and communicate effectively with larger groups. Finally, the fourth circle of influence involves much larger numbers of people who may only have indirect or occasional contact with the leader, but are nonetheless influenced by the person's skills in leading organisations and communities. These skills relate to formulating visions, planning strategically, and making key decisions in complex situations (Figure 20.1).

315

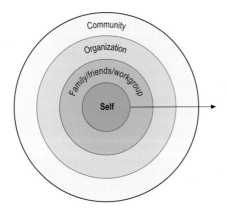

Personal sphere of influence

Figure 20.1 Personal sphere of influence

It is important to appreciate that even though different leadership skills are needed for contexts where larger and more complex organisations of people are involved, the leader of large organisations or communities (or even nations), must nonetheless possess the basic skills necessary for self-leadership and for positively influencing others during one-to-one or personal interactions.

Consider these questions: If a leader is not regarded as trustworthy and competent by those who directly interact with her or him, or if the performance and morale of people within the leader's immediate workgroup is not effective, how would it be possible for that person to be genuinely effective (or credible?) in leading a large organisation or community?

Level One: Self Leadership We have noted that effective leadership begins by having sufficient self-leadership skills or personal habits and characteristics, so as to be an effective individual and credible role model. One could call this effective personhood.

The terms authenticity and integrity are often included in the characteristics necessary for becoming an effective individual. An effective individual enjoys the unqualified respect of others. To be respected is to be admired and valued by others. It is important to lead by example.

Consider the attributes and characteristics that contribute to this sort of public image and reputation. Such approval is largely earned through one's interpersonal relationships. It begins with trust, and through acting in a trustworthy manner. A trustworthy person honours commitments and is dependable in other ways, such as through maintaining confidences. I assert here that the most important characteristic a leader (or effective person) can possess is *trustworthiness*.

An effective leader is also a responsible individual. One can interpret the word 'responsible' as meaning being 'capable to respond' or not having one's actions be at the mercy of others or external events. Thus, the effective leader has a personal orientation that enables the assumption of responsibility (being response-able) for action. When something goes wrong, effective people first ask what they could have done differently to influence a different outcome. Because they are attentive, effective individuals do not act without thought. They are goal-driven when they act, clear about the outcomes they desire to achieve. But their achievement is not pursued in a competitive or selfish manner, and never at the intentional expense of others.

Effective people are also good managers of personal resources. This not only signifies that they are capable of balancing their chequebooks, it also shows that they manage their time and energy in a manner that enables them to be effective and efficient. They keep themselves physically healthy through sound nutrition, exercise, rest and renewal. They attend to their spiritual needs and recognise the importance of balancing their lives to achieve these ends.

An effective leader is also considerate of others. This type of reputation is built over time through a consistent pattern of responsible behaviour. Being considerate means being genuinely concerned with the needs of others and demonstrating such concern with attention and compassion. The attributes of and compassion of an effective leader suggest that one listens carefully, genuinely attempts to see matters from the point of view they present, and recognises and forgives human imperfection.

A positive attitude is also important. No one wants as a leader someone whose emotional demeanour is gloomy and pessimistic. Enthusiasm is contagious, and a positive, optimistic outlook is what everyone expects when they need encouragement.

Closely related to a positive disposition is a good sense of humour. The world is full of strange events and unforeseen circumstances. Things almost never turn out exactly as planned. Therefore, expecting the unexpected and having an attitude of amusement when things go awry helps to keep things in context and reduce the tension often associated with mistakes.

People who are effective also have a personal orientation that truly wants others to succeed and to be able to create their own happiness. Thus, truly effective leaders constantly seek creative solutions that enable everyone to attain their ends.

This idea does not differ significantly from the idea of the benevolent or servant leader. The concept of groups headed by benevolent leaders is well established. Indeed, in the Tao Te Ching, a classical Chinese work of virtues and ways of living and being written by Lao Tzu, who lived 2500 years ago in the 3rd century BC, there is a chapter devoted to the characteristics of effective leaders (Le Guin 1998) (Box 20.1). This chapter clearly illustrates the principle that effective leaders win the respect of others and are not concerned with gaining recognition for their accomplishments. The personal satisfaction comes when others feel success at having attained an important goal.

Level Two: Influencing Family, Friends and The Immediate Workgroup The second set of skills pertains to those necessary for influencing those immediately around us. To be maximally effective, leaders must be knowledgeable, socially involved, enthusiastic, upbeat and organise their lives in ways that enable them to be perceived as great role models.

To be an effective leader to those around us means having the ability to teach or coach new skills and abilities. Thus, the effective leader must be knowledgeable about those matters of importance to success in the group and organisation. This means that the leaders must continually study to remain knowledgeable and well-informed.

The effective leader must also be involved socially, so as to be familiar with the issues that are on people's minds and to be compassionate when personal situations affect individuals with whom they relate on a daily basis. Part of being socially involved is to remain current on the topics of the day, including being informed about local, national and international issues and events.

Successful leaders must be able to organise people, conduct effective meetings and communicate effectively. Effective organisation begins with matching the skills and abilities of people to the tasks needed in a particular workgroup. Occupational therapists are adept at assessing performance skills and selecting challenges that are aligned with skill levels. The effective group manager must likewise fit the task to the appropriate group and assure that the necessary systems are in place to enable success in performance. Of course, a key part of success involves communicating clearly what the tasks or work responsibilities are to those to whom they have been assigned.

Box 20.1

This English translation of Chapter 17 of the Tao Te Ching (Le Guin 1998) clearly reflects an appreciation for the virtues of effective leaders

"True leaders
are hardly known to their followers.
Next after them are the leaders
The people know and admire;
After them, those that they fear;
After them, those they despise.
To give no trust
Is to get no trust.
When the work's done right,
With no fuss or boasting,
Ordinary people say,
Oh, we did it.

Le Guin U K. "The Tao Te Ching: A book about the way and the power of the way." 1998, Boston & London, Shambhala Publishing (p.24)

Communicating clear expectations is vitally important. The expected outcome must be clearly delineated along with the timeframe for completion and the expected standard of performance. Such standards must be stated in measurable terms. The consequences for failure to perform should also be defined. This does not mean punishment, rather what the consequences to the organisation will be if a particular workgroup fails to meet expectations. Explaining how the work contributes to helping the organisation meet its overall mission is an important connecting link in aligning the workgroup within the organisation. Provided with this information, a workgroup should have a clear sense of what is expected.

Communicating expectations is one part of a larger set of communication skills that an effective leader will need. In general, people in an organisation want to feel connected and informed. Thus, regular communication is a must. The best communication anticipates the information needs of the receiver and provides this in a manner that can be easily understood; i.e., clearly, succinctly and directly. In this technological age, it is too often the case that communication that should be face-to-face or at least synchronous is handled asynchronously by email or voicemail. Direct communication is efficient and effective because it enables quick clarification of uncertainty and ambiguity. The author has learned through many years experience that people can deal with the truth. While it is important to be diplomatic, civil and respectful in all communications, leaders should avoid the temptation to 'soften' or avoid unpopular messages. Where ambiguity is present, message recipients will interpret messages according to their own needs. The need for leaders to clarify previous communications may be interpreted as an example of administrative doublespeak.

Finally, the orientation of an effective leader is one of service. One of the principles of servant leadership is having a mission of serving the needs of others (Spears 1996). The mission can only be attained to its highest degree if those in pursuit of it have the encouragement, resources, direction and motivation to work toward it. Another way of imagining success as a leader is to envision the rowers in sculling. A scull is a small, light racing boat that can have as many as eight rowers, each pulling their oars (or "sculls") together in unison to move the boat down the river. The rowers are perfectly aligned. Not only are they sitting in an aligned position, one behind the other, but team members are also aligned with the group because of their knowledge of the objective, their individual roles and responsibilities, and their motivation and dedication to devote full attention and effort to the task (Figure 20.2). In a racing competition, the scull that achieves the highest degree of alignment or overall cooperation among its team members tends to be most successful, that is, to accomplish the mission of attaining distance, speed and efficiency with the best results.

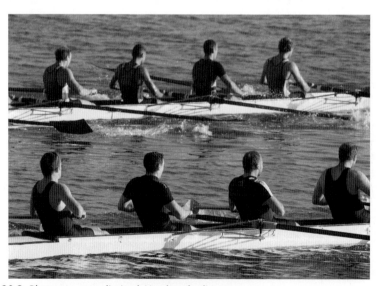

Figure 20.2 Photos to go unlimited. Used under licence

In a similar manner, the organisation or workgroup that achieves a similar level of alignment, in terms of recruiting the motivation, attention and passion around its mission by its members, is destined to be successful.

Level Three: Organisational Leadership Third-level leadership competencies add to those previously listed - the ability to effectively organise people, lead meetings and communicate with large groups. The organisation or assignment of people into workgroups is both an art and a science. It is an art in the sense that it assembles workgroups based on the tasks and objectives to be accomplished and an alignment of the people with the training, experience and skills best suited to accomplishing those tasks and objectives. Each workgroup needs an assigned leader, and the successful organisation of workgroups is at least partially dependent on the 'chemistry' of the group. Group chemistry refers to the collective personality of a group, and this may be influenced by traditions, shared values, experience and other factors. Thus, one attempts to best match people and their assigned group leaders based on both objective and subjective criteria. Some subjective decision-making is based on intuition, observation and knowledge of personality and individual circumstances.

Another skill necessary with this third level of leadership competence is the ability to effectively lead meetings. While meetings are a ubiquitous, fundamental and necessary part of organisational activities, they vary widely in their value and effectiveness based on the skills of their leaders. No meeting should ever be held without thoughtful preparation. Attention should be given to its objectives, the agenda and the actual conduct of the meeting. Effective meetings start punctually, end punctually, and focus productive discussion on agenda items carefully selected, ordered and communicated in advance. All agenda items should have clear purposes in mind (i.e., information, discussion, action) and to the extent possible, require some advance preparation from participants (Haynes 1997).

The final set of skills at this level of influence pertains to communication with large groups. With larger groups comes the greater probability that one or more persons will misunderstand a message. Therefore, clarity and care must be taken in formulating and delivering messages. One cannot become an effective organisational leader without having the skill to speak convincingly in public arenas and to provide 'off the cuff' or extemporaneous presentations when these are required. The effective leader must project confidence, because confidence communicates competence. Of course, being good at speaking is not enough. One must also perform competently in the leadership role using the skills described in this chapter.

Level Four: Influencing Communities; Being a Strategic Leader As responsibilities of the leader increase, so does complexity. The leader of a large organisation must contend with the political realities of communities, where other organisations may be competing directly or have interests or objectives that conflict or complicate goal completion. Large organisations also have communities within, because as the division of labour becomes more specialised, each division or collection of workgroups takes on its own personality and develops its own culture. The worst possible outcome in such a case is when units of the same organisation begin to compete with each other in a manner that erodes morale or interferes with alignment and efficiency. Recalling the example of sculling, it would not do if members of the same team began to compete with each other to achieve more strokes per minute, since the important objective of synchronised rowing would be lost.

Level four leadership situations require the leader to have a systems perspective, recognising that in systems, each element is connected to and affects the others. Thus, they are interdependent. Interdependence is an important concept in leadership (Senge 1990). No organisation can succeed if it does not recognise the interdependence of its units and if it fails to recognise the important relationships between organisations, neighbourhoods and cultures in society.

This fact calls to mind the important principle of seeking 'win–win' solutions (Covey 1989). In this type of solution, the goal is to resolve problems, challenges and conflicts in a manner that best enables all parties of interest to achieve their aims. Too often, in business and in life, situations are viewed as winner takes all competitions. Victories under these conditions are temporary, or obtained at a long-term cost that is not worth what is often a short-term benefit.

319

Strategic leadership situations also require careful planning, with an eye toward anticipating key trends and envisioning the future. The visioning process is key to strategic planning, since it must anticipate conditions and create bold possibilities that collectively motivate group members to align themselves in support of the imagined future. A good vision serves as the backdrop for strategic planning. Good vision statements are inspiring, succinct and focused (Collins and Porras 1991). The process of imaging the future invites creativity and good leaders have clear visions of what they hope to accomplish. An organisation's vision should be the overarching element, or mental picture, that provides the motivation for each day. In the absence of a vision, an organisation may be directionless and will certainly not be inspired. Consider these lines from Lewis Carroll:

> 'Would you tell me, please, which way I ought to go from here?'
> 'That depends a good deal on where you want to get to,' said the Cat.
> 'I don't much care where –' said Alice.
> 'Then it doesn't matter which way you go,' said the Cat.
> Lewis Carroll, Alice's Adventures in Wonderland (1865)

In the context of a vision, an organisation must carefully plan its activities and the use of its resources. This is where the functions of management come in. Being a leader and being a manager are different organisational roles. A leader focuses on the big picture, determining directions, and motivating people. A manager focuses on the operational requirements for getting the job done, such as scheduling and coordination, maintaining quality, and budgeting. In ideal circumstances, systems are designed to be sustainable. That is, the focus is on the longer-term picture rather than the immediate, so that the organisational climate is conducive to retaining and developing people (has trust), fostering creative problem-solving, and assuring that the organisation has the resources necessary to invest in its future.

Strategic leadership also seeks to gather as much information as possible about how the organisation performs compared to its peers. Organisations can always track their own performance and compare it from year to year, but this information should be supplemented with knowing how an organisation compares to leading organisations of its type. Gathering this type of information is sometimes called benchmarking, a process invented by Rank Xerox. Benchmarking identifies best practices by answering the question: 'How do the leading organisations do this process?' In this way, it promotes alternative ways of thinking about process. Two types of benchmarking can be described. In competitive benchmarking, data are collected to analyse how an organisation measures up against the competition. In collaborative benchmarking, organisations or groups cooperate to identify performance ranges and share improvements. Any process within an organisation can be benchmarked and in today's environment it is critical to be aware of the most efficient and effective ways to get the job done (Hassanali et al 2002). Benchmarking is a type of knowledge management, the modern term used to describe the sharing of information throughout an organisation to improve its performance.

Words often attributed to Goethe, but belonging to the Scottish mountaineer William Hutchinson Murray (Murray 1951: 27) seem to capture the importance of thinking boldly when creating visions: 'Whatever you can do or dream you can do, begin it. Boldness has genius, power and magic within it.'

Contemporary Views on Servant Leadership

In descriptions of leadership skills at all four levels of leadership that have been described, the notion of servant leadership has been suggested. It has already been noted that this concept dates back thousands of years and yet remains as viable and germane as it did at that time. Modern notions of servant leadership are attributed to an essay by Robert Greenleaf originally published in 1970 (Greenleaf 1991). Servant leadership is collaborative rather than hierarchical, and focuses on the leader as steward of an organisation's resources, especially its people, while focusing attention on objectives and results. Thus, the service orientation does not come at the expense of organisational success. The principles of trust, integrity and ethical practices are paramount in this approach, which has been adopted by many successful organisations throughout the world. According to Spears, the servant leader as defined by Greenleaf focuses on ten leadership characteristics: listening, empathy, awareness, healing, persuasion, conceptualisation, foresight, stewardship, community and commitment (Greenleaf 1977).

One practice often used in organisations with servant leader philosophies is 360 degree feedback. This is a type of performance appraisal that differs from the traditional top-down evaluation or even from the process where direct reports or subordinates evaluate their leaders. In 360 degree appraisals, these two approaches are combined with appraisals by one's organisational peers, thus providing a comprehensive view of how the individual is performing. Typically, 360 degree feedback processes focus on identifying areas for leadership training (Lepsinger and Lucia 1997). Hence, it can be viewed as a facet of staff development.

Strategies and Resources for Leadership Development

It is clear that one does not become an effective leader after reading a short chapter on leadership. Effective leadership requires skills that are honed over careers, requiring experience, self-development and feedback. Without objective feedback on how others perceive a leader's skills in the four levels of leadership, one cannot identify areas to focus on further development.

As suggested by Robert Greenleaf's characteristics of a servant leader, leadership development requires a commitment to self-development as well as a commitment to others. Developing leadership skills requires a willingness to seek feedback from others, to read widely and participate in formal leadership development programmes, and if possible, to seek a coach who can provide the context in which self-development is able to occur. Effective coaches help leaders through recommending useful self-development strategies and through confidential reflective dialogue that enables the aspiring leader to critically analyse their own leadership behaviours and identify and apply practices that are likely to result in more effective performance.

There are several national and international centres for leadership development of both for-profit and non-profit varieties. In addition, there are many excellent books and articles on effective leadership (see for example Covey 1989, 1992; Greenleaf 1991; and Blanchard et al 2005).

Summary

Occupational therapy settings, whether clinic- or community-based, are often staffed with large numbers of people and exist as part of larger, complex organisations, such as hospitals and systems. As such, they require effective leadership. In this chapter, we have identified four levels of leadership beginning with the self and the skills associated with each level. In describing these skills, references to the concept of the servant leader have been made, and the traditions of servant leadership and client-centred therapy have been compared. Because of their traditions and training, occupational therapists may thus be especially well-positioned to become effective leaders within the confines of therapy units or beyond. Attention to the skills and use of the resources identified in this chapter can be helpful within either context.

Further Reading

Bennis W, Gretchen MS, Cummings TG (eds) 2001 The Future of Leadership. Jossey-Bass, San Francisco, CA

Blanchard K, Fowler S, Hawkins L (2005) Self-Leadership and the One Minute Manager. HarperCollins Publishers, New York

Collins JC, Porras JI 1998 Built to Last: Successful Habits of Visionary Companies. Random House, London

Covey SR 1992 Principle-Centered Leadership. Fireside, New York

Covey SR, Merrill AR, Merrill RR 1994 First Things First: To Live, to Love, to Learn, to Leave a Legacy. Simon & Schuster, New York

dePree M 1992 Leadership Jazz. Currency, New York

Farber S 2004 The Radical Leap: A Personal Lesson in Extreme Leadership. Dearborn Trade Publishing, Chicago, IL

Gardner JW 1993 On Leadership. The Free Press, New York

Gladwell M 2002 The Tipping Point: How Little Things Can Make a Big Difference. Little, Brown and Company, New York

Google 2006 Mission Statement of Google, Inc. Retrieved at http://www.google.com/corporate Retrieved on 8/12/2006

Greenleaf RK 1977 Servant Leadership. Paulist Press, New York

Joyce W 1995 Transformation Thinking. Berkley Publishing Group, New York

Katzenbach JR, Smith DK 1993 The Wisdom of Teams: Creating the High-Performance Organization. HarperBusiness, New York

Kegan R, Laskow Lahey L 2001 How the Way We Talk Can Change the Way We Work: Seven Languages for Transformation. Jossey-Bass, San Francisco, CA

Senge PM 1990 The Fifth Discipline. Currency Doubleday, New York

References

Baer D, McEachron DL 1982 A review of selected sociobiological principles application to hominid evolution. 1. The development of group social-structure. Journal of Social and Biological Structures 5(1): 69–90

Carroll L 1871 Alice's Adventures in Wonderland. The Millennium Fulcrum Edition 3.0. (Project Gutenberg) Retrieved at: http://www.cs.cmu.edu/~rgs/alice-table.html

Collins JC, Porras JI 1991 Organizational vision and visionary organizations. California Management Review 34(1): 30–52

Covey SR 1989 The Seven Habits of Highly Effective People. Powerful Lessons in Personal Change. Simon and Schuster, New York

Covey SR 1990 Principle Centered Leadership. Simon and Schuster, New York

Dawkins R 1989 The Selfish Gene, 2nd edn. Oxford University Press, Oxford, UK

Greenleaf RK 1991 The Servant as Leader. The Robert Greenleaf Center, Indianapolis, IN (originally published in 1970)

Hassanali F, Hubert C, Lopez K et al 2002 Communities of Practice: A Guide for Your Journey to Knowledgement Management Best Practices. American Productivity and Quality Center, Houston, TX

Haynes M 1997 Effective Meeting Skills: A Practical Guide for More Productive Meetings. Crisp Publications Inc., Menlo Park, CA

Le Guin UK 1998 Lao Tzu: Tao Te Ching, a Book about the Way & the Power of the Way (a translation and commentary). Shambhala, Boston/London

Lepsinger R, Lucia AD 1997 The Art and Science of 360 Degree Feedback. John Wiley & Sons, New York

McNamara C 2006 Free Management Library. Located at http://www.managementhelp.org Retrieved August 9, 2006

Murray WH 1951 The Scottish Himalayan Expedition. JM Dent, London

Spears L 1996 Reflections on Robert K. Greenleaf and servant-leadership. Leadership & Organization Development Journal 17(7): 33–35

Trivers RL 1971 The evolution of reciprocal altruism. Quarterly Review of Biology 46(35): 35–57

Practice education: skills for students and educators

21

Christine Craik

Highlight box

- Practice placements are an influential element of occupational therapy education.
- Students and educators have different perspectives and understanding these are key to successful placements.
- Varied models of placement will increase and will be essential to prepare students for new ways of practising occupational therapy.
- Preparation, a shared appreciation of supervision, understanding the assessment process and dealing effectively with problems are central to successful placements.
- Reflection on what has been learned from the placement is an essential skill for educators and students.

Overview

Practice placements are central to occupational therapy education and they have a profound influence on occupational therapists. Practice placements and practice placement educators, usually shortened to practice educators, are the current terms used in the UK although fieldwork education and fieldwork educators and clinical practice and clinical supervisor have been employed previously and may still be used in other countries. All therapists experience practice placements as students and many later become practice educators. Despite this shared experience, the perspectives of students and educators are different and understanding these viewpoints is fundamental to success on placement. Occupational therapy education is based on blending academic study and practical proficiency and so the concept of practice placements appears straightforward. However, the real world of practice is full of challenges and understanding the regulatory background and requirements of practice placement education is important.

The global expansion of occupational therapy into different areas of practice has led to new placement models and more are likely to emerge in the future. Whatever the setting, the components for successful placement education remain the same; careful preparation, shared understanding of supervision, clear awareness of assessment procedures and the ability to deal effectively with problems if they arise.

Introduction

Unique impact of practice placements

Most occupational therapists reflecting on their education will evaluate placements not only as the most influential and enjoyable feature but also the most challenging and anxiety-provoking. They will describe a 'good' placement as one with a supportive and knowledgeable educator able to encourage and inspire learning. This may be recalled as a life-enhancing event which can change forever their perception of an area of practice or client group. It frequently confirms career choice and later may influence the area of specialist practice. Conversely, for a smaller number of therapists, a 'poor' placement with a critical and demanding educator can have the opposite effect. Therapists will recall feeling unsupported and deskilled and determined never to work in that area of practice or with that client group. These feelings are often strongly held and long-lasting and can shape the subsequent action of therapists as practice educators. Therefore, practice placements are a unique aspect of occupational therapy. All therapists encounter them during their education, many therapists later becoming practice educators and some go on to a career in occupational therapy education.

Differing perspectives

These different groups have different perspectives and priorities. For students the desire to get the right placement with interesting clients and the prospect of meeting their learning objectives are paramount. Sometimes students are so focused on these that they can appear self-centred to busy educators who have to juggle a range of demanding tasks, only one of which relates to student learning. Educators have a primary duty of care to their clients whose needs and safety are paramount. So a student may want to practise a specialist assessment with a patient but the educator may judge that the student is not ready to do this and it might be detrimental to the patient. The student may feel frustrated and concerned that the occasion will not occur again.

So, for everyone to achieve the most from practice placements, trying to see issues from alternative points of view will reap benefits for those directly involved, the profession itself and, most importantly, for our clients. This chapter is structured to explore issues from these different perspectives and the examples also illustrate them in this way.

Aims of practice education

Practice placements are a simple concept. They provide the chance for students to learn and practise aspects of their profession under the direction of an occupational therapist. A series of placements in different settings with a range of clients provides varied learning opportunities and the process of reflection on the learning assists students to develop their clinical reasoning skills. Interspersing periods of placement with academic study encourages links between theory and practice. Then examples from practice provide material for further enquiry and reflection in the academic setting. However, the complexity of the real world of practice adds an unpredictable dimension to practice placements.

The regulatory framework

To manage the complexity of practice education, it is influenced and regulated by organisations within the profession at international and national levels, by national regulatory organisations and by national and local education institutions.

World Federation of Occupational Therapists

The World Federation of Occupational Therapists (WFOT) sets overarching standards for education, including practice placements. They have to be transparent enough to constitute standards but be flexible enough to be implemented in countries with established traditions of occupational therapy education and in countries where the profession is developing. A key requirement is that students complete sufficient time on placement to integrate theory and practice and a minimum of 1000 hours is normally expected (Hocking and Ness 2002). However, there is growing questioning of its evidence base (Walters 2001). Changing to a competence- or outcome-based assessment of what students have learned as a result of being on placement, rather than counting the numbers of hours spent with specific client groups, is likely to be the focus of continuing debate.

Occupational Therapy Associations

Nationally, Occupational Therapy Associations endorse the WFOT standards and may have additional requirements. In the UK standards are based on the College of Occupational Therapists (COT) Curriculum Framework (2004a) and Pre-Registration Education Standards (COT 2004b). These standards are comprehensive and auditable and relate to the provision of placements, the education and support of practice educators, the assessment of placement education and health and safety on placements. The College of Occupational Therapists has a process of Accreditation of Higher Education Institutions that deliver occupational therapy programmes to ensure that they meet its standards (COT 2005a).

Similarly in North America, the American Occupational Therapy Association sets standards of education including those for practice placements. These are revised every 5 years with the most recent version published in 2006 (AOTA 2006). These now reflect the move of the profession, in the USA, to Master's level education. Universities wishing to provide occupational therapy education must adhere to these standards and they are evaluated at least every 5 years to ensure compliance. In Canada, all programmes will be at Master's level from 2010. The Canadian Academic Accreditation Standard was revised in 2005 (CAOT 2005a). Although this document includes placement education, there is separate guidance for placements including the guiding principles, responsibilities of the partners involved in placement education and a method of profiling placement sites (CAOT 2005b).

For information about other countries, the World Federation of Occupational Therapists website, http://www.wfot.org, provides links to national associations. For European countries, the website of the European Network of Occupational Therapy in Higher Education, http://www.enothe.hva.nl, provides valuable information especially in countries where occupational therapy is in the early stages of development.

Health Professions Council

Many countries also have an independent regulatory organisation. In the UK, it is the Health Professions Council, established in 2002 to replace the Council for Professions Supplementary to Medicine. As its rationale was to strengthen regulation to protect the public from incompetent practitioners, the education of practitioners is fundamental. It has published Standards of Proficiency (HPC 2003) and Standards of Education and Training (HPC 2004). It approves programmes of education in higher education institutions to ensure that students are prepared to become competent occupational therapists eligible to apply for registration and thus a licence to practice as occupational therapists in the UK. Therapists, educated in one country, who want to practice in another country will have to meet its regulatory requirements.

National Education Standards

Occupational therapy education must also meet the national standards of the country in which it is delivered. Achieving this has signalled the acceptance of occupational therapy as a subject in mainstream education, alongside other more established disciplines. In the UK, under the auspices of the Quality Assurance Agency for Higher Education (QAA), occupational therapy and other allied health professions have developed Subject Benchmarks (QAA 2001a). These along with a Code of Practice for Placement Learning provide a national standard against which occupational therapy is measured (QAA 2001b).

Stakeholders in occupational therapy education

It can be seen that there are many stakeholders in occupational therapy education and they all influence the organisation of practice placements. Ensuring education is relevant for the needs of the health and social care sectors and user and carer groups are also important.

The role of individual universities

Universities providing occupational therapy education are responsible for interpreting these multifaceted regulations and designing a programme to meet them. The programme will be scrutinised by these organisations for initial approval and it will be subsequently reviewed to maintain that approval.

Academic staff, who provide guidance on practice education for students and practice educators, have to be mindful of these external standards as they are responsible for ensuring that students and practice educators adhere to them. So suggestions from students or practice educators to change aspects of a placement, which may appear reasonable to them, may be rejected by university staff as they breach the complex maze of standards.

Implications for students and practice educators

Potential students should ensure that the university where they plan to study conforms to the relevant regulations. Once registered on a programme, students are responsible for being familiar with information about the programme and practice placements.

As important partners in the education of students, practice educators will want to check that the universities, whose students they supervise, comply with relevant regulations. The university will provide information about their approach to placement education and their requirements of occupational therapy services and individual educators.

Universities will have handbooks, guidance, newsletters and, increasingly, web-based services to provide this. Many universities will provide briefing sessions and training for educators. In the UK, there have been systems of training and accrediting practice educators for some years (Craik et al 2004) and there is now a national scheme of accreditation (COT 2005b). With increasing emphasis on continuing professional development, therapists are encouraged to view achieving recognition for placement education as a useful way of providing evidence of this.

Models of practice placements

Traditional placements

The World Federation of Occupational Therapists requirement to complete 1000 hours of supervised practice is usually achieved through a number of placements in a range of settings, with different clients. Placements are often several weeks long with students spending all of the week on placement and the College of Occupational Therapists recommends that the final placement should be at least 8 weeks long (COT 2004b)

However, throughout the world, different placement patterns are being devised to meet the needs of individual countries. Occupational therapy is a developing profession, resulting in more students being educated than there are therapists to supervise them so imaginative ways are being created to provide learning opportunities for students.

Role-emerging placements

During the 1990s role-emerging placements, in settings where there was little or no occupational therapy input, were advocated in the UK (COT 1994) and were described in Canada (Bossers et al 1997). A decade later, Wood (2005) surveyed occupational therapy programmes in the UK, distinguishing between non-traditional placements where supervision is provided by an occupational therapist and role-emerging placements, a non-traditional setting where no occupational therapist is employed. These models occur most often in the voluntary or independent sector. Twenty-one of the 24 programmes, who responded, used these new models. While lack of traditional placements was one reason for their development, many benefits were noted including students establishing a clear professional identity, improving problem solving, thinking skills and creativity. However, students could feel isolated and anxious and they created additional work for the universities in preparation for the placement and support for the student and supervisor (Wood 2005). Based on this work, further guidelines are available for these placements (COT 2006).

Occupational therapy managers have noted further benefits in generating opportunities for the profession to emerge in a new setting, potentially creating new posts for occupational therapists; however, expecting students to act as advocates for the profession in this way may be too challenging (Fisher and Savin-Baden 2002). The managers thought that role-emerging placements should be elective noting that they encouraged independence and self reliance in students but they were concerned that they would not develop an occupational therapy identity (Fisher and Savin-Baden 2002).

Totten and Pratt (2001) describe the placement of a student in a project for homeless people. Weekly supervision was provided by an academic who was also available for telephone discussions. Initially, the student established relationships with staff and clients before embarking on an activity project with clients. Choosing a project that could be completed by the end of the placement was emphasised to ensure that the clients did not feel let down when the student left. Although initially introduced as an elective placement, all second year students in this institution now have a placement in the non statutory sector.

Collaborative/2:1 models

A collaborative model, where one educator supervises two students, elicited comment from occupational therapy managers concerned about the additional workload for educators, the potential limitation of learning opportunities for the student, competitiveness between students and the availability of support if problems arose during the placement (Fisher and Savin-Baden 2002). However, Martin et al (2004) used interviews to compare the experience of 11 occupational therapy students and their six educators while undertaking 1:1, 2:1 and 3:1 placements. While all models had advantages and disadvantages, the 2:1 model was preferred. The multiple models provided more peer support and peer learning opportunities but sufficient clients had to be available. The 1:1 model offered more time for the student to spend with the educator but could lead to dependence on the educator. In multiple models, it was important to ensure that educators allocated sufficient time for the students. Irrespective of the model, planning was essential.

Interagency model

Fisher and Savin-Baden (2002) proposed an interagency model, where a therapist working in a mainstream setting would collaborate with staff in an independent or voluntary setting and share supervision so that the student would gain experience in both settings. This could increase the number of placements and might reduce the concerns about role-emerging placements. This concept would work best when the staff involved were already working together.

Future models

The delivery of health and social care is changing rapidly throughout the world and the profession has developed in different directions in different countries. As pre-registration education aims to prepare 'occupational therapists for lifelong, safe and effective practice within the global marketplace' (COT 2004a: Section 1.2), universities have a responsibility to use a diversity of placement models to prepare students for this. Some universities

Vignette 21.1

Susanne was looking forward to her final placement in a mental health setting and she was allocated to a voluntary organisation offering support to people with dementia and their carers. She was reluctant to accept it, as it involved working some evenings and weekends and, as there was no occupational therapist working there, supervision was to be provided from the university. After discussing it with university staff, she went to the placement. She found it challenging but the experience of explaining occupational therapy to colleagues and clients reinforced her belief in the profession and she relished the freedom from the formality of her previous hospital placements. She did well, achieving a high grade. Her reflective diary written during the placement recounts how much she had learned. At interview for her first post, her description of that learning and the flexibility and adaptability she demonstrated were just what her prospective employer was looking for. She was offered the post.

may offer students placements overseas but this requires complex arrangements and is not always feasible. Not all students will have these opportunities, but exchanging information about them at university shares the knowledge gained.

Students should regard an alternative placement as a chance to encounter new and innovative ways of working, which are likely to become more common and may lead to employment prospects, rather than a poor substitute for a traditional placement. In the future, placement educators and occupational therapy managers will need to appreciate the benefits gained by graduates through undertaking these placements and not take the short-term view that they have had insufficient traditional experience.

The placement experience

Preparation

Expectations

Part of the apprehension students may feel about placements relates to the range of settings in which they can be placed. The expectations of working in a busy city centre unit assessing elderly people with medical conditions who are ready for discharge home will be very different from a community unit for adolescents with learning difficulties. Davys et al (2006) highlight the challenges for students' behaviour, and especially personal appearance, as they move between the expectations of university and placement. They also noted that occupational therapists and academics have no universal view of what is an acceptable professional dress code. Similar differences may be apparent in relation to punctuality, priorities and professional behaviour.

General placement information

Fortunately information is available to assist students and educators. For example, the Code of Ethics and Professional Conduct (COT 2005c) provides guidance on professional behaviour. Universities will have different ways of providing general information, perhaps through a placement handbook or via a formal agreement or learning contract. Whatever method is used, it will outline the roles of the student, the educator and the university. It should state what is required for students to meet the learning outcomes of the placement, the criteria and methods for assessment and arrangements for supervision.

Students are responsible for understanding university guidance, regulations and information about placements prior to embarking on their first one. They should read the information provided and attend preparatory lectures or briefings as practice placements have different requirements from other academic parts of their programme. Students in doubt need to check written material or ask university staff, not fellow students, for advice.

Practice educators, especially those who have students from more than one university, should check the requirements of the university and not make assumptions or rely on their memory of what they did on previous occasions. Many of the challenges on placement could be avoided if students and educators had been more aware of procedures, assessments and regulations.

Specific placement information

Ideally, allocating an individual student to a specific placement and educator will occur well in advance of the placement, allowing time for preparation. But, as demand for placements exceeds supply (Craik and Turner 2005), these arrangements may happen at short notice, limiting time for preparation and organisation.

Practice educators are encouraged to have plans in place for students in their setting including orientation to the placement, hours of work, travel arrangements, suggested pre-placement reading, dress code, an outline timetable and other relevant information. Providing this information in advance allows students to prepare for individual placements. Where possible, a pre-placement visit, allowing the student and educator to meet, can be a useful way of answering questions and relieving anxieties.

If offered, students should try to visit and certainly should be familiar with the advice provided by their educator. Creating good communication between students and educators, as early as possible, will do much to avoid the difficulties that can occur on placement as a result of poor communication.

Reflection on previous learning

Universities and educators will expect students to go to a placement having reflected on previous learning, perhaps through a statement of expectations or areas to develop on the forthcoming placement. For students this is challenging. How much should they reveal of their learning style, experiences on previous placements, academic performance or personal circumstances? Universities and educators want to help students learn and this information assists them arrange a placement to facilitate individual learning. However, students may want to start each placement afresh with no reference to previous ones. While this may appear to have advantages students are usually best to tell their educator about previous difficulties and the resultant growth in self awareness is a valuable skill to acquire.

Reluctance to self disclose is perhaps most apparent with disabled students. In the UK, the Special Educational Needs and Disability Act (2001) requires the education sector to make reasonable adjustments to ensure that disabled students are not disadvantaged. This extends to placements but depends on students disclosing relevant information to the university and placement educator. Many universities have developed systems which involve discussion with the university, educator and student prior to the placement to negotiate adjustments. When this takes place it usually works well with everyone involved being full informed, aware of potential challenges and ready to respond positively should they occur.

Vignette 21.2

Peter is a mature student with many years experience as an assistant in a health-care setting. He has found academic study challenging and he had feedback about his poor writing skills both at university and on his first placement. Uncomfortable about this, he does not mention it in his learning needs before his second placement. At the beginning of the placement, his educator explains the style of report writing required and provides an example. This method has worked well with previous students. However, the next week the educator tells Peter that his report writing is not up to standard and asks him to do it again. During the next weeks Peter tries hard but is still not meeting the standards expected but he now feels that it is too late to ask for extra help. It is only when the lecturer from university visits half way through the placement that the issue is fully recognised. The educator is able to provide extra guidance on report writing and Peter responds well but the situation could have been avoided if Peter had been more forthcoming initially.

Supervision

Relationship between the student and educator

In an opinion piece, a UK student describes the relationship between the student and educator as pivotal to the student's success on placement (Dean 2006). She considers that supportive educators, enthusiastic about the profession, can have a profound influence on students but that educators are often unaware of their power. In responding, Lawson-Porter (2006) accepts the importance of the relationship but suggests that students also have power to make judgements about the educator and service. As both have much to gain or lose, they share responsibility to work at the relationship and contribute to the quality of supervision.

Guidelines

The recommended minimum for formal supervision is one hour per week (COT 2004b). This is an occasion for the educator and student to spend time together planning learning opportunities and discussing the student's abilities. Individual universities will give guidelines about the level of supervision the student can expect and practice educators are responsible for facilitating this. Differing viewpoints on what constitutes supervision, and how to achieve it, can cause misunderstandings between students and practice educators.

Definitions

Students are likely to have less experience of formal supervision than educators and they will view it in the formal definition of a process which takes place at a pre-arranged time with a clear agenda and outcome. This expectation can limit their view of less formal types of supervision that experienced practice educators may have evolved. Students may not recognise the informal comments on planning an intervention or how they could improve their performance, which take place outside a formal session, as supervision.

Process

Where universities have supervision guidelines these should be followed. In their absence, there are books and articles which can be referred to. However, the essence of supervision is clarity of purpose agreed between the student and educator and a willingness to engage in open discussion about pertinent issues. Both parties need to prepare for supervision and to allow sufficient time in a private setting to discuss these issues and then to confirm in writing what has been agreed and what action is to be followed by both parties. Recording supervision avoids ambiguity and provides verification if differences of opinion materialise.

Assessment

Purpose

Students have to demonstrate that they are familiar with the occupational therapy process and can perform its components at a level appropriate to their stage of education. University requirements for each placement will explain the aims of the placement, the expected learning outcomes in terms of knowledge and understanding, cognitive skills and professional skills, the main topics to be included, the learning and teaching strategies to be used and the assessment methods which will enable students to demonstrate the learning outcomes.

Practice educators will have to convert these general, academic requirements into more specific, practical tasks to be achieved in that location with their clients. They have to plan how students can move from observation through guided performance to independent action and how they will assess their performance. Often this is devised as a series of weekly tasks, usually agreed in advance with the student. It is essential that students are aware of how and when they will be assessed.

Process

Each university will have a system of assessment and students and educators should be familiar with this, but assessment should not dominate the placement. Students are naturally apprehensive about being judged and may feel that they are under scrutiny throughout the placement which can lead to performance anxiety when they feel that they can do nothing right. However, educators are responsible for verifying that future practitioners are competent, so their assessment needs to be robust.

Openness between the educator and student is helpful but may be difficult to achieve. Sensible advice for educators is to give regular feedback, at least weekly, to make students aware of their progress and any remedial action required. However, like most advice, it is easier to give than to act on. Many educators are reluctant to comment on poor performance, especially early in a placement, preferring to wait until the student settles into the placement to see if performance improves. But, with no feedback, students are unlikely to make progress and can feel aggrieved if they later learn that they have not been functioning as expected and have less time to improve. Sensible advice to students, who consider that they are not receiving sufficient feedback, is not to assume that everything is going well but to invite constructive criticism. This advice is also easy to give but difficult to follow.

Outcome

Most students will meet the placement learning outcomes but a small minority will not. In most cases, a student who fails one placement will be allowed another attempt in a similar setting but a second failure may have serious consequences. Therefore, any student at risk of failure should be informed in advance and given opportunity and support to meet the learning outcomes. Many universities advise involving an academic from the student's university for advice in situations of potential failure. This can help to clarify assessment criteria and procedures and may lead to an alternative outcome. However, educators and academics must be aware of their responsibility as gatekeepers of the profession's standards in deciding whether a student passes or fails.

The university's assessment criteria are the basis for grading a student. Whatever system is used, assessment should be made in relation to these. These are usually transparent and students should be able to judge their own performance and some settings encourage students to do this as part of a formal process. Some placement assessments have a pass/fail structure, while others have a more complex scheme of grades, marks or percentages. Although this is helpful to students, there are concerns that these assessment criteria remain subjective and that it may be easier to obtain a high mark in some placements or from some educators. Where placement grades contribute to the overall performance on the programme, there has been criticism that they inflate the final grade obtained and students can become too concerned with gaining a high grade.

Problems on placement

Identification

While most placements progress smoothly to a successful conclusion, some do not. Early recognition of a potential problem is important and can allow the educator and student to discuss this. If both agree that there is a problem, then planning remedial action and evaluating its effectiveness may lead to resolution. More challenging are situations where only the student or the educator believes that there is a problem and this is when involvement of academics from the university is advised.

Action

This may involve clarification of expectations or regulations or a more active role. University academics can then engage in dialogue with both the student and educator. This is best accomplished through a visit to the placement but if this is not possible, telephone discussion or video conferencing may be alternatives. As many difficulties relate to communication between the educator and the student, the academic will often speak to them individually to establish the nature and extent of the problem. However, if resolution is to be attained, then a discussion with all three is necessary to agree an action plan. This will usually include a timescale and possibly a further meeting. In many situations this strategy will be sufficient to enable resolution and for the student to pass the placement. If it does not then the student may fail or the placement may be finished early.

Whatever the outcome, the educator and the student may benefit from writing an account of events, which can be the focus of their future reflection and learning. Sometimes a more formal debriefing may be useful.

Reflection

Reflection on learning during the placement is the final stage for the student and one which students may neglect in the rush to get on with the next part of the programme. But reflection is necessary to make the most of the experience, to link it to previous knowledge and use it to prepare for future academic and placement studies. For educators too, reflection is helpful to prepare for future students and to provide valuable insight to their professional performance. These reflections can be an important aspect of continuing professional development and give added value to the process of student supervision.

Vignette 21.3

Anita is in the fifth week of placement and feels that she is not doing well and will fail. At her weekly supervision session her educator never praises her and is full of criticism or 'points for improvement' as she calls them. Anita contacts the university to explain the situation and ask for a visit. On the visit, the university academic first listens to Anita's account and then she speaks to the educator who says that Anita is doing very well, is quick to respond to her suggested 'points for improvement' and should achieve a high grade. The educator is astonished when she hears of Anita's concerns. When all three discuss the situation, Anita acknowledges that her educator has given her positive feedback but only informally, often immediately after an intervention session. The educator recognises that in formal supervision she has concentrated on 'points for improvement' as she has already given Anita positive feedback. The situation is quickly resolved once the educator and student understand the other's viewpoint and agree to more open discussion.

Summary

Practice placements are a valuable learning opportunity not only for students but also for educators. Willingness to see the other peoples' perspective, which is an essential component of effective occupational therapy, is also important for successful practice education. Educators and students who can apply this skill in the practice setting will gain benefits for themselves, the profession and their clients.

References

American Occupational Therapy Association 2006 Accreditation Council for Occupational Therapy Education, Standards and Interpretative Guidelines http://www.aota.org/nonmembers/area13/docs/acotestandards806.pdf accessed 27th October 2006

Bossers A, Cook A, Polatajjko H et al 1997 Understanding the role-emerging fieldwork placement. Canadian Journal of Occupational Therapy 64(2): 70–81

Canadian Association of Occupational Therapists 2005a The Canadian Academic Accreditation Standard http://www.caot.ca/pdfs/GuideComplete.pdf accessed 27th October 2006

Canadian Association of Occupational Therapists 2005b Canadian Guidelines for Fieldwork Education in Occupational Therapy http://www.caot.ca/pdfs/CGFEOT_2005%20reved.pdf accessed 27th October 2006

College of Occupational Therapists 1994 Standards Policies and Proceedings 166 Statement on Fieldwork Education: Recommended requirements for the accreditation of fieldwork educators, College of Occupational Therapists, London

College of Occupational Therapists 2004a The College of Occupational Therapists curriculum framework for pre-registration education. College of Occupational Therapists, London

College of Occupational Therapists 2004b Standards of Education. Pre registration Standards. College of Occupational Therapists, London

College of Occupational Therapists 2005a Accreditation of pre-registration programmes in occupational therapy. College of Occupational Therapists, London

College of Occupational Therapists 2005b Guidance on the accreditation of practice placement educators' scheme (APPLE) http://www.cot.co.uk/newpublic/about/pdf/apple_guidance.pdf accessed 25.8.06

College of Occupational Therapists 2005c College of Occupational Therapists Code of Ethics and Professional Conduct for Occupational Therapists. College of Occupational Therapists, London

College of Occupational Therapists 2006 Developing the occupational therapy profession: providing new work-based learning opportunities for students. College of Occupational Therapists, London

Craik C, Turner A 2005 A chronic shortage of practice placements: whose responsibility? British Journal of Occupational Therapy 68(5): 195

Craik C, McIntyre A, Gallagher M 2004 Accreditation of practice educators: an expectation too far? British Journal of Occupational Therapy 67(9): 404–409

Davys D, Pope K, Taylor J 2006 Professionalism, prejudice and personal taste: does it matter what we wear ? British Journal of Occupational Therapy 69(7): 339–341

Dean A 2006 The power of the educator. Mental Health Occupational Therapy 11(1): 4

Fisher A, Savin–Baden M 2002 Modernising fieldwork, part 2: realising the new agenda. British Journal of Occupational Therapy 65(6): 275–282

Health Professions Council 2003 Standards of Proficiency; Occupational Therapists. Health Professions Council, London

Health Professions Council 2004 Standards of Education and Training. Health Professions Council, London

Hocking and Ness 2002 Revised minimum standards for the education of occupational therapists. World Federation of Occupational Therapists, Perth

Lawson-Porter A 2006 The influence of the student. Mental Health Occupational Therapy 11(2): 40

Martin M, Morris J, Moore A et al 2004 Evaluating practice education models in occupational therapy: comparing 1:1, 2:1 and 3:1 placements. British Journal of Occupational Therapy 67(5): 192–200

Quality Assurance Agency for Higher Education 2001a Benchmark Statement: Health Care Programmes. Occupational Therapy, Quality Assurance Agency for Higher Education, Gloucester, UK

Quality Assurance Agency for Higher Education 2001b Code of practice for the assurance of academic quality and standards in higher education Section 9: placement learning. http://www.qaa.ac.uk/academicinfrastructure/codeOfPractice/section9/default.asp accessed 25.8.06

Special Educational Needs and Disability Act 2001 http://www.opsi.gov.uk/acts/acts2001/20010010.htm accessed 25.8.06

Totten C, Pratt J 2001 Innovation in fieldwork education: working with member of the homeless population in Glasgow. British Journal of Occupational Therapy 64(11): 559–563

Walters B 2001 Radical action for radical plans. British Journal of Occupational Therapy. 64(11): 517–518

Wood A 2005 Student practice contexts: changing face, changing place. British Journal of Occupational Therapy 68(8): 375–378

Further reading

Alsop AE, Ryan S 1996 Making the Most of fieldwork education: A practical approach.Nelson Thornes, Cheltenham, UK

Clinical supervision skills 22

Jenny Strong

Highlight box

- Supervision is an active process where the skills, knowledge and practices of a therapist are enhanced.
- All occupational therapists can benefit from supervision.
- Ideally, supervision should occur on a regular, monthly basis.
- The ultimate recipient of the benefits of supervision should be the patient. There are also benefits for the individual therapist, including support, and the organisation, such as staff retention.
- The use of supervision agreements and agendas can help both the supervisee and the supervisor to make the maximum gains from supervision.
- Within supervision sessions, multiple learning methods are recommended, including discussion, appropriate observation of practice, reading and role-play.
- Supervision training is beneficial.

Overview

In this chapter, clinical supervision will be defined, and the elements of clinical supervision elucidated. What clinical supervision is not will be briefly mentioned, as will the differences between supervision and mentoring. The perceived benefits of clinical supervision for occupational therapists, the organisation and the clients will then be described. While there are many models of supervision, the model this author has successfully implemented as part of a multidisciplinary collaboration in a mental health setting will be presented. The evidence in support of clinical supervision will be outlined. Skills, procedures and guidelines for enhancing clinical supervision will then be described. Examples of clinical supervision in action will be presented throughout the chapter.

Historical context

Within occupational therapy, considerable attention has been given to the clinical supervision of students undertaking clinical placements (see, for example, Strong et al 1996, Hummell 1997). The other area of practice where clinical supervision has traditionally been available has been in mental health, where workers of many disciplines have sought supervision (see Spence et al 2001). More recently, supervision for new graduate occupational therapists (Jacobs 1994) and occupational therapists working in isolated, rural and remote locations has become prominent. For example, Lee and Mackenzie (2003), identified that the availability of support/supervision was the most common factor assisting in the transition of new graduates starting work in a rural setting. Cusick and her colleagues (2004) examined priorities and problems for new graduate occupational therapists entering acute care hospitals. The need for quality supervision was highlighted as critical for assisting these new graduate occupational therapists to function in the acute care clinical role, and to assist with staff retention.

Professional associations worldwide have developed standards and position papers about supervision and mentoring. For example, in 2000, OT Australia Inc published its national policy on mentoring and supervision, in tandem with its personal accreditation scheme. The policy identified the need for new graduate occupational therapists and therapists newly arrived in Australia to gain a minimum of 20 accreditation points from the 'receiving mentoring or supervision' category during the cycle of accreditation. Practitioners with more than 2 years of experience were not mandated supervision/mentoring, but could still gain accreditation points.

In this chapter, the contention is made that the benefits of clinical supervision are to be had in all areas of practice, and for occupational therapists of all levels of clinical experience. Of course, one size does not fit all. New graduates will need more frequent and possibly directive supervision than occupational therapists with many years experience working in a particular area. Occupational therapists moving from one practice area to another may also require more frequent supervision. Experienced practitioners also have much to gain from supervision.

As we reflect on our experiences as occupational therapists, it will be clear that supervision, when and where it occurs, does not just happen. For occupational therapists working within mental health facilities, there is a rich tradition of supervision, both within the work setting and privately. Supervision denotes a considered, planned, and resource-intense interaction, usually between two people, over a period of time. It can be considered as having a set of functions, core tasks and processes. As Rich (1993) commented, supervision is characterised by 'the development of a supportive supervisory climate and a base of staff professional skills and values, enacted through a cycle of observation and discussion, and directed towards the delivery of quality client services in accordance with organisational and professional values' (p. 172).

It should also be clear that supervision is different to mentoring, although some supervisors provide the encouragement and professional development support that we might typically expect to receive from a mentor. They provide this support and encouragement *in addition to* other roles and functions they perform as supervisor.

Supervision

Supervision has been defined as a 'working alliance between two or more professional members where the intention of the interaction is to enhance the knowledge, skills and attitudes of at least one staff member' (Spence et al 2001: 136). Spence et al (2001: 136) asserted that the main aim of supervision was 'to optimise the service provided to clients, in line with the goals, expectations, and ethical and professional standards of the organisation and profession concerned (Proctor 1994; Rich 1993)'. Within supervision, clinical practice issues, administrative/organisational issues and personal support issues are worked on (Spence et al 2001).

What supervision is not …

It is important to understand that supervision is not therapy (Jones 1998, Yegdich 1999, MacDonald 2002). The goals of supervision and therapy are different, as is the focus of the interaction (Yegdich 1999). In supervision, the focus is upon the supervisee's work with their patients, while the focus of therapy would be the well-being of, in this case, the supervisee (Yegdich 1999). Keeping the clients centre-most is critical for supervision. For example, it is not appropriate for supervision to become a time where the supervisor helps the supervisee with his personal problems. In circumstances where the supervisor ascertains that the supervisee has personal problems which are impacting upon their ability to perform his work, the supervisor should advise the supervisee to seek professional help for their problems. Where such facilities exist, the supervisor may also recommend the supervisee attends the organisation's occupational health department for assessment and support.

Supervision is not a time for the supervisor to dazzle the supervisee with their brilliance, or unload their own issues. The focus must be on the supervisee and her work. Supervision is not a time for a general chat about life. Nor should it become a conversation where either party complains about the professional practices of other staff.

Having a clear supervision agreement and basing supervision upon a model of practice helps ensure focus upon the real business of supervision.

Differences between mentoring and supervision

The example that comes easily to mind of a mentoring relationship is one of a more experienced occupational therapist (or other more senior health professional) providing general career guidance, emotional support and staff development for a more junior occupational therapist. Reflecting on my own career, I was fortunate to find life-long mentors through both my early involvement with the occupational therapy professional association, my university academic mentors who continued to be significant in my professional life long beyond my graduation ceremony, and my clinical practice environments. These women and men were dedicated and selfless in the mentoring relationship. Rather than dealing with specific clinical cases as should occur in supervision, they assisted me to see the generality of practice, the thematic issues in practice, the burning questions for myself and the profession, and the key issues for scholarly practice. At a time when few of my peers were embarking upon post-graduate studies, they nurtured and supported my dreams and visions, and challenged me to dig deeper to achieve more, more for me as an individual therapist, and in so doing, more for the profession and for my patients.

How did these mentoring relationships differ from clinical supervision? In a number of ways:

1. These mentoring relationships developed, seemingly organically. They were not mandated; they were not set up by external parties. Perhaps they were serendipitous. However, with hindsight, I am sure that there was some intention on the part of my mentors to act as a mentor.
2. These mentoring relationships were of a voluntary nature. I went into these mentoring relationships because I wanted to, and my mentors entered into the relationship with me because they wanted to.

3. Some of my mentoring relationships dealt with a single theme, e.g. gaining skills in grantsmanship or career development.
4. The matters I discussed with my mentors, and my learnings, were never reported on to another person. They were our privately constructed business.
5. The methods of learning mostly involved verbal communication, although with writing and grant writing, written communication and feedback was crucial.
6. Many of these mentoring relationships were external to the work environment in which I was situated.

Several agencies (see, for example, The University of Queensland http://www.uq.edu.au/hupp/index.html?page=25415&pid=25173, accessed 24/04/2006) make a clear distinction between performance management and mentoring, with the key element being that mentoring is a private, non-reporting relationship. Mentoring is something which is entered into on a voluntary basis, on both the part of the mentee and the mentor. Supervision, on the other hand, is not an optional matter; it is a requirement of many workplaces.

Benefits of supervision

Strong et al (2003) in their study of supervision practices for occupational therapists, psychologists, social workers and speech pathologists (hereafter referred to as allied health professionals) working within a large mental health service, found that allied health professionals perceived five main benefits from supervision. First and foremost was the view that supervision provided important professional development and support for workers. Such support was seen as affirming and greatly valued by participants. Furthermore, the provision of such support was seen as a useful way of enhancing job satisfaction and reducing job burnout.

The second perceived benefit found in the study (Strong et al 2003) was that supervision provided an important means of ensuring the competence of allied health professionals, and hence assisted with the provision of best practice for clients. This quality assurance function was seen as working through the provision of feedback and direction to supervisees on their practice with particular clients. The delivery of evidence-based outcomes to clients was highlighted as an important benefit of such quality assurance.

Third, the allied health professionals saw supervision as helping them learn about the organisational culture and practices of a workplace. Supervision was also seen to assist in the preservation of disciplinary identity, especially given the interdisciplinary nature of much of the work. Finally, allied health professionals saw that supervision was beneficial because it assisted them to learn new skills and further develop their clinical reasoning.

Using a similar methodology of focus group interviews with school guidance counsellors in a large education service, McMahon and Patton (2000) found that supervision was perceived as providing support to individual counsellors, as reducing professional isolation, as providing opportunities for debriefing, as assisting in accountability, providing professional skill development, and helping induct new counsellors into the profession. Thus it seems the benefits of supervision are similar, regardless of professional grouping.

Vignette 22.1 provides an example of how supervision can assist a newly graduated occupational therapist in her work.

Skills and procedures for effective supervision

Good supervision does not occur by osmosis. It requires a positive attitude and commitment on the part of the organisation, the supervisor and the supervisee. Along with such commitment, there are requisite resource implications, especially relating to time and training. Having a clear model of supervision in the organisation, and a written policy, is very, very important.

Vignette 22.1

Supervision with a new graduate

Let me give you an example of how supervision might help a new graduate occupational therapist to enhance her outcomes with the children and families she is currently working with. Let's call the therapist Lisa. Lisa is in the first 6 months of her first job, in a Child and Youth facility. Her caseload includes a number of children aged between 7–12 who are school avoidant, and falling behind in their schoolwork. One of her clients is 9-year-old Jane, who comes to therapy with her mother Nina. Lisa dreads these therapy sessions: each time, Jane and her mother end up shouting at each other, before Jane storms out of the room and won't come back. This has happened three times now, and Lisa knows she's not made any progress. But she doesn't know what to do.

Lisa brings this case to her monthly supervision session. Her supervisor asks her what her goals for therapy are. Who is she providing therapy for? Lisa thinks she's trying to help Jane to improve her performance at school and to help her get on better with her Mum. That is why she has been seeing them together. As she talks it through with her supervisor, Lisa sees how she can better structure the therapy sessions, so she works alone with Jane on her performance skills. She also schedules time to meet with the Mum, to explain the things she's doing with Jane, and to reinforce the Mum's efforts to support Jane.

At the next supervision, the supervisor asks Lisa how her client Jane has been getting on. And Lisa is able to report about the gains that Jane has been making. She's glad she raised it in supervision last month. She almost hadn't mentioned it, as she was feeling she was such a hopeless therapist, and she didn't want her supervisor to know how bad she was.

Lisa's initial hesitancy to 'expose' her ignorance to her supervisor is not an uncommon feeling. Many clinicians have expressed vulnerability in supervision where the supervisor has line management authority. However, because she and her supervisor had developed a supervision agreement, and she understood that the supervision was not a punitive thing, she had the confidence to raise the issue.

There are a number of concrete ways that individual occupational therapists can enhance existing supervisory relationships or, in the absence of a supervisory relationship, establish beneficial working alliances in the workplace. The best first step is in developing a supervision agreement (or contract) with your supervisor. It is also useful to have an agenda for each supervision session; this time is precious, so aim to maximise it. It can be useful to have some understanding about your preferred learning style, and that of your supervisee (Kolb 1984). A variety of methods for learning in supervision can be used, including self-review, chart review, audio-tape or video-tape review, or real-time observation, and role play methods. These are things you can discuss in your introductory session, when you are drawing up your supervision agreement. The best, most effective supervision is not confined to verbal learning.

It is recognised that supervision can be adapted to meet different needs and contexts. Things which should be considered include the level of experience of the supervisee, the nature of the work tasks, the resources available to support supervision, the size of the staff, and the location of the workplace. Supervision may be individual, or peer-based. It may involve face-to-face sessions, audio/visual, teleconferencing sessions or email contact.

The supervisor needs to be clear on their role as a supervisor, and ideally to have received training in supervision.

We will now consider each of these aspects.

A model for supervision and the role of the supervisor

Having a model for supervision can assist both the supervisee and supervisor to gain clarity about the supervision process. It assists all to have a clear understanding about the purpose, content, and rights and responsibilities of all parties. Concurrent with an acceptable model of supervision, there needs to be a policy that resources and supports this use of staff time to promote positive outcomes for the patients or clients and the ongoing professional development of the staff.

A model of supervision should be built on a belief that supervision is a desirable and valued activity that enhances the quality of clinical practice, improves client outcomes and supports staff who may be working in difficult circumstances.

The model which we have used in our supervision work in a large mental health workforce is called the 'flexible working alliance approach' to supervision (Kavanagh et al 2004); see Figure 22.1. The model has a triad of participants: supervisor, patient/client and the supervisee, and a triangle of supervisor functions. These functions are:

* managing service delivery, ensuring implementation of statutory and agency policies and procedures, monitoring the quality and quantity of work, prioritising and decision making about what work is to be done
* focusing on the therapist's work through a detailed consideration of individual pieces of work, as distinct from the monitoring of service delivery. It includes instructing or advising the therapist about appropriate strategies, modelling professional behaviour and practice, consulting in the context of solving clinical and ethical problems, evaluating the effectiveness of particular approaches based on observation, records of interviews and discussion and providing support
* facilitating the practitioner's professional development by focusing on staff development and the socialisation of staff into the work place (Hughes and Pengelly 1997: 40–58).

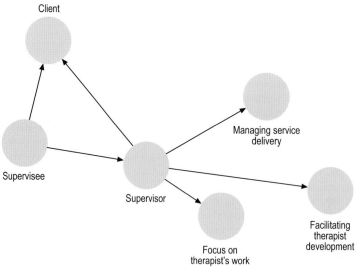

Figure 22.1 A model of supervision, highlighting the importance of the client, the supervisee and the supervisor, in addition to the supervisor's responsibilities in managing service delivery, focusing on the therapist's work and facilitating the therapist's professional development

The supervisor needs to be mindful of the focus upon the needs of the client, the needs of the supervisee, and the needs of the organisation. For example, if the supervisor focuses exclusively on only a few pieces of the supervisee's work, she may neglect to ensure that the needs of all clients are being met and an assessment of the worker's professional development needs may be inaccurate. The model highlights how different aspects of the work are linked and may be in tension with each other. This tension may manifest itself as conflict, for example asking an under-prepared therapist to take on tasks because of a high demand for services.

The triadic nature of the model illustrates that supervision involves an interaction between functions, tasks and outcomes. In any supervision session choices are made about what to focus on (Hawkins and Shohet 1989). Effective supervision requires that all functions and all participants are eventually attended to, though at any one time the supervisor will need to focus on one or two functions or participants.

A supervisor will need to adapt her personal responses, and the use of other resources, depending on:

- the supervisee's personal goals, current work challenges, abilities and learning styles
- the quality of the relationship between the supervisee and the supervisor
- the characteristics of individual clients and clients as a group
- the organisational structure of the team
- the resources of time, money and communication media, etc. available
- the supervisor's abilities and professional background and current organisational priorities.

Supervisors need to have the following core skills:

- the capacity to form relationships with a range of people from different disciplines
- well-developed problem solving, negotiation, advocacy and conflict resolution skills
- the capacity to articulate their approach to practice within their discipline
- the capacity for self reflective practice, and
- the capacity to form evidence-based assessments of the other's practice and to use this assessment to inform future decisions.

Supervision agreement

It is very helpful for the supervisee and supervisor to develop and use a supervision agreement (or contract) (see Figure 22.2 for an example). First and foremost, the agreement will identify the goals of the supervisory relationship. This should involve making a detailed list of the knowledge and skills that the supervisee and supervisor would like the supervisee to develop in the supervision sessions. Goals might include:

- Developing expertise in working with patients who acquired brain injury
- Understanding the implications of deficits of awareness on functional goal-setting with patients
- Becoming skilled in managing agitation in patients.

It will be useful for this list to be reviewed regularly, and renegotiated as the needs and skills of the supervisee change over time. In developing this list, it can be useful for the

From 1 January 2007 – 30 June 2007

Agreed goals of supervision:

1 To gain experience in working with individuals with chronic pain
2 To become competent in using a variety of different assessment tools
3 To become competent in formulating occupationally focused treatment goals
4 To develop expertise in working with so called difficult patients

Structure of supervision:

1 To occur once per month, on third Thursday from 2-3pm, in interview room 2
2 Resources required will be the interview room, the 60 minute time period, video player and screen on occasion, support to enrol in next scientific meeting on pain
3 Preparation as mutually agreed to occur
4 Preparatory agenda to be set up at the conclusion of each monthly session, it can be modified by mutual agreement
5 Supervisor will be available between sessions if required
6 Discussions/case materials to remain confidential between 2 parties, except in situation where supervisor has concerns about the safety of patients or supervisee. If this occurs, the supervisor will advise the supervisee of his need to disclose
7 A variety of methods to be used in supervision, including verbal discussion, listening to audio-tapes or watching video-tapes of client sessions, use of direct observation, role play and article review

Records:

1 Monthly notes, as per Figure 20.3 to be kept
2 Both supervisor and supervisee to keep a copy of these notes
3 These records to be used for personal use, and for review at end of supervision period
4 Records to be stored in the supervisor's filing cabinet for a 12 month period

Evaluation of supervision:

1 Preferred process will involve review of original goals and progress made from perspectives, with comparison between supervisor and supervisee
2 To occur in month 5, or sooner if either supervisor or supervisee request a review

Signed by: AJ Supervisor and AT Supervisee on 08 August 2006

Figure 22.2 Supervision practice agreement between AJ Supervisor and AT Supervisee

supervisee and supervisor to independently write a list, and then compare lists to arrive at a set of mutually agreed goals. If at this time, it appears that there are some skills required which the supervisor does not herself/himself hold, then the mechanisms and resources for gaining these skills should be identified.

The structure of supervision should then be documented. Matters such as the frequency of supervision, time available and location need to be explicitly stated, for example, supervision will occur on the third Friday of the month in office X from 2–3 pm. The sorts of notes that will be made of the sessions, and who has access to those records will be identified. A set of sample supervision session notes are contained in Figure 22.3.

The format of the supervision sessions will also be documented. For example, case notes will be reviewed, training videos and role-plays will be used, in addition to verbal discussion of cases. Acceptable reasons for non-attendance at supervision will be discussed and agreed upon. (Note: being too busy with clinical work is generally, but not always, a non-defensible reason for cancelling supervision.) The mutual obligations of both supervisor and supervisee should be discussed and documented. These include matters around confidentiality, especially when the supervisor is the line manager for the supervisee. Also, the level of preparation required for supervision sessions by both supervisor and supervisee should be indicated. Establishing the use of agendas can also be a useful part of this agreement. The agenda planning can be included as part of the notes of supervision, as illustrated in Figure 22.3. The supervision agreement should indicate when and how the supervision will be reviewed.

Between AJ Supervisor and AT Supervisee

Date: 10 August 2006
Topic: Working with difficult patients, especially angry, hostile patients, when seen both individually and in a group

Discussion revolved around the reasons why some patients present as difficult, and its impact on therapy.

Discussion about possible antecedents to patient anger, including being unjustly hurt, being misled, violation of norms, attacks on ego integrity, or being unjustly treated.

Discussed use of of a process approach, which develops rapport using active listening, a thorough assessment and developing a therapeutic alliance with the patient.

Role played use of process approach with 'an angry patient'

Agreed action: Supervisee to read chapters by Large et al (2002) and DeGood & Dane (1996) and article by Fernandez and Turk (1995)

Agenda items for next session: the patient who somatisizes
Preparation required: Supervisee to consider examples from patient load, and outcomes of therapy

Signed by ....and..

Date: 10 August 2006

Figure 22.3 Sample of monthly supervision notes and agenda planning

There are times when a therapist's supervisor is also the line manager of a service. This can place pressure on both the supervisee, who may think 'but I can't let him know I am having difficulty with my therapy with clients, or I might be put on performance review', and the supervisor, who may be juggling demands to increase caseload and client outcomes versus supporting a new member of the team find his feet with his clinical cases. This is definitely a case where developing clear expectations and boundaries for supervision and building them into a supervision contract can be so useful.

It should be stated that many points in the supervision agreement will not be open to negotiation (Hughes and Pengally 1997). This is not a contract between equals. However, it is important for building the trust in the relationship that the supervisee's views are carefully considered in formulating the supervision agreement.

The supervision agreement which will be developed needs to be based on relevant policies that exist in the organisation, including policies on the aims and functions of supervision, resources to carry out supervision, including time, space, absence of interruptions, the status of records of supervision, provision for situations where the supervisory relationship breaks down, rights and responsibilities of supervisor and supervisee, confidentiality and its limits, and evaluation and reviewing supervision and the role of supervision in staff appraisal.

Situations that may arise in supervision

Some supervisory relationships proceed without a hitch, and the agreed goals of assisting the supervisee to become a more competent practitioner are realised. In other cases, situations may arise in supervision which challenge either the supervisor or the supervisee. For example, the situation might arise where the supervisor notices that the supervisee is very defensive, and resists participating in the supervision, right from the first session when they met to draw up a supervision agreement. The supervisee attends his supervision sessions, but seems to be responding only on a superficial level. In this case, the supervisor needs to consider whether the supervision relationship is contributing to the supervisee defensiveness, and if so, attempt to build a greater level of support and trust. The supervisor would highlight this issue, and indicate how it was hampering effective supervision. In one case where a supervisee was upset that the supervisor had been promoted to a position for which the supervisee had also applied, it was necessary to obtain a different supervisor, as the deep-seated resentment limited any progress.

In another case, the supervisor became aware that the supervisee was engaging in unethical practice. She was able to discuss this problem with the supervisee, and review both the professional and organisational ethical guidelines for practice. Sometimes, the correct ethical stance is not directly clear to therapists. As a young graduate I worked with patients with brain tumours, and their families, over extended periods of time. In one instance, I became close to one patient who came for weekly therapy almost up until the time of her death. I wanted very much to attend her funeral to pay my respects to her and her family. Unfortunately, I did not have a supervisor to discuss this issue with. Supervision was not an accepted part of the landscape in my work environment at this time. I decided not to go to her funeral, as I worried it was unethical to do so. I did not want to get personally involved, and misconstrued attending a funeral with getting personally involved. With hindsight, my decision would have been different. I certainly did not do anything unethical. However my interpretation on my code of ethics was not totally sensible at that time.

Another situation that might arise is where the supervisor and the supervisee have different theoretical orientations. For example, an occupational therapist may have begun work in a pain management unit, where the prevailing theoretical orientation is the cognitive-behavioural approach. His supervisor is a strong advocate of cognitive-behavioural-based therapy, while he has a much more humanistic, client-centred approach. Rather than argue over which approach is better, in supervision the pair agreed to respect both approaches after the supervisor reframed the questions to consider what was in the particular patient's best interest.

Supervision training

As may have been gleaned from earlier sections, the skills for effective supervision do not just appear by serendipity. This has been both our experience (see Spence et al 2001, Strong et al 2003, Kavanagh et al 2004), and that of other workers (see Hancox et al 2004). Ideally, both supervisors and supervisees can be trained, so that both have the skills and attitudes to make supervision work best for them and their patients. MacDonald (2002) has suggested the importance of adult learning principles in supervision training. Training programmes have been developed by multiple authors, and for multiple purposes. For example, Kavanagh et al (2004) developed a 2-day supervision training programme for allied health professionals, nurses and medical staff working in a statewide mental health service. Hodgins et al (2005) developed a model of supervision to be provided to rural general practitioners working with clients with mental health problems. Jones (1998) developed a seminar to prepare nurses for clinical supervision, while Hancox and her colleagues (2004) developed a clinical supervision training programme for nurses working in the mental health service in one Australian state.

Evidence in support of supervision

In 2001, as part of a supervision project with allied health professionals in a large mental health service, Spence and her colleagues observed that there was minimal evidence in support of supervision, despite a plethora of literature and a general agreement among practitioners that supervision was of value. 'It is not clear whether supervision actually produces a change in clinical behaviour, nor whether it produces benefits in terms of client outcome' (Spence et al 2001: 135). Other researchers concur with the paucity of empirical evidence on the impact of supervision (Holloway and Neufeldt 1995, Freitas 2002).

Several authors have observed the difficulties in evaluating the effectiveness and impact of supervision (Freitas 2002, Worrall et al 2006). Issues such as lack of comparison groups, the lack of random assignment of supervisors and supervisees to experimental groups, small sample sizes, and drop-out rates have all been observed in the research literature (Ellis et al 1996, Spence et al 2001). Furthermore, attempting to determine the impact of supervision on client outcomes raises issues with client confidentiality and confounding life events that may have a bearing upon outcomes.

It is proposed that the effectiveness of supervision can be best considered through the lens of the tripartite model of supervision illustrated in Figure 22.1. Using this model, one can ask 'what is the impact of the supervision on?':

- the supervisee – their perceptions of its value, their job satisfaction, morale, intention to stay in the organisation, and their actual delivery of services to clients
- the client – their clinical outcomes, and their satisfaction with therapy, and
- the organisation – the perceptions of service directors, staff retention data, and the absence of critical incidents.

Key findings from available studies will be considered from these different viewpoints.

Supervisee studies

McMahon and Patton (2000) utilised a focus group methodology to ascertain the value of clinical supervision for school guidance officers in a large education authority. A randomly selected group of 51 guidance officers reported that supervision assisted them to develop their skills, for personal development, to debrief, to counteract the effects of geographical and/or professional isolation, to assist in induction of new staff members and to help with accountability. These findings were similar to those by Strong et al (2003) reported earlier in this chapter.

Teasdale et al (2001) surveyed 211 nurses about the impact of clinical supervision, using both written questionnaires and qualitative comments on critical incidents. Results compared supervised and non-supervised nurses. It was found that supervised nurses felt part of a more supportive organisation, coped better at work, and felt that they had better access to support than non-supervised nurses. These findings were particularly notable in more junior nurses.

In a state-wide mental health service study of 272 allied health staff, using a Supervision Attitude Scale, Kavanagh et al (2004) found that staff perceived the benefits of the supervision in terms of managing their own stress levels and in debriefing, rather than a specific improvement in their own skills.

Studies by Christie et al (1985) of occupational therapy students, and Kadushen (1974) of social work supervisees, found that inexperienced practitioners preferred the supervisor to observe their practice, to provide skills training and to be available to assist them when and if they had difficulties.

Organisation studies

Kavanagh et al (2004) examined the perceptions of service directors regarding the benefits of a state-wide supervision training programme for allied health professionals. Seventy-eight percent of the Directors of all community mental health centres in Brisbane reported a positive impact of the project on the clinical effectiveness of their staff, while 64% reported a positive impact on staff morale. 'Directors reported that they perceived that the quality and standard of allied health practice had improved' (Kavanagh et al 2004: 18).

Client studies

As noted by Spence et al (2001: 144), 'there has been very little research to determine whether supervision is actually effective as a method of enhancing the best practice of clinicians and of maximizing client outcomes.' Some researchers have reported that clients are more likely to attend therapy sessions more often with therapists who have been receiving more frequent supervision (see, for example, Burgoyne et al 1976, Steinhelber et al 1984). While this does not indicate better client outcomes, it is suggestive of some positive impact of supervision upon the clients. Clearly, more work is needed in this difficult area.

Conclusions

While the research evidence is still not in about the benefits of clinical supervision, there are many indications that the provision of clinical supervision can have benefits for the individual therapist, the organisation and most importantly, the clients. It is recommended that occupational therapists' embrace the concept of supervision, across all areas of practice. Training in the provision of supervision is helpful, as good supervision does not just happen. Practical strategies such as developing a supervision agreement, and using agendas for supervision, should be used. Using a variety of learning methods in supervision is also strongly recommended.

Acknowledgements

I thank my colleagues, Prof David Kavanagh, Prof Jill Wilson, Prof Susan Spence, and Prof Linda Worrall, with whom I have spent many hours learning about supervision. Most of the ideas raised in this chapter were learned and/or crystallised with these good colleagues and friends over the past decade. I acknowledge the financial support of Queensland Health which enabled us to develop and evaluate a supervision training programme for the mental health services in Queensland Australia. Queensland Health is the copyright holder of all the reports delivered on the outcomes of this project. Some findings from the studies are referred to in this chapter.

References

Burgoyne RW, Santini S, Kline F et al 1976 Who gets supervised? An extension of patient selection inequity. American Journal of Psychiatry 133: 1313–1315

Christie BA, Joyce PC, Moeller PL 1985 Fieldwork experience: I. impact on practice preference. American Journal of Occupational Therapy 39: 671–674

Cusick A, McIntosh D, Santiago L 2004 New graduate therapists in acute care hospitals: priorities, problems and strategies for departmental action. Australian Occupational Therapy Journal 51: 174–184

deGood DE, Dane JR 1996 The psychologist as a pain consultant in outpatient, inpatient and workplace settings. In Gatchel RJ, Turk DC (eds)

Psychological approaches to pain management. A practitioner's handbook, pp. 403–437. Guilford Press, London

Ellis MV, Ladany N 1997 Inferences concerning supervisees and clients in clinical supervision: an integrative review. In Watkins CE Jr. (ed) Handbook of psychotherapy supervision, pp. 447–507. Wiley, New York

Ellis MV, Ladany N, Krengel M et al 1996 Clinical supervision research from 1981 to 1993: a methodological critique. Journal of Counselling Psychology 43: 35–50

Fernandez E, Turk DC 1995 The scope and significance of anger in the experience of chronic pain. Pain 61: 165–175

Freitas GJ 2002 The impact of psychotherapy supervision on client outcome: a critical examination of two decades of research. Psychotherapy: Theory, Research, Practice, Training 39: 354–367

Hancox K, Lynch L, Happell B et al 2004 An evaluation of an educational program for clinical supervision. International Journal of Mental Health Nursing 13: 198–203

Hawkins P, Shohet R 1989 Supervision in the helping professions:an individual, group and organisational approach. Open University Press, Philadelphia, PA

Hodgins G, Judd F, Kyrios M et al 2005 A model of supervision in mental health for general practitioners. Australasian Psychiatry 13: 185–189

Holloway EL, Neufeldt SA 1995 supervision: its contributions to treatment efficacy. Journal of Consulting and Clinical Psychology 63: 207–213

Hughes L, Pengelly P 1997 Staff supervision in a turbulent environment: managing process and task in front-line services. Jessica Kingsley Publishers, London

Hummell J 1997 Effective fieldwork supervision: OT student perspectives. Australian Occupational Therapy Journal 44: 147–157

Jacobs J 1994 Clinical supervision. An international issue. American Journal of Occupational Therapy 57: 488–499

Jones A 1998 Getting going with clinical supervision: an introductory seminar. Journal of Advanced Nursing 27: 500–506

Kadushin A 1974 Supervisor–supervisee: a survey. Social Work 19: 288–297

Kavanagh D, Wilson J, Worrall L et al 2004 A research evaluation of professional supervision and mentoring of health professionals in the mental health service. A collaboration between the University of Queensland and Queensland Health. Reports 7–14. Brisbane, Australia

Kolb DA 1984 Experiential learning: experience as a source of learning and development. Prentice Hall, Englewood Cliffs, NJ

Large RG, New F, Strong J et al 2002 Chronic pain and psychiatric problems. In: Strong J, Unruh AM, Wright A et al (eds) Pain textbook for therapists. Churchill Livingstone, Edinburgh

Lee S, MacKenzie L 2003 Starting out in rural New South Wales: the experiences of new graduate occupational therapists. Australian Journal of Rural Health 11: 36–43

MacDonald J 2002 Clinical supervision: a review of underlying conceptual developments. Australian and New Zealand Journal of Psychiatry 36: 92–98

McMahon M, Patton W 2000 Conversations on clinical supervision; benefits perceived by school counsellors. British Journal of Guidance & Counselling 28: 339–352

OT Australia Inc 2000 mentoring/supervision policy paper. Available: http://www.uq.edu. au/hupp/index.html?page=25415&pid=25173

Proctor B 1994 Supervision: competence, confidence, accountability. British Journal of Guidance & Counselling 22: 309–318

Rich P 1993 The form, function and content of supervision: an integrated model. The Clinical Supervisor 11: 137–178

Spence SH, Wilson J, Kavanagh D et al 2001 Clinical supervision in four mental health professions: a review of the evidence. Behaviour Change 18: 135–155

Steinhelber J, Patterson V, Cliffe K et al 1984 An investigation of some relationships between psychotherapy supervision and patient change. Journal of Clinical Psychology 40: 1346–1353

Strong J, O'Reilly M, Elliot Schmidt R et al 1996 Clinical supervisors' training for rural occupational therapists. A University of Queensland and Rural Health Support, Education and training (RHSET) funded project, Australia

Strong J, Wilson J, Kavanagh D et al 2003 Supervision practice within a large allied mental health workforce: exploring the phenomenon. The Clinical Supervisor 22: 191–210

Teasdale K, Brocklehurst N, Thom N 2001 Clinical supervision and support for nurses; an evaluation study. Journal of Advanced Nursing 33: 216–224

Worrall L, Wilson J, Kavanagh D et al 2006 Reported effects of supervision on clinical practice – an initial descriptive study. Clinical Supervisor, revision submitted

Yegdich T 1999 Lost in the crucible of supportive clinical supervision: clinical supervision is not therapy. Journal of Advanced Nursing 29: 1265–1275

Index

C

357